# KILLER LOOKS

## THE FORGOTTEN HISTORY
## OF PLASTIC SURGERY
## IN PRISONS

*Zara Stone*

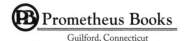

Prometheus Books

Guilford, Connecticut

**Prometheus Books**

An imprint of Globe Pequot, the trade division of
The Rowman & Littlefield Publishing Group, Inc.
4501 Forbes Blvd., Ste. 200
Lanham, MD 20706
PrometheusBooks.com

Distributed by NATIONAL BOOK NETWORK

British Library Cataloguing in Publication Information Available

**Library of Congress Cataloging-in-Publication Data**

Names: Stone, Zara, author.
Title: Killer looks : the forgotten history of plastic surgery in prisons /
   Zara Stone.
Description: Lanham, MD : Prometheus, [2021] | Includes bibliographical
   references and index. | Summary: "In this highly original and highly
   researched book, Zara Stone draws on the intersectionality of
   socioeconomic success, racial bias, the prison industry complex, and the
   fallacy of attractiveness to get to the heart of how appearance and
   societal approval creates self-worth, and uncovers deeper truths of
   beauty bias, inherited racism, effective recidivism programs, and
   inequality"— Provided by publisher.
Identifiers: LCCN 2021013133 (print) | LCCN 2021013134 (ebook) | ISBN
   9781633886728 (cloth ; alk. paper) | ISBN 9781633886735 (epub)
Subjects: LCSH: Prisoners—Medical care—United States. | Surgery,
   Plastic—Social aspects—United States. |
   Criminals—Rehabilitation—United States. | Physical-appearance based
   bias—United States.
Classification: LCC HV8843 .S86 2021  (print) | LCC HV8843  (ebook) | DDC
   365/.667—dc23
LC record available at https://lccn.loc.gov/2021013133
LC ebook record available at https://lccn.loc.gov/2021013134

♾️™ The paper used in this publication meets the minimum requirements of
American National Standard for Information Sciences—Permanence of Paper
for Printed Library Materials, ANSI/NISO Z39.48-1992.

# CONTENTS

# READER'S NOTE

Throughout this book, the terms "cosmetic surgery," "aesthetic surgery," and "plastic surgery" are used interchangeably when referring to procedures like face-lifts and nose jobs. This is reflective of the historical and current use of the terms and displays the blurring between medical and cosmetic work. To change the terms would be to dismiss the language used and its natural fluctuations. In regard to the data, I've referred to available figures for plastic surgery procedures in the United States and elsewhere while recognizing that they are far from perfect.

Regarding the many types of surgical operations described in the book, I have chosen to simplify the technical terms and refer to the procedures by their colloquial names; a rhinoplasty becomes a nose job, a rhytidectomy a face-lift, and so on.

As with any history book that addresses racism and inequality, much of the language in the source material is problematic. In most instances, I have replaced this vernacular with "Black" and "Latino" as more acceptable terminology. In places where this is not appropriate, I have used italics or quotation marks to denote direct speech.

Throughout the book, you'll find terms like "inmates" and "offenders," and I want to acknowledge that these words are no longer widely used in regard to individuals who have come into contact with the criminal justice system. Such labels dehumanize and stigmatize people, creating marginalizing stereotypes that impede their reintegration and rehabilitation process.

I want to stress that this is a work of nonfiction. Every character that appears in this book once lived and breathed and walked on this earth. All narratives and dialogue are constructed from personal communication, interviews, diaries, books, archival collections, magazine and newspaper articles, journals, government reports, and radio and television broadcasts, and, where possible, personal recollections have been fact checked for accuracy. Some quotes have been trimmed for narrative clarity and brevity. On occasion, some words have been added for additional clarification (for example, replacing "we" with "plastic surgeons").

Factual details regarding building design, weather, and other details have been confirmed via multiple historical sources and are accurate to the best of my knowledge. In a few instances, the personal details of the former inmates have been changed to protect their privacy. In those cases, their last names have been chosen to reflect the ancestry of the person in question.

*Content note*: Due to the nature of the historical events and conditions described in this book, the content engages with ableism, racism, disfigurement, sexism, drug addiction, marginalization, mental health issues, and body shaming, which readers may find emotionally and intellectually challenging.

# INTRODUCTION

It is amazing how complete is the delusion that beauty is
goodness.—Leo Tolstoy, 1890

New Faces for Convicts—*New York Times*, 1927

There is no question as to the advisability of plastic surgery
where said features are so repulsive or ugly to interfere with
life adjustment.—Federal Bureau of Prisons, 1967

Early Wednesday morning on December 6, 1967, the daily frost still glisten-
ing on the trees as the city's homeless dismantled their cardboard shelters
to a chorus of sirens, the doors to the Montefiore Hospital and Medical Center
conference center in the North Bronx swung open.

In ones and twos and threes, braving the six- to twelve-mile-per-hour gusts
of wind sweeping through the Bronx, seventy-odd besuited professionals, a
mix of sociologists, psychologists, corrections workers, and plastic surgeons,
trickled in. One of the first to arrive, heavily bundled against the chill, was Ellis McDougall, the director of corrections for South Carolina, followed by the
assistant surgeon general, Dr. Ernest Siegfried, fresh off the Washington, D.C.,
commuter train. Attendees came as far afield as California and Washington State
and as close as a ten-block radius.

These white men—only two of those gathered were women and all were white-presenting—had gone to this effort for one reason only: the inaugural Montefiore Conference on Correctional Plastic Surgery. This three-day event was the world's first scientific conference about utilizing prisoner cosmetic surgery as a recidivism tool. People respond better to the beautiful, the attendees reasoned; would remaking inmates' faces curb future criminal tendencies?

In strode the answer to their questions, Dr. Michael L. Lewin, a sturdy, striking man with thick brown hair that was just beginning to gray at his temples, who headed up Montefiore Hospital and Medical Center's plastic surgery division.

For the last three years, Lewin had codirected the Surgical and Social Rehabilitation (SSR) project, an experimental study conducted with Rikers Island inmates. Funded with $254,000 from the U.S. Department of Health, Education, and Welfare, the SSR investigation was rigorously designed and included a control group, work training, and counseling in addition to free cosmetic surgery.

The reason for the governmental go-ahead for Lewin's surprising surgeries was born of necessity; during the last decade, the U.S. prison and jail population had skyrocketed, with prisons so flooded that convicts often slept three or four to a one-person cell. In New York, 68 percent of ex-cons re-offended within three years of release.[1] The city's jails were brutal; deaths were common, with violence and abuse a daily occurrence. What little medical care existed was shoddy, its personnel understaffed, and few programs offered inmates the chance to find a new path upon release, which contributed to inmates returning to prison multiple times. This revolving door of crime was untenable. Hence, the administration's exploration of preventative pathways.

Lewin stepped onto the stage and the room hushed. He smiled at the audience, cleared his throat, and assumed the lecturing tone he used with his residents for his address. "We live in an era when social medicine assumes increasing importance," he said. "Plastic surgery services offer the promise of becoming an important adjunct in the social rehabilitation of the public offender."

I'm not talking about functional plastic surgery such as reconstructive breast surgeries or cleft palate treatment, which fall under medically necessary plastic surgeries, he clarified. What was up for discussion here was face-lifts, liposuctions, nose jobs, chin implants, scar removal, and more—the majority of operations falling squarely in the cosmetic sphere.

The hypothesis was that improving an inmate's appearance would have a twofold effect, Lewin explained. The hope was that the societal benefits awarded the conventionally beautiful would increase their employment and relationship prospects, and the positive response to their appearance would increase their self-esteem and lower the rate of re-offense.

Inmates who were interested in receiving plastic surgery volunteered by filling out an application slip and dropping it in one of the submission boxes placed inside Rikers Island's jails. Volunteers had to clear a number of physical and psychological tests to enter the study. We vastly underestimated prisoner interest, Lewin admitted. He'd thought that a few hundred might apply, but so far, they'd screened more than 9,300 men. He flipped his glasses down onto his nose. "So. Our findings."

The Rikers Island experiment was not the first time that American prisoners had received free plastic surgery as a recidivism treatment. The practice of re-modeling the physical features of criminals—or assumed criminals—dates back to the turn of the twentieth century.

Most of these early surgeries stemmed from the burgeoning concept of ra-cial science, which conflated certain physical traits with low intelligence, poor health, and criminality. Here, surgeons carved up the faces of Black, brown, and Jewish people, reshaping ears, noses, and breasts in an attempt to correct the so-called disease of "ugliness of nonwhite races."[2] Over time, these operations evolved from deracializing features to focusing on improving an individual's attractiveness.

In January 1910, Henry Solomon, New York's prison commissioner, published a report that advocated providing free plastic surgery for the state's criminals. "Often a man's physical condition makes it easier for him to steal a dollar than to earn one," he told the *New York Tribune*.[3] "The relationship of physical defects to crime is generally not appreciated. We readily see how physi-cal distress might conduce to crime."

The press took Solomon at his word. "Surgery on Criminals: New York Of-ficial's Plan to Remove Bad Streaks" was front page news in the *Chattanooga Daily Times*.[4] "Surgery to Help Convicts" reported the *Baltimore Sun*.[5] The headlines were inflammatory, but their contents were sympathetic; wanting to appear socially acceptable was easy to understand.

This outlook wasn't an anomaly; historically and to the present day, people have instinctively understood the societal benefits of conventional beauty. Even the word "beauty" is studded with emotional landmines, the term so deeply commingled with the language of our culture. A scroll though the synonyms and related words listed in the Merriam-Webster dictionary exemplifies this;

"beautiful" receives "fair," "good," "lovely," "elegant," "flawless," "personable," "charming," and "lovesome," whereas "ugly" is paired with "monstrous," "grotesque," "hideous," "homely," "vile," "repellant," "revolting," "awful," "disgusting," "sickening," and "nauseating." The correlations between appearance and personality traits, and the de facto assumptions inherent in those terms, are reflective of how the beauty bias permeates today's social and cultural mores.

Correlations between criminality and appearance have persisted over centuries—and society's insidious, instinctive response to beauty, and the lack of it, harms some of its most vulnerable. Beauty is a valuable currency in society. The benefits the conventionally good-looking receive include higher salaries at work, better service in bars, and shorter sentences in court. They're fined 174.8 percent less for serious misdemeanors, and they're convicted less. The beauty premium begins at birth. Attractive preschoolers get more one-on-one time with their teachers, attractive middle schoolers get more flexibility with their grades, and when they act out, they're more likely to be called "high spirited" than badly behaved. Overall, attractive students score higher on tests, all the way through university.[6]

"I like to think that eventually people won't care anymore about looks, but I don't think this will happen in my lifetime or yours," Daniel Hamermesh, a beauty economist and global research director of the IZA Institute of Labor Economics, informed me. It's more than a social construction; studies show that that babies as young as nine hours old will track the most attractive person in the room.[7]

Beauty privilege is real, and it's *real* uncomfortable.

There are many signifiers of one's attractiveness beyond the attributes that are distributed at birth. Well-cut clothes, gleaming hair, glowing skin, and straight teeth—even eyelash length!—all play a part in the impression of someone's overall attractiveness. Generally, these are socioeconomic privileges, available only if one can access health care, hairdressers, cosmetics, and unguents. Privileges—thanks to historic discriminatory practices against Black and marginalized communities—have created an unbreachable wealth gap.

What we think of beauty, then, is a combination of genetic luck and economic and social status, which perpetuate a circular economy of beauty privilege. This works in reverse as well; less access to health care and retinols can result in rotting teeth and age-spotted, wrinkled skin. Without care, easily treatable wounds can leave scars and broken noses may set crookedly. Taken to the extreme, one may have a scarred, wart-filled face with blackened teeth and a crooked nose, the eponymous bogeyman or witch from children's stories, the archetypal bad guy.

Small wonder, then, that the cosmetic surgery space is booming—people recognize the benefits of the beauty premium and are angling to get some of that special sauce for themselves. In 2019, the American Society of Plastic Surgeons reported that they performed some 18.1 million cosmetic surgery procedures. Americans spent approximately $16.7 billion on self-beautification, their surgeries ranging from face-lifts to nose jobs, calf implants, and nonsurgical fillers, a 77 percent increase since 2005.

In the age of the influencer, the emphasis on physical attractiveness is heightened more than ever. The relationship between the way a person looks and his or her bank balance has never been clearer. By seeking improvement, one is seeking to raise one's status. However, the ability to successfully self-improve surgically directly corresponds to one's place on the socioeconomic ladder. Cutting costs can have horrific consequences, from bursting breast implants to death; a 2019 investigation from the Center for Health Journalism reported that fourteen women died in Florida after receiving Brazilian butt lifts.[8]

The majority of surgical improvements and the benefits that go in hand with them are reserved for those with disposable income. In 2019, Black and Hispanic Americans (who generally earn less than white Americans), accounted for 20 percent of all cosmetic surgeries in America.[9]

At the bottom of the socioeconomic ladder falls prisoners, with approximately 30 percent of all inmates growing up below the poverty level, according to a 2018 report by the Brookings Institution.[10] The poverty-to-prison pipeline encompasses education; 70 percent of all state prisoners lack high school diplomas.[11]

The wealth gap continues once incarcerated; don't expect the American prison system to exact a high level of medical care or compassion. In 2016, Texas State prisons provided seventy-one dentures, total, to its 149,000 inmates—chewing wasn't considered a "medical necessity" by officials.[12] In 2017 an Arizona inmate with skin cancer was given Tylenol and taken to a dermatologist but not to an oncologist. He was refused sunscreen and did not receive radiation therapy. He died shortly thereafter.[13]

Incarceration itself is famously hard on the body. The incarcerated experience almost five times as many head injuries as civilians. An analysis of intentionally caused facial fractures inside Louisiana penitentiaries found that injuries via "slock" (a padlock in a sock) had doubled between 2011 and 2019. A 2017 study of inmate health care in New York City found that facial trauma accounted for 33 percent of all inmate emergency room visits,[14] compared to 0.7 percent of the general population.[15]

When released, many ex-cons struggle to gain employment due to hiring biases against former felons and find their criminal records preclude them from many positions. "Uglier" ex-cons have an even harder time of things, their physical appearance adding to the prejudices stacked against them.

Which brings us to the current 68 percent recidivism rate[16] within three years of release, according to a 2018 Bureau of Justice Statistics report.

A lot of attention has been given to the problem of recidivism and the benefits of being beautiful, but these have rarely been addressed at the same time. For many, the combination of the two produces confusion; the history of prison plastic surgery has been heavily buried, so much so that few of the (unaffiliated) plastic surgeons, criminologists, or prison historians I consulted were aware of its history. Its existence is America's dirty little secret.

Starting in the early 1920s and lasting well into the mid-1990s, more than five hundred thousand face-lifts, chin implants, nose jobs, breast implants, liposuction, and other cosmetic surgeries took place in jails and prisons across America, with thousands more occurring in lockups across Canada and Britain. For the most part, these surgeries weren't experimental or residency training programs; they were bona fide cosmetic surgeries.

Prisons welcomed these programs, viewing the face-lifts, nose jobs, chin implants, and so forth as rehabilitative, acknowledging the benefits inherent with perceived "pretty privilege." This was a surprising move, given the racial and social turmoil of the mid-twentieth century, as the battle for equality and civil rights swept America, and Black bodies were shunted into cells. As ideas about crime became more racialized, a deeper emphasis was placed on imparting long-lasting social change. The correctional investment in inmate beautification was seen as a recidivism treatment, akin to the investment in prisoner education and reentry programs.

No one is more disenfranchised than criminals, reasoned the officials—and likely no one could benefit more from these programs. This state-sanctioned, taxpayer-covered mass beautification was part of a larger push for prisoner rehabilitation by President Lyndon Johnson, spurred by the civil rights movement and postwar rehabilitative ideals, alongside the growing acceptance of using psychology and sociology to treat people.

But starting with President Nixon's administration and continuing deep into the Carter, Reagan, and Bush years, there was a major overhaul in policy. The administration moved away from the medical model of crime, whereby it was a disease that could be treated, to viewing offenders as "incurable" and necessary to lock away for the public good. The rehabilitative ethos was replaced by punitive sanctions, and the government passed hard-line edicts that discriminated against minorities. Cosmetic surgery was slowly phased out as money was diverted from educational and reentry programs into building more cells, leaving few options for inmate improvement. Pell grants for prisoners were eradicated. By 2001, approximately $57 billion was spent on incarcerating Americans,[17] a 493 percent increase since 1982.[18] The political "tough on crime" approach birthed our "incarceration nation"—today, America houses approximately 22 percent of the world's prisoners.

It was seven more years before President Obama was elected, and prison reform finally returned to the political and social agenda. When he left office, there were concerns that President Trump wouldn't continue his work. The answer to this is complex; in 2018, President Trump signed the First Step Act to reduce the number of federal prisoners and prepare them for reentry. He also supported prisoner education initiatives. However, President Trump's push for stronger border sanctions and funneling money into private prisons has mitigated that impact.[19]

Even so, these changes add to the slow but steady shift back toward the rehabilitative-minded ideals of yesteryear, and President Joe Biden's campaign promises, if followed through, could result in significant changes. Biden vowed to fully support the Safe Justice Act, a criminal justice reform bill, to develop a $20 billion grant program for state prevention programs, to cancel incarceration for drug use alone, to decriminalize cannabis, to eliminate private prisons, and to "end the criminalization of poverty" by removing cash bail. His campaign page declares he has a "national goal of ensuring 100 percent of formerly incarcerated individuals have housing upon reentry."[20]

On October 17, 2019, the city council of New York approved plans to close Rikers Island. Of all the city's jails, Rikers Island in particular has acquired a reputation for brutality and human rights abuses. Inmates sleep in rat-infested cells and are regularly served rotten food and tortured with solitary confinement. The idea, today, that the prison *ever* offered its residents free cosmetic surgery is laughable. Here, inmates are lucky if they receive access to showers, menstrual products, and sewage-free cells.[21] Still, the symbolism of abolishing the jail and its abusive systems is indicative of a new wave of reforms sweeping America as people seek to address the historic inequalities and racist laws that have criminalized addicts and Black and brown people. COVID-19 related crises have put the closure of Rikers Island on hold, but the promise to close remains.

There are still too many people in prisons. In 2017, the number of people imprisoned for drug-related charges was 1,007 percent higher than in 1980.[22] In 2020, America housed approximately 1.4 million men, women, and children in correctional institutions.

To make real progress, the country needs to address its troubled history, a reeducation that will prevent the problems of the past from reoccurring. A cosmetic excision will not create the change necessary for progress.

The socioeconomic gap between the haves and the have-nots has never been more prominent, with the world sharply segregated on religious opinion, political discourse, and personal liberties. It's time to reevaluate the contribution of appearance bias in today's criminal justice system and how it intersects with race, economic privilege, structural inequalities, and the prison industrial complex.

Through the narratives of plastic surgeon Dr. Michael Lewin and other pivotal characters involved in the prison plastic surgery programs, this book spans the myriad surgical programs available in the twentieth century. Through the lens of identity, beauty, and privilege, I examine the benefits and pitfalls of these programs and the ethics of performing medical work on a disenfranchised population.

At its heart, this is a story about the power the prison system wields over those in their care, but it's also about the socioeconomic power the beautiful wield—and how this problematic power has shaped society today.

# 1

# BABY BLUES AND THE
# BAD MEN BIRTHRIGHT

On January 23, 1953, Dr. Michael Lewin painfully watched eight-week-old
John struggle for air inside the neonatal intensive care unit at St. Joseph's
hospital in New Jersey.[1] The baby's tiny fists clenched with every labored gulp,
each breath followed by a grunting inhale that left the child trembling and limp.
John's face was purple with the effort, his skin dripping with sweat. The tips of
his fingers and toes were blue, an early sign of gangrene.

Fourteen hours earlier, John had started crying and rocking, his father, a
twenty-one-year-old veteran, told Lewin. His wife was worried, but the baby's
temperature was normal, so he'd suggested letting him cry himself to sleep. He
was sure it was just typical newborn behavior, he'd told her. They'd just wait it
out. The wailing continued. Four hours later, dime-sized red blotches appeared
on his pudgy legs. He squirmed when his mother touched them and cried
louder. The spots spread to his arms and marched across his face, sprinkling
his skin like confetti.

John's cries grew more piercing, his tiny feet and hands drumming in his
crib, his body squirreling from side to side. His mother picked him up, but he
was so frantic that he almost wormed his way out of her arms. She looked at her
husband and he nodded. It was time to go to the hospital. They covered him
with blankets to keep out the January chill,[2] but his temperature kept rising; he
was 101 degrees on admission. Alarmed, nurses fast-tracked his case straight to
Lewin, the hospital's on-call specialist and attending plastic surgeon.

Lewin gravely probed John's skin with gloved fingers. The baby was hot to the touch, which suggested a rising fever, but his blood pressure was plummeting, and his restlessness and gasping were signs of shock. All symptoms pointed to acute meningococcemia, a particularly nasty virus in the meningitis family with a high mortality rate.

He looked down at John, so small in his bassinet, his heart twisting. No matter how long he worked in hospitals, sick babies were always the worst. They were so vulnerable, their tiny lives so easily snuffed out, all their potential lost in an instant. He prescribed a course of penicillin, instructing the nurses to administer two hundred thousand units every three hours, plus a vitamin and cortisone drip. The balance of chemicals in the child's system was critical; there needed to be enough fluid to keep his body functioning, but not so much that it overloaded his system.

In the waiting room, John's parents squeezed each other's hands as they waited for news. His mother, a dark-haired eighteen-year-old, alternated between nervous and suspicious looks at the hospital staff. She'd been in America[3] for four months now and spoke little English—she relied on tone of voice and body posture. The nurse's friendly but efficient mannerisms filled her with fear. She loved John with a fierceness that shocked her. The minute he'd nuzzled against her, warm and sticky and soft, she knew she'd fight to the death for him.

He was her first child, and his tiny hands and trusting fingers had forced her to acclimatize to this strange American world. For his sake, she'd gone out and made connections in her new community.[4] But here, surrounded by scrubs and white men and beeping machines, she was helpless. Eyes closed, she prayed for his recovery, murmuring Saint Gerard's prayer over and over: "Listen to us who are pleading for our sick child. We thank God for the great gift of our son and ask Him to restore our child to health if such be His holy will. This favor, we beg of you through your love for all children and mothers."

Her prayers didn't work. John's health continued to decline, his heart rate spiking to a thundering two hundred beats a minute. The red rash on his skin thickened and crusted and the ends of his fingers and toes blackened. His stomach distended so far that Lewin could trace the edge of his liver and spleen with his thumb. The child barely looked human anymore, with wires snaking into his body and black and red patches obscuring his face. Would he even last the night? Lewin wondered. He went home troubled.

But John was a fighter. He survived the night, then another, and by day three, his IV was removed so he could drink unassisted. His skin however was another matter entirely. On day four of his recovery, his nose collapsed, the bridge folding in on itself like damp cardboard. A putrid yellow fluid seeped out, which the nurses gently wiped away. Over the next few days, the gangrenous skin on his face and body was gently sloughed off, and the raw skin covered with a surgical compress. With his temperature stabilized, Lewin gently applied skin grafts to his cheeks and operated on John's ragged upper lip, knitting the edges back together. But his nose was a problem. The infection had destroyed most of it, leaving a gaping hole in the center of his face—a problem that only plastic surgery could fix.

Lewin decided to follow the rulebook for this "faceless tot"—standard procedure was to wait a few years before performing plastic surgery on infants, the reasoning being to limit the number of operations performed. "My inclination was to discharge the child from the hospital and delay further elective surgical intervention for at least a few years," he recorded[5] in his daily notes. As John grew, his nose would need continual reshaping to match the changing contours of his face, and Lewin didn't want to put the boy through any unnecessary pain.

Satisfied with the child's recovery, Lewin smiled down at the baby. His breaths came in regular bursts, his body had regained that childhood chubbiness, and his movements were relaxed. What a difference eight weeks had made! From a sickly little thing, John was now a charming—if odd looking—child, gurgling at the nurses and rolling around in his crib as he grew familiar with the limits of his body.

The following day, as Lewin tackled the overflowing paperwork in his office, Dr. Onver Mahadeen from the pediatric ward knocked on his door. He entered looking flustered, and Lewin sat up in his chair, concerned. Mahadeen was in charge of John's day-to-day care and had assisted Lewin with John's surgical recovery. He respected the pediatrician's work ethic and his principles—on top of his hospital duties, Mahadeen was a regular consultant for local law enforcement agencies, assisting to curtail infant abuses, as well as guest lecturer regarding the importance of infant immunizations.[6] He was usually unflappable.

There's a problem with John, he told Lewin.

"Really?" Lewin was confused. John had seemed fine yesterday. "He's recovering well, I thought, at least he was when I last checked."

"It's not about his health, well, not really . . ." Mahadeen paused. "It's his parents."

"His parents?"

"They won't take him."

"Won't take him?" Lewin didn't understand what Mahadeen was saying. "Won't take him where?"

"Not where . . ." Mahadeen sighed. "At all. They say that they won't take him home with them. They can't be reasoned with."

"I'll speak with them. I'm sure we can sort something out."

He found the baby's parents a mess of bewildered emotions, oscillating from joy, thanks to their child's survival, to intense loathing because of his beat-up body and destroyed face. John's father looked anywhere but at his son, and although his mother rocked him in her arms and cooed to him in Italian, she angled him away from her and averted her eyes so as not to see the hole where his nose should be. "Mimmo, mimmo," she whispered.

It's a blessing John survived at all, Lewin told them, stressing that his survival had never been assured. He can breathe! He can eat! He can sleep! He looked the father in the eye as he spoke, hoping his words would get through to him. I understand that he might look a little beat up to you now, but I promise that's a temporary state. When he is old enough to cope with the stresses of an operation, I will personally fix his nose, at no cost to you.

But the parents wouldn't budge. "Taking him home is not an option," John's father said, raising his voice for emphasis. "He doesn't come back with us until he looks human." He refused to discuss alternatives.

Dr. Mahadeen was furious. What kind of parents would refuse to take their own child? Their own recently sick child. They weren't fit to be parents, he raged. The pediatric team was in an uproar. They'd never had a problem like this before. Parents wanted to take their sick kids home, that was just how it worked. Lewin agreed with Mahadeen's sentiment—how could you reject your own child?—but he couldn't help sympathizing with the parents' plight.

On December 31, 1949, three-quarters of a million people descended on Times Square, New York, to watch a four hundred-pound wrought-iron ball drop seventy-seven feet[7] to ring in the new decade.

January 1950 heralded in a decade of progress, with easy access to cures for once-terminal diseases like polio, a booming economy, and growth in spending power that led to 77 percent of U.S. households owning televisions.[8] Life was so good that novelty items like Mr. Potato Head[9] became a state-wide obsession, raking in $4 million in sales in its first year.[10] However, many of the divides and discrimination from earlier decades remained. President Harry Truman's bid for sweeping social reforms, including universal health care, higher minimum wages, and civil rights reforms, was thwarted by the Republican Party.[11]

In the 1940s, more than a million people immigrated to the United States, a mix of war refugees and dreamers clamoring for the opportunities that the United States represented. But by the early 1950s, mass immigration was linked to the rising crime in cities, and Italians in particular were under fire. Their bad reputation dated back to the turn of the century.

"Certain kinds of criminality are inherent in the Italian race," reported the U.S. Immigration Commission in 1911. "In the popular mind, crimes of personal violence, robbery, blackmail, and extortion are peculiar to the people of Italy." These beliefs stemmed from the idea of inherited and innate criminality, which swiftly worked its way through America in the late nineteenth and early twentieth centuries, falling broadly under the eugenics umbrella.[12]

A key proponent of the "inherited criminality" movement was Italian criminologist Cesare Lombroso, born in 1835, a short, portly man with narrow wire-rimmed glasses, drooping white whiskers, and a box-cut beard.[13]

Lombroso grew up in northern Italy in a Jewish household. His father worked as a tradesman, and his mother supported his interest in classical literature and science. Early on, he was fascinated by scientific theories and awestruck by Charles Darwin's work. He read Darwin's scientific reports and his book, *On the Origin of Species by Means of Natural Selection*, over and over again. This fascination with the inner workings of the body drew him to a career in medicine, first as a doctor for Turin's military in 1859, then as a professor for the local college, and in 1871, he was appointed chief of staff for the local asylum. He oversaw a large staff, worked in diagnostics, and advised on the correct treatments for his patients, as well as consulted at local prisons.

This work gave him a chance to test some of his anthropological theories on human subjects, namely that criminals could be identified by their physical attributes.

His breakthrough came in 1872, when Giuseppe Villella, a renowned bandit and escape artist, died in jail at age sixty-nine.[14] Lombroso started Villella's postmortem the same way he began every autopsy, with the careful removal of the skin via scalpel and the ribs with a bone saw and precisely measuring the deceased's skull and chest cavity. Lifting Villella's head, he was surprised to find a large indent at the back of his skull; similar, he thought, to the apes that he'd dissected in medical school. Was Villella a throwback to more primitive humans, an atavistic dangerous type?

He cut into his scalp, pulling it gently away from the skull with forceps. A depression in the center of the occipital part of the skull appeared, to his eye, to more closely resemble the skulls of rodents and lemurs than primates. Perhaps people with similar physiognomy shared the same characteristics, he thought. If his assumption was correct, identifying such people early on could save society much grief, he concluded.

Something about this concept connected with him. It felt right, somehow, like he'd struck upon the answer to the bigger question of how society manages to breed criminals. "At the sight of that skull I seemed to see all of a sudden, lighted up as a vast plain under a flaming sky, the problem of the nature of the criminal," he later wrote.[15]

He grew more and more interested in his theory and became obsessed with proving it.[16] In the months that followed, he took intricate skull and body measurements from anyone who would let him, including his family, students at the local university, and his extended network. The only requirement was that his subjects be "honest and moral women and men." Using his initial research as a starting point, he then designed an array of instruments to assess everything from skin sensitivity, pain response, blood pressure, and even truthfulness.[17] His toolkit assembled, he visited every local prison in the region, coaxing thousands of inmates to sit for his measurement tests. He compared their data to his "moral" control group, meticulously recording any differences in his notebooks.

Some criminal traits, he discovered, were specific to gender: 15 percent of female offenders had jutting brows compared to 8 percent of "moral" women, and 20 percent of inmates displayed forehead anomalies, whereas the control group of women clocked in at 6 percent. "The criminal woman is a true monster," he wrote in his 504-page book, *La Donna Delinquente: La Prostituta E La Donna Normale* (*The Delinquent Woman: The Prostitute and the Normal Woman*). "Honest woman are kept in line by factors such as maternity, piety and weakness; when a woman commits a crime despite these restraints this is a sign that her power of evil is immense."[18]

For men, jug ears, large ears, and excessively long arms correlated to criminal behavior. In a rare touch of poetry, he labeled these signifiers as "the stigmata of degeneration."

Lombroso also found that the convicts had lower brain weights, which he believed related to their intelligence. "The maximum brain weight in healthy women is greater than that of criminals," he wrote. To him, this suggested that intelligence—and the corresponding lack of it—was key to understanding people's behavior. After all, if you're born evil and stupid, you couldn't be blamed for actions for which you are genetically predisposed—but you could be prevented from committing those offenses.

His resulting metric created a photofit of the born criminal type: dark, hairy, with overly large foreheads. These traits served a double purpose, as they were also key indicators of nonwhite heritage, in addition to "criminality." By packaging these features as reprehensible, Lombroso classed large swathes of people as detestable based on their physique rather than their actions.

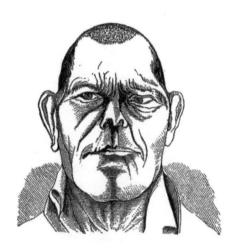

**1. P. C., brigand de la Basilicate, détenu à Pesaro.**

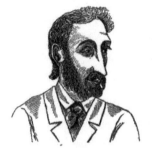

**2. Voleur piémontais.**

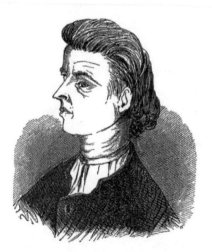

**3. Incendiaire et cynède de Pesaro, surnommé *la femme*.**

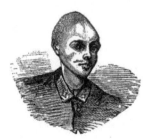

**4. Misdea.**

Sketches illustrating criminal types by Cesare Lombroso. *Courtesy Wellcome Library, London*

The hypothesis that criminals could be recognized before they'd robbed or raped someone was a comforting proposition to the people in power. Lombroso's work was embraced by the U.S. eugenics movement, which approved of his warped take on Charles Darwin's theories and used his ideas to double down on "breeding out" bad characteristics from people. This "social Darwinism" was used to justify racism and conservative politics and to dissuade reform. Numerous eugenicists advocated for mandatory sterilization for the mentally ill and the disabled, imposed discriminatory marriage restrictions, and even forced abortions on undesirables. Many American universities including Harvard and Stanford[19] dedicated programs and lectures to Lombroso's work and the broader study of eugenics.

As a direct result of these early eugenics policies, the 1924 U.S. Immigration Act set quotas on immigration.[20] Southern Italians,[21] with their dark hair and broad jaws, were viewed as the most dangerous migrants in Europe, and their entry was severely restricted. Senators based their decision on a mix of Lombroso's work and the well-publicized behavior of U.S.-based Italian terrorists; in 1919 an anarchist group mailed bombs to U.S. politicians and judges and in 1920 bombed Wall Street, killing 30 people and injuring 143.

It wasn't till 1952 that the Immigration Act was revamped, and Italians once more moved to the United States in large numbers. Although the borders opened up, negative sentiment remained. Despite the evolving laws, the majority of immigrant Italians ended up in ghettoized city enclaves and were the first to be suspected by police in times of trouble.

This was the world that baby John was born into when he took his first breaths in November 1952. Given the historical context, Lewin believed he understood (but did not approve of) John's parents' reluctance to take him home.

At St. Joseph's hospital, the staff were at a stalemate. One week passed. Then another. And another. Little John languished in the pediatric ward, his nurses friendly but unable to give the infant their full attention. Occasionally his parents stopped in for a visit, but they were resolute: fix him or he stays here.

"We have to do something!" one of Lewin's nurses said, almost in tears. "That poor baby."

A memo appeared on his desk, then another. Baby John was taking up valuable bed space. His condition was stable, and he wasn't receiving treatment from the specialists. He needed to go. The hospital didn't have the facilities to keep him indefinitely. Staff called in social services, but it was no help. "He just has too many needs for us to cater to right now," the social worker apologetically told Lewin. "We wish we could help, but he needs so much care." The social worker didn't say that he couldn't be housed because of his appearance, but Lewin knew that young babies were generally placed with families.

The memos kept coming. John was four months old now and hitting all his developmental goals; he could hold up his head and chest, roll from front to back, smile, recognize people, and his cries had evolved into babbles. He needed personal attention; someone to play with him, to introduce him to new colors and shapes, and to help him navigate his strange new world. The nurses and doctors did what they could—he'd become something of a pet—but a hospital wasn't the right place to raise a baby. The hole in his face was jarring, but the staff felt his innate sweetness more than made up for his odd looks. They appealed to his parents again, pointing out that his appearance was temporary. They stayed firm; they'd made their position clear.

Lewin puzzled about the solution to this problem. The current situation wasn't sustainable. There had to be something he could do. He leafed through the sheaf of notes in John's file, searching for an answer. A number of photographs of John's face were included, and he held them up to the light, angling them one way and then the other. Perhaps this was the answer he'd been looking for.

Using a mixture of latex, acrylic, and water, Lewin and the pediatric team carefully crafted a miniature nasal prothesis for John. This was a temporary solution that would have to be regularly reworked, but it was one that he thought the parents might accept. Carefully, he attached the prosthesis to the inside of the remainder of John's nose, then stepped back to check his handiwork. John's immediate reaction was displeasure. His hands turned into fists scrabbling at his face, and he started wailing, louder and louder, shaking his head left and right to dislodge the prothesis. Lewin hoped that John would get used to it, but when he wouldn't stop crying after an hour, he reluctantly removed it.

Undeterred, he tried another approach, this time using adhesive to secure the false nose to the skin on John's cheeks. John wailed again, but successfully removed the annoying addition by vigorously rubbing his "nose" against the bed until it detached, leaving a small piece of beige rubber in his crib.

Maybe the size is wrong, suggested a nurse. They went back to the craft table and created a smaller proboscis. Lewin tried again, using a stronger adhesive the second time around. John was restrained during the procedure and until the glue had fully dried. But a few hours later, he'd wiggled it off again. He looked rather smug, Lewin thought. He didn't have a solution that stuck.

He tried talking to John's parents about this but struck out again. St. Joseph's staff was getting creative with their opinions of the couple. They had a right to be angry, but Lewin felt saddened rather than enraged. John's parents were almost children themselves; his mother still had puppy fat, his father a smattering of acne. In a just world, they might have found themselves going on dates and studying for college classes instead of caring for another life and trekking to the hospital most weeks. But life wasn't fair, and John's tiny, lonely, disfigured face was the source of so much pain for everyone because of the couple's concerns about being viewed as different. Lewin didn't approve of their actions, but he knew all too well what it was like to be young, poor, and different, especially in New York City.

Mieczyslaw Lewin was born in 1909 in Warsaw, part of the Russian partition of Poland, and lived under the uneasy rule of a country surrounded by aggressors. His parents were Jewish; his father worked in the lumber industry and his mother was a homemaker who loved the arts and took Lewin and his older brother to the opera and orchestra recitals regularly. His brother was indifferent to these outings, but Lewin loved the culture and the ceremony involved.[22] He enrolled in piano lessons but couldn't get the hang of it. His fingers fumbled at the keys and he hated practicing. He quickly realized that he preferred enjoying music passively rather than performing.

His uncle ran the town's main pharmacy, and as a treat, he'd let Lewin mix and wrap powders for prescriptions. He marveled at the supplies and the many colored bottles and pills. At school he excelled in religious studies, history, drawing, and physics and rated satisfactory for French, Latin, mathematics, and philosophy. He thought about joining his father's business, but trips to the lumberyard quickly disenchanted him. Maybe I'd be better off working in medicine, he wondered. At school, his best subject was religion, with his work graded as excellent, whereas he was marked as "good" for physics and chemistry, along with drawing and history. However, he knew that if he applied himself, he could improve his marks and then build on that training in medical school.

The looming war didn't make that easy. Poland, which gained independence in 1918 in the aftermath of World War I, had instituted numerous restrictions on medical training for Jewish students, making it impossible for Lewin to study there. So Lewin moved to Switzerland when he was eighteen years old to attend the Medical School of Zurich—it was more expensive than Warsaw, but it was his only chance to get qualified. His parents were sad to see him go but supported his decision; they wanted him to have the best education possible. He was especially drawn to surgery, impressed by how a delicate operation could have instant beneficial results.[23]

Lewin graduated in 1933 and was eager to return home, but his parents advised against it. Poland was now heavily anti-Semitic, they warned, and he might not be allowed to practice medicine if he returned. Saddened by this news but resolute in his desire to treat people, Lewin looked farther afield for his next position. He settled on New York City, as his uncle, the renowned plastic surgeon Dr. Jacques Maliniac, was based there. To fit into American culture, he changed his name from Mieczyslaw to Michael, hoping it would help with his assimilation. He'd heard that Americans struggled with foreign-sounding names and wanted everything to run smoothly. He never used Mieczyslaw again.

Dr. Maliniac helped him land an assistant residency position at Beth Israel Hospital in Manhattan's East Village. The work was unpaid but provided him with free accommodation and meals. Two or three nights a week he attended English language classes to develop his vocabulary and eliminate his accent.

New York City was overwhelming to twenty-five-year-old Lewin, with its bafflingly tall buildings, bright billboards, and banks of television screens broadcasting the latest fashions and music. It felt like he'd stepped into the Land of Oz. All the women seemed incredibly sophisticated as they trotted around in their tailored crepe suits and figure-hugging jersey knits, with their finger-waved hair swishing behind them.[24] But the glitz of New York felt a million miles away from him, with his shabby clothes and shabbier English. He lived there, but he felt like he didn't belong, as if he was marked as different, as alien, to everyone he met.

It was awkward simply to exist, a struggle to complete basic activities like buying a bus ticket or ordering himself some American fries. With each halting word, he felt that he was drawing attention to himself, his otherness, his un-American-ness. He hated how his Jewishness was mentioned as a slur; even when ignored, it remained ever present in the eyes of his peers and his professors. At one of his language classes he met Berta, a twenty-nine-year old social worker and adult educator, but he couldn't afford to treat her. He wanted to take her to the finest places, but he had to settle for picnics in Central Park that she prepared and rowing her round and around Central Park Lake. After Beth Israel, he worked at his uncle's plastic surgery practice for a couple of years and saved up for months to buy her a ring. Even so, the diamond was tiny. They married in 1940 in a small City Hall ceremony. He was happy to have met her, but he still felt judged and dismissed; he'd noticed people wrinkle their noses at his shabby shoes and laugh at his accent.

Some still did, surely, even now, but not to his face, not anymore. Not now that he was the senior plastic surgery attendee at St. Joseph's Hospital, as well as at two more local hospitals, plus a private clinic in Manhattan. These roles were

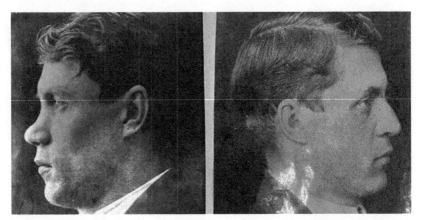

Before and after nose surgery on San Quentin inmate. *Courtesy Anne T. Kent California Room, Marin County Free Library*

born out of sweat, long hours, and his burning desire to fulfill the American dream in an America that was slow to recognize him as one of its own.

He didn't approve of John's parents' behavior, but he found it easy to see how their circumstances might have led them to believe that they had no alternative. Standing out from society involves pain, finger pointing, and a sense of otherness. People who didn't fit society's perceived norms can be subjected to rejection and ridicule. Parenting a baby when barely out of your teens with little income was a momentous task in itself; to do so with a child that likely would draw negative attention and cruelty with every breath seemed impossible.

Even so, Lewin felt strongly that a loving home with two supportive parents would provide John the best start in life. Lacking that, the only option left was social care, where John would grow up shuttled from institution to institution, taunted and bullied for his unusual appearance. John would become a statistic, another number on a form in a social worker's office. With that kind of start in life, Lewin reasoned, this sweet little boy likely would grow into an angry, resentful teenager, leading to its own set of problems.

He read the news; the papers highlighted the growing number of juvenile delinquents and the problems they caused. The number of these problem children locked in reformatories seemed to increase daily.[25]

Public consensus about the problem was mixed. The *Times-Advocate*, a small paper in Escondido, California, published two poems on the topic, a month apart.[26]

A juvenile delinquent, I now would say,
And I am sure it is,

A modern term, that's being used
For what we did as kids

rhymed thirty-six-year-old Velva Hulen, expressing her displeasure at how youths were being labeled. A rebuttal from Mrs. J. E. Joy followed.

There are Gods laws and mans laws, to guide us all along
A juvenile delinquent son, is a youth who has gone wrong.[27]

Notwithstanding the syntax, current research suggested that children who lacked positive parental influences were more likely to commit crimes, especially as adults. This problem didn't affect just big cities; earlier that year a local paper, the *Chatham Press*, published an impassioned column on the subject.[28] "Delinquency springs from seeds sown in the home," it chastised. "It is up to the parents to see that [children] are properly educated." Even Lewin's local rotary club was up in arms about teenage crime, with a never-ending roster of speakers discussing the role of parenting in delinquent behavior.[29]

Lewin didn't want that to become John's future. His parents really did love him, he knew. Lewin saw their eyes soften as they held him, and he had watched them wait, white faced and barely eating during the week that John's life hung in the balance. They could give him a good home, a loving one, a place where he could flourish and grow into the man he was capable of becoming—if only they could see the big picture. However, John's physical appearance first needed to be acceptable to his parents so they would take him home.

The problem gnawed at him. At home, he couldn't concentrate on his wife's conversation, smiling absentmindedly at her while he took deep drags of his pipe. He exhaled slowly as he considered the remaining options. He couldn't in good consciousness operate and build John a new nose, just to subject the child to a painful surgical readjustment when he outgrew it four months later.

Hmm. Outgrow it. Outgrow it. . . . He stood up quickly, accidentally flicking ash onto the floor in his haste. He walked to his study, retrieving a number of thick, bound journals from his shelves and thumping them onto his desk. He thumbed through the volumes, becoming more excited by the minute. Maybe, just maybe. . . . He pulled out a crisp sheet of paper from his desk tray and wrote in his scrawling blue script: "Can I ask you—." If this plan was going to work, he needed all the help he could get.

Several weeks later, Lewin reshelved his journals in despair. He'd reached out to everyone he knew—and others who they'd recommended—and they'd all said the same thing. They were sorry, and they wished they could help, but they had no records of any similar operation performed on a child this small. Lewin scanned the latest letter again, hoping that somehow, some new piece of information would appear on the page.

"If it were practicable, all such cases should be fitted with an artificial piece until the face is fully grown," wrote Dr. Thomas Kilner, a London-based plastic surgeon, in response to Lewin's inquiry. Kilner was considered a global expert on infant operations. "Even if expense was no object, as the infant grew up, no child would ever tolerate the wearing of such an appliance and there would be constant trouble when school days began," he continued. "It is however, in my opinion, quite wrong to condemn a child to go about so sadly disfigured, partly for its own sake and partly for the sake of the parents who have to see it all day and every day for years. I have therefore proceeded to reconstruct a nose as early as three years."

Three years! That was a lifetime for John. Lewin shook his head, resigning himself to the fact that there were no answers to be had. He was going off script; there was no rulebook for his plan.

It took some explaining for John's parents to understand the situation, and Lewin still wasn't sure they fully comprehended what he was attempting by the time he started operating. John was eight months old by now, a lively infant prone to wriggling out of the nurses' arms and speeding around the wards on his chubby hands and knees till he was recaptured. An operation was far from ideal at his age, but Lewin had weighed the benefits of surgery. In the end, he felt that the challenges involved with operating on an infant were offset by the problem of caring for him during the intervening time.

Based on the assumption that John's new nose would not be his final nose, Lewin worked toward a future concept of what John would look like in a year, rather than at the present time. Under light anesthesia, he detached a slice of skin from John's abdomen, leaving one flap still attached in order to maintain the flap's blood supply. A month later, he attached the flap of skin to John's forearm, and a little time later, to his face.

Once the additional piece of skin had latched on to its new blood supply, Lewin freed John's arm from its brace and reshaped the skin flap into a nose. He was cautious with his work, operating seven times in order to complete it, ending when John was a year old.[30] Finally, John's face was fully formed again—

with an elephantine schnozz. "I Cyrano de Beregarc'd him," Lewin told the nurses, with a shy but pleased smile.

The effect was comical. John looked like a half-drawn cartoon caricature, a miniature Jimmy Durante. But he was physically complete. "He'll grow up to his nose," Lewin told his parents. They stared at their child, stunned into silence by his new appearance. His mother looked bewildered as she rocked him—but she did look him straight in the eyes for the first time in months.

"I'll see him again in a few years; the hospital work isn't done yet," Lewin told them. Every few years he adjusted the child's nose until he became an adult.[31]

For now, it was up to his parents to care for him as best they could. Lewin's gamble was a success; the parents accepted this compromise and took John home with them. There were cheers throughout the ward when they left as a family unit. Lewin's plan had worked.

The national papers covered the story, sans pictures, due to patient privacy. "Surgeon gives tiny baby new nose," commended the *Boston Globe*.[32] "Baby's lost nose replaced by long one," bandied the *Miami News*.[33] "Baby given new nose so parents will accept him," remarked the *Record*.[34]

"In spite of the shortcomings the main goal was accomplished, namely acceptance by the family and community," Lewin recorded in his clinical notes.[35] Their acceptance continued; on checkups, he observed their devotion to John, almost as if nearly losing him had made them love him all the more.

This matter settled, Lewin could return to work as usual, he thought. He didn't need any more drama. Then a letter arrived on his desk, postmarked Sing Sing Correctional Facility, Ossining, New York.

# 2

# SING SING PRISON
# AND PLASTIC SURGERY
# SOCIAL WORK

Every time Michael Lewin passed through the Corinthian columns that bracketed Grand Central Terminal, he paused to take in his surroundings. In 1953, four thousand light bulbs kept the station unnaturally bright for the 560,000 or so folk who frequented it each day. People of all ages and economic backgrounds mingled together as they weaved across the pink marble floor, so intent on their destinations that few looked up to view the 2,500 stars painted on the ceiling. Fragments of conversations drifted Lewin's way; he caught snatches of German, French, and his native Polish from among the throng. Smiling, he made his way to the platform and boarded the Metro-North train.

As it chugged out of Manhattan, he took a long drag on his pipe, releasing the cherry-flavored smoke in one smooth exhale. The forty-four-year-old watched the landscape turn from gray to green, globs of nature brightening his view as the skyscrapers receded. It took forty minutes to get to Ossining, a small village in Westchester County, the train snaking its way along the banks of the Harlem River before curving upstate along the Hudson. En route Lewin passed Yonkers, home to America's first golf course, and Sleepy Hollow, the town made infamous by Washington Irving's gothic horror story, before the train pulled into Ossining station.

Ostensibly a sleepy commuter town with a population of sixteen thousand people[1]—around 1 percent of the population of the Bronx—Ossining's unhappy claim to fame had gained it worldwide attention. Since 1826, it was home to the notorious Sing Sing prison. It was a short distance from the station to the prison, and Lewin decided to walk, enjoying the chance to stretch his legs after the train ride. The prison was uphill, an architectural design choice that made it loom ominously over approaching visitors. Towering redbrick cell blocks peeked inscrutably over the twenty-four-foot concrete walls[2] enclosing the fifty-five-acre maximum security facility.

Lewin had never visited an inmate before and wasn't sure what to expect. The little he knew of prison life was gleaned from movies and newspapers, which dramatized inexcusable acts and broadcast tales of violence and misery and hardened good-for-nothing cons.

He knew that these reports were likely to be exaggerated or at least that they represented the worst of the worst, and, alongside these monsters, there were sure to be some small-time crooks. But Sing Sing inmates had a particularly nasty reputation; right now the prison housed Julius and Ethel Rosenberg, the New York couple convicted of espionage for leaking nuclear secrets to the Russians. Two years earlier, the Lonely Heart Killers had fried here, their electrocutions splashed all over the *Daily News*[3] and the *New York Times*.

Lewin checked in with the uniformed guards at the iron front gate who gestured him inside, cranking the gate open with a hellish screeching sound. He passed a few more checkpoints before an inmate in gray pants and a white shirt arrived to escort him to the prison hospital, driving him up the hill inside the prison van. They stopped outside a four-story block made of the same red brick as the other buildings.[4]

Built in 1928, the hospital's architects had designed each floor to cater to different needs. The pharmacy and the eye, ear, nose, and throat clinic were on the first floor; psychiatrists who provided full intake assessments were on the second floor; and the third floor held patient wards and isolation rooms for contagious diseases.[5]

The fourth floor was for surgery and was equipped with two scrub rooms, two operating rooms tiled in white, a room for sterilizing equipment, and a recovery area for patients. Lewin tried his best to keep his face relaxed but couldn't help peering into the rooms he passed, trying to get a sense of the space. The barred windows and shackles attached to some of the beds were a constant reminder that a patient's liberty—and health—was no longer his own.

Overall, he thought the hospital's facilities were on the small side—especially for the number of men it served—and it was stocked with outdated equipment and worn benches and tables. It was significantly more provincial than he was used to, but his time in the U.S. Army had trained him to adapt to difficult environments.

What an unpleasant place to live, he thought. Out the window, he glimpsed the prison's large football and baseball fields—leftovers from the reforms of

Warden Lewis Lawes, who served from 1920 to 1941, the inmate told him, warning him that the current warden, Wilfred Denno, a man who bemoaned the end of corporal punishment to the press, did not hold with such luxuries and ruled the 1,700[6] or so souls under his control with a firm hand. When Denno took charge of Sing Sing, he immediately canceled all football games (baseball was still allowed) and cut down on amenities. Whereas Lawes believed that every man had the potential for goodness, Denno publicized his belief that a proper upbringing and judicial use of the lash had a more lasting effect on men than education or exercise.

⌒⌒

A few weeks earlier, Lewin had written to Warden Wilfred Denno, requesting the opportunity to meet and possibly operate on twenty-two-year-old William Ricci, recently admitted for first-degree manslaughter. Ricci was his former patient, he explained, and he'd appreciate the chance to finish his treatment. To be precise—though there was no need to go into this with Warden Denno— Lewin had inherited Ricci's case when his mentor, Dr. Morris Smith, died in 1950.[7] One of Smith's last requests was that Lewin continue treating Ricci, a pro bono patient born with a harelip and cleft palate.

Lewin found Ricci to be a typical dead-end kid raised in a one-parent household and brought up in poverty. His mother died when he was seventeen. Ricci had little interest in his education and few prospects for his future; he wasn't even pleased that Lewin would continue Smith's work. Nonetheless, Lewin dutifully started repairs on his face. Fixing a cleft lip and palate was a process; Ricci needed at least three surgeries, each building on the last, each new operation reliant on how well the scars had flattened as they healed. In Lewin's experience, it could take three or four operations just to make the boy's lips look even, and his palate needed to be tweaked a few times so as to improve his speech.

Ricci was an awkward patient, often disappearing for months at a time and rarely keeping his appointments. His lackadaisical approach and inconsiderate behavior irritated Lewin. This was not how his patients were supposed to behave!

Still he persisted, sending letter after letter to Ricci, encouraging him to reschedule and finish the process. Lewin had respected Dr. Smith a great deal, and the old surgeon's kindness and mentorship was not something he took lightly. Smith had been one of the people who were there for him in 1945, on the day he got the dreadful news from Warsaw that his parents had died in a ghetto. Lewin treasured people who were kind to him and did his best to honor

# PLASTIC SURGERY RESULTS

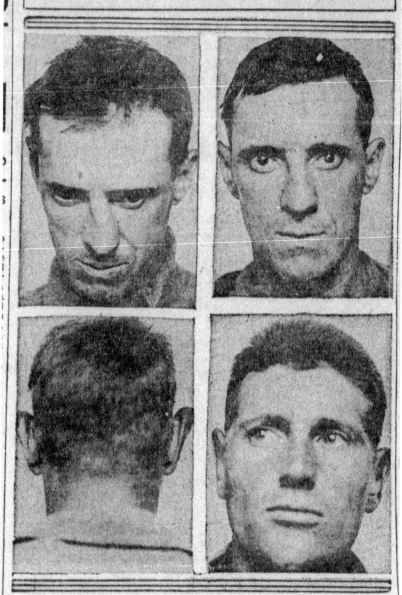

Here are two examples of how San Quentin surgeons are "making over" auricular and nasal defects of prison inmates. Above, on left, a convict's nose before the operation. On right is shown the straightened nasal organ. Below, a felon's ears "before and after."

Plastic surgery results from San Quentin prison, California, 1921. San Francisco Examiner, *July 3, 1921*

Smith's request. But his letters returned unopened; the boy had vanished despite his incomplete surgery.

Two years passed before he heard from Ricci again. Now a resident in Sing Sing Correctional Facility, he wanted Lewin's help once more. Lewin folded and refolded Ricci's letter in his hand. That boy had been trouble from the start, and it looked like that would continue. He had no experience with prisons and wasn't even sure that the boy's face would be operable, but he wrote back to Ricci, promising he'd try. Warden Denno was surprised but intrigued by Lewin's letter and agreed to let him visit and tend the boy, with the proviso that any surgery took place in the prison hospital at no charge to the prison.

Lewin shifted awkwardly in his hardback chair as he waited for the guards to escort Ricci in. The door creaked open, and Ricci stepped inside, a wide smile brightening his sallow face when he saw the surgeon. His expression stretched his skin into a twisted mess of tissue, exposing chipped and broken teeth. The boy was five feet eight but seemed to have shrunk, looking very small and young in his prison scrubs. Lewin instinctively curled his shoulders to make his five ten height less intimidating.

It was immediately clear to him that Ricci's condition had worsened, in no small part due to the number of appointments he'd missed: his face now classed as a "resident deformity." He'd also busted his nose, his septum deviating sharply to the left, no doubt caused by a fistfight or something similar.

Once admitted to the facility, prison protocol had shuffled Ricci through the production of inmate processing at Sing Sing's classification center. Around 70 percent of prison admissions throughout the state arrived in Ossining to be weighed, prodded, and psychologically tested before being assigned to an appropriate institution.[8] For two weeks, Ricci was held in the classification unit undergoing the prison orientation. His personal effects were recorded and locked away, and he was outfitted with the white shirt and gray pants that made up an inmate's uniform. His mug shot was taken, first from the front and then from the side, and he was fingerprinted, weighed, measured, and prodded by the medical staff. They recorded his eye, skin, and hair color on the intake register. Under "distinguishable marks," they'd noted his harelip, the twisted bow of skin that snaked across Ricci's upper lip and nose.

He'd been a model inmate so far, the prison doctor told Lewin, noting that Ricci was polite, quiet, and didn't give any trouble. His behavior had been graded an "A" on the receiving blotter. But he rarely smiled and seemed antisocial.

Lewin gestured for Ricci to sit down so he could examine him. Leaning forward in his chair, he ran his thumbs and index fingers gently across the boy's face, pressing gently but firmly to gauge the shape of the bone below. The boy's face still could be saved, he realized, but the procedures and aftercare would be challenging. But with Ricci confined to Sing Sing, he'd at least be able to finish his work this time around.

Lewin kept his questions short and to the point—Does this hurt? What about this? How does it feel when I do this? He didn't ask Ricci about his crime, but, lulled by Lewin's familiar presence and calm brown gaze, Ricci volunteered details, his words tumbling over each other in a way that would have amazed the arresting officers.

"It was the teasing," he told Lewin. "It . . . it got to be too much."

He wasn't dumb, he explained. He'd always known he looked different from the other kids, that he was the ugly mug in the crowd. Ever since he could remember, his scars, snaggled lip, and stutter had made him the butt of every joke. The other kids called him monkey boy, pig face—name a slur, and he'd heard it. Even adults joined in sometimes. This happened everywhere: in the classroom, in the streets, at the movie theaters. He couldn't get a date. Even the idea was laughable; what kind of girl would touch him? He pushed down his feelings of inadequacy and self-loathing, refusing to address them. What was the point? But he got by, he said, even if it wasn't on book smarts. He was good with his hands, he said, and he'd proved himself on New York's docks, unloading crates and barrels without complaint. Among the smoke and grime of the port, he'd built himself a life, made friends. He drank whiskey with his coworkers in the cheap bars that ringed the port. It wasn't much, but it was his.

But then, around 3:00 a.m. at a New Year's party, his friend Jack started teasing him, mimicking his slurred speech and rolling his eyes. Ricci told him to stop, but that just spurred Jack on. There was a roaring in his ears. It felt like he'd been punched—a deep, visceral pain. Something in him snapped. Everything he'd repressed for so long came out, fueled by the mocking laughter. Bang! Jack was dead, just like that, with three shots in his chest, and the laughter had stopped.[9] He hadn't even realized his gun was out till it was too late. Now his life, what little it was, was over, he said morosely.

Or was it? With Lewin's help, maybe he could change, he said. Lewin nodded sympathetically. He'd heard variations of this tale a thousand times. The circumstances and the characters changed, but the story was a classic, a sad history of alienation, disenfranchisement, and lookism, parceled along with poverty and poor parenting. "I can help," he told Ricci. "But I'll need you to follow my directions properly this time." Ricci nodded.

Ricci's first surgery took around four hours, during which Lewin painstakingly excised the scar from his last surgery and reshaped his nostrils into symmetrical tunnels. Using a cartilage graft, he rebuilt his septum, employing a scaffold of cartilage, so his nostrils stood as distinct entities. He gave extra attention to his soft palate muscle, suturing it till it lay smooth, so Ricci wouldn't struggle as much with his speech. Ricci was groggy when he woke up and initially afraid to look in the mirror. When he finally lifted his eyes to the glass, his eyes widened involuntarily.

Thirty years earlier, Ricci's operations would have looked very different. With plastic surgery in its infancy, as many people died in hospitals as at home. During World War I, soldiers with devastating wounds—faces blown off, bones crushed, skin shredded and burned—crowded military hospitals in vast numbers, their beds filled as soon as they died.[10] Teams of surgeons struggled to find solutions to horrific injuries, drawing inspiration from multiple disciplines, consulting with dental specialists to prevent rebuilt jaws from collapsing and dermatologists to investigate the use of skin tissue to cover burns. Postwar, these doctors offered apprenticeships to junior doctors so their new skills could be shared.

Many of these surgeons turned their attention to disfigurements in general—children with cleft palates and burns, as well as the lucrative private practice of beautifying socialites and the Hollywood elite. For the average person, plastic surgery remained a novelty, but surgeons, filmmakers, and writers found that women craved these Cinderella stories.

For many, it was personal. The economic slump of the growing Depression had forced vast numbers of women into the workforce, and many found increased self-image awareness as part and parcel with the bright city lights. It wasn't surprising to be judged based on appearance—for most, this had been part of life since they were old enough to recognize beauty, but it felt a lot more immediate when ensconced in an office. No longer hinted at, here the segregation was clear: the slim and symmetrical white girls were sent to the front desk, the Black and homely girls to the backroom. For now, plastic surgery was out of reach, but many wondered how their lives might change if somehow they could afford it.

Some of these plastic surgeons turned their newfound talents on the prison population. Eugenic thinking might be consigned to history, but that didn't mean that prisoners couldn't benefit cosmetically from the scalpel. And certainly, injuries were rampant in prisons, with incidents two or three times that of the general population, and surgical treatment often required.

"Crime we know to be a real social or economic malady," stated the 1921 New York Department of Correction report.[11] "While we do not believe that medicine, psychiatry or surgery play the only role in the rehabilitation of the criminal, much can be learned from the medical men." Sing Sing, under Warden Lewis Lawes's guidance, embraced this philosophy. Warden Lawes implemented thorough health checks for the inmates and increased the number of medical staff.[12] For him, the link between inmate health and behavior was clear; providing inmates access to quality medical treatment was no longer purely functional—health care served a rehabilitative purpose too.

Since the early 1930s, plastic surgery had been included in Sing Sing's medical care. "We restored self-esteem to men whose hideous appearance had made them bitter, resentful and antisocial," Dr. Amos Osborne Squire, then Sing Sing's chief medical officer, revealed in his 1935 memoir, *Sing Sing Doctor*.[13] One inmate was particularly memorable, Squire recalled, a brawler who'd arrived with an "almost completely demolished" nose. Squire got creative with his beauty doctoring, carving out a slim slice of the man's left rib and grafting it onto his face for support, resulting in a "perfect Grecian model." Once released, the inmate never returned to Sing Sing.

More operations followed, but throughout the 1930s and 1940s, the New York Department of Corrections drew little attention to this unusual incarceration benefit.

"It's been done occasionally in the federal service," New York's Corrections Commissioner Austin MacCormick told the media in 1934.[14] "You find a case every now and then of some man with a busted nose or disfiguring scar who looks like a broken-down pug and complains he can't get a decent job because of his appearance." When pressed for information, he described the case of an inmate who'd arrived with a large scar on his face, a slash that ran across his cheekbone to the curve of his jaw. His injury was caused by a car accident, but at first glance, it looked like a stab wound. "It made him look like a very rough character—but he was not convicted for a serious crime," MacCormick explained. "It would handicap him when looking for a job, especially if his prison record was known. He would feel he was carrying a brand for life." In all cases, he stressed, the idea was to make the men presentable to society, not to make them Hollywood stars.

# REFORM SURGERY

Convict's Face Remodeled in Hope of Changing Character

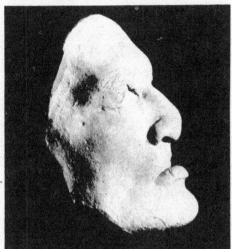

A new face has been given to Convict 25578 of Stateville Prison, Joliet, Illinois, in hope of giving him a new, non-criminal character. Convict 25578 was born with roofless mouth and a misshaped nose lacking septum, had few teeth because of a missing gum line. These handicaps were blamed for an attitude toward life which made him a problem child, an adult criminal, now serving his third term. Above is a mask of his old face.
International News Photos

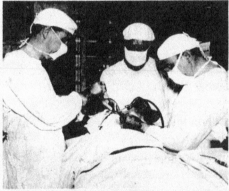

In a two-hour prison operation performed by Dr. John Pick, Chicago plastic surgeon, the face of Convict 25578 is remodeled.

Dr. John Pick provides plastic surgery
to a twenty-two-year-old convict
at Stateville Prison, Joliet, 1947.
*International News Photos*

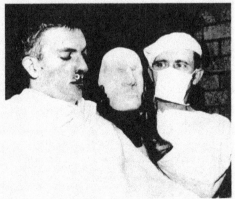

After the operation, Dr. Pick holds up the face mask for comparison with the 22-year-old convict's new features. Nose has been shaped to ordinary proportions, upper lip built out to improve appearance of mouth. Buttons are for holding lip in place until incisions heal.

ober 19, 1947

The press didn't appreciate his efforts with New York's prison population.[15] "Making Angel Faces?" asked the *Lancaster Era*'s headline.[16] "Shall We Remodel Criminals or Remodel Prisons?" questioned the *Courier*.[17] "Beauty Clinic for Thugs!" screamed the *Charleston Daily Mail* and the *Hartford Courant*. "NY May Beautify City Jail Inmates," reported the *Daily Capital News*.[18] One reporter was so amused, he composed a ditty.[19]

Handsome does as handsome is becomes a newer guide
And criminals to be reformed must first be beautified.

Thanks to the hyperbolic headlines, an embarrassed MacCormick was forced to issue a statement clarifying that "hardened criminals" were ineligible for plastic surgery work. The fuss faded away but resurged every couple of months; it was too juicy a topic for the press to leave alone. The public loved it as well or, more accurately, loved to hate on every new report of cosmetically altered criminals.

⌒⌒

In 1948, one case in particular seized the nation's attention, that of the so-called "Ugly Burglar," John Glaefke of Cleveland.[20] Glaefke was arrested as he tried to steal a gum-dispensing machine from a local sweet shop. In a court hearing, he told the judge that he'd been driven to crime because of lifelong social shunning from his peers.[21]

His tale of woe started when he was small—in school, he said that his classmates avoided him. "I'm the ugly duckling of my family," he said; his three sisters and one brother were all conventionally attractive. He'd always been friendless—people always rejected him.[22] He'd asked out one girl only to be told, "I wouldn't be seen dead with you!"[23]

He dreamed about getting plastic surgery, viewing an operation as the only way to make friends. "I thought I could get a better job and meet some nice girls," he told the court. "I'm so ugly no one cares for me."[24] But with no money, at twenty-three years old he turned to theft and stole a typewriter from a school.[25] He was arrested and sent to the reformatory, where the other inmates shunned him, he said. At twenty-eight, he was drafted into the army, and the same thing happened; no one wanted to know him. "His flat nose, wide nostrils, thick lips, and protruding ears combined to make him so ugly that GIs wouldn't associate with him," the court reporter wrote. Depressed, Glaefke tried to drown himself and was discharged.

The judge exchanged glances with the court psychiatrist and probation officers. Looking at Glaefke's disjointed features, they could see the truth in his words. "His head was enormous, his ears huge and protruding, his eyes hooded and sullen, his nose grotesque, splayed, twisted like an animal's, his mouth a monstrosity."[26]

His story moved the public, and two local surgeons volunteered their time and expertise. Over the next couple of months, Glaefke had free plastic surgery and oral work worth approximately $3,000, with three hospital visits and numerous medical appointments. His out-of-pocket cost was $35 for denture materials.

. "I'm still no Adonis," Glaefke shyly told reporters, but he was happy with his slimmed down nose and lips. The boost in his confidence enabled him to hold down a job, and he had started night school. "He is a changed man," his probation officer declared. "It is almost unbelievable."[27]

Talk show hosts debated the "ugly burglar" conundrum, and columnists penned op-eds about Glaefke's transformation. His story was covered by *Time* magazine.[28] The public was so intrigued by his tale that two years later, when Glaefke got married, the newspapers covered it—"Wedding Bells Ring for Ugly Burglar," read one headline.[29] The *New York Times* opted for a simpler, "Ugly Burglar Married."[30] They printed photographs of Glaefke with his new bride, the pair beaming behind a four-tier wedding cake.[31]

Dear Dr. Lewin,

I am very sorry that I didn't thank you for coming up and operating on me like you did. I didn't realize it until the day after the operation and I felt very bad about it. . . . The nose and the lip came out very nice. . . . All the civilian nurses at the hospital said what a good job you did. All my friends say that I talk better than I did before the operation. I want to thank you again for all you have done for me. . . .[32]

—William Ricci, c/o Sing Sing Correctional Facility

Lewin returned to Sing Sing multiple times during the next few years, always accompanied with a fully equipped doctor's bag. Ricci stayed true to his word. For once, he was a perfect patient. He followed Lewin's postoperative instructions to the letter, changing his bandages at the correct intervals, and spent hours practicing his pronunciation to help mold his refashioned palate.

Back in the city, Lewin couldn't get Sing Sing out of his head. While walking down the crowded Manhattan sidewalks or on his knees, pulling up tomatoes in his garden, images of the men at Sing Sing would surface in his head. His four-year-old daughter and six-year-old son tugged at his arms for attention, "Daddy, Daddy!" Distracted, he smiled at them, trying to put the prison work behind him. Family time was such a pleasure. "We like that there's roamin' room," his son confided, stretching his pudgy arms wide to encompass their backyard. "All children should be raised like this."[33]

It was the first time his kids had enjoyed a backyard. During his conscription in the war effort, they'd moved from

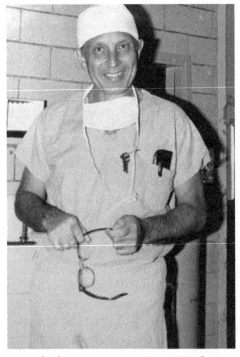

Dr. Michael Lewin in surgery, circa 1962. *Courtesy of Michael L. Lewin Papers, 1927–1994, PS 16, Harvard Medical Library, Francis A. Countway Library of Medicine, Boston*

place to place, never putting down any real roots. His modest house in Tenafly, New Jersey, was his son's first real home, a home where the grass was green and his parents literally put down roots in the garden. In summer, slices of tomato, freshly picked, were served at dinner. Lewin agreed with his son—this *was* the way to live. The way all kids should live. But his boy didn't know how lucky he was or how hard Lewin and his wife had worked to give him this. Children like Ricci hadn't had it so good.

Ricci's mother, the only nurturer he'd known, was dead. He'd had to fight for everything in his life. He'd had no one looking out for him, no one teaching him right from wrong. It was almost a surprise he hadn't been jailed earlier. Who could blame him with that kind of start in life? It was hard surviving in America when you were poor and alone; Lewin knew that for a fact. What would have happened to him if his uncle hadn't helped set him up in New York? Lewin couldn't see himself succumbing to crime; his parents had been very firm about right and wrong—but who could say what a man would do when he'd run out of options? Now that he was in a position of privilege, he wanted—no—he needed to help those less fortunate.

It wasn't just Ricci who needed help. On his visits to the prison he'd seen so many injured men, men with backstories that were likely similar to Ricci's, he realized. Men who had fallen on bad times, who had been dealt a rough hand, or who simply suffered violence or prejudice by virtue of being born with Black or brown skin.

Lewin was shocked by the high number of disfigurements he'd seen while cursorily walking around the hospital. Men with jug ears, noses crooked, flattened, and twisted, faces scarred and burnt, and among that, an abundance of obscene tattoos: crude drawings of genitals and curse words scarred across inmates' shoulders and backs. The prisoners were far more scarred than the general population. He'd known this on paper—medical journals from the *British Medical Journal* to the *Rocky Mountain Medical Journal* and the *Plastic and Reconstructive Surgery Journal* regularly covered inmate health care—but he hadn't fully comprehended it till seeing it in person.

Lewin wanted to do more for the inmates but he had so many time commitments—every week he was traveling between hospitals in New Jersey and New York while trying to build up his private practice in Manhattan. But just because he was busy didn't mean he couldn't spare some time—and, perhaps, even convince other plastic surgeons to help as well.

"How about we send some New York plastic surgeons to the prison every week," he proposed to Warden Denno. "We could schedule specific days and times, and it would take the pressure off your medical team." He was careful not to sound dismissive of Denno's staff—the prison occasionally performed plastic surgery but, lacking the specialist knowledge of Lewin and his peers, their results were of varying success. Lewin was emphatic that he could change that. We'll work with your protocols, we'll comply with everything necessary, he said.

Denno agreed—as long as it didn't cost anything.

Lewin never asked the inmates what crimes had brought them there. He didn't want to know. He would treat them regardless, if they asked for his help. And so many needed help—every time he visited, he stayed later and later, aware that there would always be patients he wouldn't have time for. And these inmates needed him, he felt. He could see it in their eyes, in the way that they held themselves once he'd worked on them: like new men ready to face the world. "Their motivation is to free themselves from their self-conscious occupation with their deformity," he wrote.[34] He rarely saw an inmate he'd worked on return to the prison.

He thought of his work there as plastic surgery; treating Ricci's cleft palate so that he could speak and eat better was a purely functional operation, just as fixing a depressed nose or weak chin helped patients function better in society. However, inmates rarely drew distinctions between cosmetic and plastic surgery; surgery was surgery, but Lewin's surgeries made them feel better about themselves.

Due in part to Lewin's work at Sing Sing, the American Correctional Association added a section on plastic surgery to the 1954 *Manual of Correctional Standards*, a hefty 451-page volume that had been distributed to every jail and prison in the United States since 1946.[35]

Their revision highlighted the correctional association's new approach to criminal reform. "Plastic and other types of elective surgery to correct or reduce disfigurements of the body, especially repulsive facial disfigurements, has a definite place in the rehabilitation of prisoners," it stated. "Such corrective measures tend to reduce feelings of inferiority, encourage greater self-confidence, and make it easier to obtain and hold a job."

The manual advised that plastic surgery be teamed with psychotherapy and "limited to cases in which genuine benefits may be anticipated." The push to rehabilitate offenders came from the top down. As the behavioral sciences grew, the concept that one could "treat" offenders like those with physical ailments such as cancer became the dominant outlook on prisoner care. In 1949, the U.S. Supreme Court promoted this perspective. "Retribution is no longer the dominant objective of the criminal law," it declared.[36]

Averell Harriman, the New York State governor, followed Lewin's work with interest. "We Americans have, in general, no taste and not much natural talent for prisons. Our belief in liberty makes us just not good at repression," Harriman told the delegates at the National Probation and Parole Association Conference.[37] "We know that there are some types of persons who have committed antisocial acts who can be rehabilitated. Medical treatment, including plastic surgery, often helps change a man's whole viewpoint. We need new knowledge—penitentiaries do not make men penitent and reformatories do not reform."

# 3

# CRIME'S CINDERELLA COMPLEX

Facelifting Helps Criminals—*Bedford Daily-Times Mail*, 1958[1]

U.S. Crime Rate Tied to State of Economy—*Democrat and Chronicle*, 1959

In 1958,[2] Michael Lewin was offered the position of chief of plastic surgery at Montefiore Medical Center, a 1,400-bed hospital in north-central Bronx[3] sandwiched between the Williamsbridge Oval Park and Woodlawn Cemetery. His title was something of a misnomer, as Montefiore had no plastic surgery programs in operation, and initially he'd be the chief of himself. The role entailed building the department from scratch while developing a training program for medical residents. It was a challenging enterprise made more difficult by the fact that the rival teaching hospitals of Columbia-Presbyterian and Mount Sinai had long-established trainee programs and were many students' first pick.

Lewin accepted the job immediately. He'd never shied away from hard work, and there was a certain cache attached to building something from the ground up—if he was successful, of course, which was not guaranteed. Still, he felt good about his decision—he'd long appreciated the values held by Montefiore Medical Center, which paralleled his own. Since 1884, the hospital had provided free treatment to anyone in need, whereas care at most other hospitals came with a bill. Accordingly, for many New Yorkers, medical care was accessible only to the middle class and above, a concept Lewin disagreed with. Good health shouldn't belong to the wealthy.

Montefiore Medical Center also took a progressive view on social care and health in the city, a legacy that went back decades. It was one of the first hospitals to run a social work clinic and had accepted Black trainee doctors since the 1930s, despite protests and resignation threats[4] from staff and patients. Lewin felt proud that he'd be working somewhere so inclusive, but mostly he was just happy to have a full-time job.

His career, like many others, had been sidetracked by World War II—requisitioned by the government as an army surgeon, he'd moved his family from New York to California to Massachusetts and then finally back to New Jersey. He'd had scant time for research during this period. The time spent away from formal institutions had hurt his prospects; he'd been trying to get a full-time position at a teaching hospital since 1945, but he kept getting rejected in the final stages of the interview process.[5] Not every surgeon was so unlucky; those with moneyed backgrounds and deep networks found work, but he had only his uncle. Frustrated, he'd called in every favor he could think of, asking numerous respected surgeons to write letters of recommendation. Many obliged, but it hadn't been enough, especially with the struggling economy.

Lewin adjusted to the life of the freelance surgeon but found it unsettling to travel to a different hospital every few days. It felt like he never really belonged anywhere. And he missed research—there were so many facets of surgical techniques that he wanted to explore, but without a hospital backing him, that was all but impossible. He'd asked the chiefs of staff at both Barnert hospital and St. Joseph's hospital if he could run a plastic surgery training program there, but they both rebuted him with well-meaning lectures about how there was no money for plastic surgery in public hospitals.

"I can appreciate your difficulties getting started in New York City," Dr. Jerome Webster, the director of plastic surgery at Columbia-Presbyterian Medical Center wrote him. "There is no position available now." Dr. Webster couldn't offer him a job but, impressed with Lewin's tenacity, he recommended him to Montefiore's medical director. "He is a brilliant plastic surgeon . . . an unusual type of person whom I think has a great deal to offer," Webster wrote. Finally, all of Lewin's efforts had paid off, and as the new chief of plastic surgery, he could start implementing some of his ideas and realizing his research dreams.[6]

Montefiore assigned Lewin to a dark, cramped office on the top floor of the main hospital wing, a temporary measure while they renovated an adjacent building, he was told.[7] Lewin and his secretary walked to the new site to check it out. He was impressed; his new digs were in a tidy three-story redbrick house with ivy trailing across the windows and pink and yellow shrubs on the front lawn. It's like moving from the East Side to Park Avenue, he told his secretary who smiled back at him. They counted the days until they could move into the new office. Two weeks later, around eleven at night, he got a call. "There's been a fire in your new office, and the entire floor has collapsed," he was told. Renovations would be pushed back a few months.[8] He sighed. Of course, this would happen.

One of the first things Lewin did in his new role was to formalize his work at Sing Sing. He outlined his goals for an official prison plastic surgery program; he wanted it to be a fully cooperative enterprise in which the prison medical staff selected patients they believed could benefit from plastic surgery, who then would be evaluated for suitability by Lewin's senior residents. It was win-win, he thought; the inmates would get their much-needed treatment and his residents would have the opportunity to flex their skills on a variety of cases. No condition was ruled out, he noted. Mashed-up noses, receding chins, facial scars, fat removal—it was all on the table.

With a steady stream of plastic surgery residents arriving each year, hopefully he had enough manpower to effect real change at the prison. Ideally, the residents would make the drive one or two days a week. Lewin's proposal was signed off by Albany Corrections Commissioner Paul McGinnis, Attorney General Louis Lefkowitz, and Sing Sing Prison's Chief Medical Officer Dr. Harold Kipp.

Warden Denno's two stipulations were that Lewin's team utilize the existing medical facilities and that they would not incur extra cost. Lewin quickly grew to regret those terms; after a few visits, it was clear that he needed more equipment on site. Residents brought their own tools, but even so, there was much they still needed. Lewin purchased the necessary equipment and invoiced a few hundred dollars to New York State. "But that's it," he promised Denno, who was displeased by the small sum. "With this, we should be covered!"

There were always more inmates requesting surgery than there were residents, due in part to the statewide shortage of qualified medical professionals in prison. Staffing had always been a struggle for the corrections field, but the volume of inmates had grown to record-breaking proportions.

Throughout the 1950s New York crime rates had spiked, with a 157 percent increase in arrests since the turn of the decade and the number of robberies and rapes climbing each year. The state now had the largest prison population in America.[9] Much of the blame was apportioned to Italian immigrants and Black people, who started to fill the state's jails and prisons. With every arrest and news report about the crime problem, racial tension mounted, and a general sense of unease percolated the smog-filled air. The city air itself was toxic, the noxious fumes burning the eyes and throats of citizens, resulting in an upswing of emphysema and bronchitis-related deaths. The dank subways were plastered with warnings for riders to watch their valuables, and violence was so common on the graffiti-ridden trains that police were assigned to guard the newly designated women-only cars.[10]

In response, New York City's mayor, Robert Wagner, announced a war on crime, but his well-intentioned mandate led to the already overcrowded prison system becoming an even bigger dumping ground for petty criminals. Truck hijacking grew 200 percent, and around 50 percent of all arrests were drug related.[11] Racial and xenophobic prejudices split the city even further; despite the 1954 Brown v. Board of Education victory, school desegregation was slow, and civil rights crusaders were increasingly discontent with the progress they were making.[12] Unemployment was high, and out-of-work twentysomethings sat on stoops and filled the parks, seething about the divide between the have and have-nots.[13]

Correspondingly, huge amounts of money were poured into correctional and social welfare services, a large percentage of which was dedicated to research, much of it building on work of earlier decades. New York City's corrections commissioner, Judge Anna Kross, appointed in 1954, was a key proponent of this method. "We need more education," she told the press.[14] "If there's really a desire to end crime in the country it could be done—by women. The men can't do it—they have proved that."

Sixty-eight years old, Kross, whom newspapers described as "diminutive and gray haired," had a keen sense of justice and fairness, and she wasn't afraid to ruffle feathers.[15] She'd entered corrections from the courtroom, leaving her role as a family court judge to assume the mantle of rehabilitating New York's criminals, bringing with her a keen sense of how unjust the city could be to its low-income residents, especially women and minorities. Her goal was to make the jail system more humane and rid it—and the department—of the corresponding dungeon-like associations.

It was a hard task. New York's corrections department had a big public relations problem, with notoriously poor conditions, deaths while in custody,

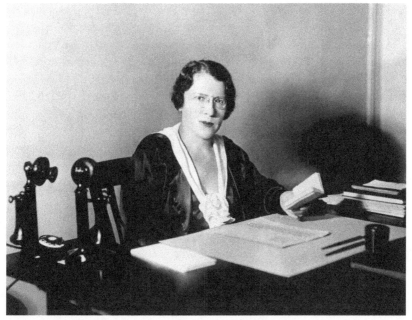

Judge Anna M. Kross seated at her desk, New York Criminal Court, circa 1939. *Courtesy Municipal Archives, City of New York*

and escapes—"14 Escape in One Week!" crowed the *Gazette*; "9 Prisoners Saw Their Way Out of Jail," another paper reported.[16]

Clearly, punitive measures hadn't been effective at quelling crime, and Kross had a different approach in mind. "We must abandon the notion that we are merely jailers or keepers," she wrote in an impassioned letter to New York Mayor Robert Wagner on her first day of work. "I was struck with the imposing realization that the key phase of our obligation, rehabilitation, has been superficially administered. There's little or no social case work being done. We must do a better job of human engineering."[17] Kross's appointment was viewed with reservation by much of the city's old guard, used to doing things their way and uncomfortable with a woman in charge. But Mayor Wagner was firm, and additional support from Eleanor Roosevelt, who publicly praised Kross's commitment to justice, helped establish her authority.[18]

Kross started by inspecting the jail facilities, visiting them one by one, always with a neat little hat perched atop her perennially pin-curled hair. She favored unique designs; at the Brooklyn House of Detention she wore a black bonnet covered in daisies, and for her official portraits she switched between a feathered pillbox hat, a yellow Juliet cap, and a black mesh cloche hat.[19]

Overwhelmingly, she found the jails in a sorry state; shabby, damp, and frequented by mice and lice. They're an embarrassment to the state, she declared. "The physical facilities of the Department had been permitted to deteriorate to a dangerous stage. . . . There must be a provision of adequate and proper facilities for detention and rehabilitation," she wrote in her annual report.[20] Horrified by the unsanitary conditions, she instituted some sweeping departmental changes, which included building better shower facilities and mess halls to instituting educational programs.

From now on, all corrections officers must be formally qualified, she insisted; when she became commissioner, the officers didn't even need to furnish a high school diploma! Accordingly, the lack of qualifications went hand in hand with low pay, which meant there was a constant shortage of candidates, let alone good ones. Correctional staff must be paid better, she asserted—they deserved a salary in line with other professional jobs. The starting salary for a correctional officer rose from $3,565 in 1954 to $6,000 and change by 1959.

Next she tackled the problem of inmates themselves. They had far too much time on their hands, she noted, and idleness led to bad behavior. Their energy needed to be funneled into productive channels, outlets that would enable them to thrive on release. Rehabilitation was key to curbing re-offenses, she asserted to the department, appointing New York's first director of rehabilitation in 1957. His job was to prepare inmates for a life outside of jail, and she encouraged and signed off on funding proposals for training programs ranging from baking and woodworking to beauty school.[21]

This led to news stories about the city's "crime finishing schools," where felons whiled away the day playing bingo and living in luxury. She rebutted that fiercely. "We need the cooperation of the public to understand that it is not mollycoddling. We have embarked now on a pioneer effort that I hope every local jail—we don't call these jails anymore—under my tenure, we have changed the term 'city prison' or 'jail' to 'detention,'" she told congressmen at a senate meeting.[22] Despite intense questioning, she remained firm about her work. "A commissioner is supposed to just sit behind closed doors and have somebody else do the work," she said. "But I will come at an unorthodox hour at night, either in the women's house of detention or any one of our prisons because I believe you cannot understand this problem except as you know it personally."[23]

Many psychiatrists posited that crime was really a personality disorder caused by a variety of social and psychological influences. Personal appearance was often directly attributed to crime, they argued. But their thesis differed from the Lombrosian theory of predetermined criminality based on inherited features. Criminality isn't innate, they argued, offering instead a nuanced analysis of the role of an attractive appearance in society. Kross believed that better health care, education, and psychiatry could stop inmates from re-offending, but she was short-staffed on all accounts.

⌒

Michael Lewin wasn't a big fan of movie theaters—he preferred Broadway plays to tawdry Hollywood movies—and he disliked the way that movies cast people into such narrow roles. For example, there were those Walt Disney movies that children were so fond of. Every time a new one was released at the local multiplex, the posters would go up, showing the slim white princess surrounded by her posse. There was Sleeping Beauty, drawn in repose, her golden locks flowing around her and her red lips parted, waiting for her white savior. In the backdrop of the poster was the villainous, green-skinned Maleficent, surrounded by her dark squat goons, some with snouts and others with beaky noses and buckteeth.

At least in *Sleeping Beauty*, the othering was merely hinted at; in Disney's *Cinderella*, it took center stage. He was grateful his daughter had been too young to go when it was released. Of course, it was good that poor, downtrodden Cinders had evolved into Cinderella, with the world now fully appreciating her kindness and her beauty. Poor little Cinders had to deal with her evil stepmother and ugly stepsisters, Drizella and Anastasia, who took advantage of her good nature. Drizella and Anastasia were portrayed as large-bodied girls, drawn with lumpy, asymmetric faces and ungainly movements.[24] It rankled him to see such caricatured representations of people.

Naturally, every little girl rooted for Cinderella (so sweet, so beautiful, even with soot on her face) and wished for the downfall of her enemies. *Cinderella* was Disney's biggest hit so far, raking in three Academy Award nominations.[25] Cinderella personified goodness, the ugly sisters, villainy. This concept—what is beautiful is good and what is good is beautiful—began to take hold during the early 1930s in New York.

This era introduced Disney to the mainstream, its cutesy animated films emphasizing that certain body features were seen as more desirable and "good"—a philosophy echoed by television shows and magazine covers. The premise was hardly unique; in Shakespeare's *Richard III*, the playwright depicted the villainous Richard as a hideous monster with a hunchback and clubfoot.[26] Popular children's tales were full of blonde, blue-eyed children's battles against wart-filled witches and scar-faced men. But movies coalesced these tropes, the moving picture presenting them as fact rather than fiction.

The messaging was clear: ugly people can't be trusted, and only the beautiful are worthy. The genesis of this sentiment had roots in Biblical texts. In Leviticus 21:18, God placed restrictions on who was allowed into the holy temple. "No man who has any defect is to come near: no man who is blind, lame, facially disfigured, or deformed, or a hunchback or a dwarf, or one who has a defect in his eye or eczema or scabs." Ugliness would "profane" God's sanctity. This concept was repeated over and over, sprinkled throughout all texts; in Samuel, Absalom, the third son of King David, is introduced as the handsomest man in all of Israel. "From the top of his head to the sole of his foot there was no blemish in him."[27] In Daniel, only "youths in whom was no defect, who were good-looking, showing intelligence in every branch of wisdom, [and] endowed with understanding and discerning knowledge"[28] were suitable for the king's court.

The biblical emphasis on appearance was echoed by modern-day leaders; in 1941, the U.S. government declared the production of lipstick a "wartime necessity," which allowed factories manufacturing beauty products to remain open, instead of retooling for the war effort, such was the lipstick's impact on morale.[29] This affirmed the notion that everyone valued a pretty girl—or guy. One brand even launched a "War, Women, and Lipstick" advertising campaign, suggesting that wearing lipstick was patriotic.[30] The attention to appearance permeated popular culture.

Small wonder that the plastic surgery industry was booming, thought Lewin. In 1949, fifteen thousand Americans had plumped for cosmetic surgery interventions.[31] In 1958, it was closer to two hundred and fifty thousand. Nose jobs, facelifts, and breast surgeries were especially popular, as more people realized the socioeconomic and psychological benefits of being more attractive.

For the most part, plastic surgeons embraced this, leaning in with informational videos that espoused the life-changing effects of their work. "The burden of an outsized inheritance need be suffered no longer," announced a plummy British voice as the camera zoomed in for a close-up of a woman's nose then cut to a plastic surgeon leaning in with his tools. "Gone is a bridge of size, and she faces life transformed!" The camera cut back to the beaming woman, now with a slender, ski-slope-straight nose.[32]

Across the United States researchers had labeled this premise "appearance psychology."[33] Many were investigating this newly formed field, hoping to unearth some larger sociological and psychological truths about behavior. Much of the information available was anecdotal—Florence Monahan, a social worker and former warden of California's state prison for women at Tehachapi,[34] was vocal about her belief that attractive girls were convicted less frequently than their uglier peers. "Even social workers accustomed to dealing with all types often find it difficult to think of a normal, pretty girl as being guilty of a crime," Monahan wrote in her memoir. "Most people, for some inexplicable reason, think of crime in terms of abnormality in appearance, and I must say that beautiful women are not often convicted. The jury sees to that!"[35]

One of the first data-driven studies on lookism came out of the University of Nebraska.[36] Psychologists corralled 175 students and gave them photographs of inmates from the state penitentiary.[37] The students were asked to match the inmates to a variety of criminal offenses, including rape, arson, embezzlement, and manslaughter. They wanted to see if specific crimes denoted a certain "look" or "type" of person. The results were uncanny; more than 70 percent of the students successfully matched the convicts to their crimes. Other studies came out; overwhelmingly better-looking people were found to get higher paid jobs, better opportunities, better sentences in court, and significantly lower fines.

Society's acceptance of this philosophy had certainly been a driving factor for William Ricci, Lewin knew. Ricci's lived experiences of rejection directly related to his crime.[38] But Ricci had embraced his second chance. Released early for good behavior, he'd settled into a new life in Manhattan, working as a longshoreman again and rebuilding a relationship with his estranged younger brothers. He still looked like himself—but better. No further appointments with Lewin were scheduled, but he sporadically checked in with the surgeon, for old times' sake.

"I'm getting married," he told Lewin during a brief visit to his wood-paneled private office on Broadway. Her name was Marie, he told him; he'd met her through a friend, and she was a sweet good-natured nineteen-year-old. And she was beautiful, he said bashfully, with clear soft skin and tumbling brown hair. He'd told her about his past, but she didn't care, he told Lewin. What mattered most to Marie was who he was now.[39] "This would never have happened without you," he said. "Thank you."

A big proponent for research into appearance bias came from Ralph Banay, a well-respected prison consultant and the former director of Sing Sing Prison's Psychiatric Clinic. During Banay's tenure, he became convinced that a prisoner's appearance played a major role in his behavior—but his problems were societal, not predetermined. "Throughout the ages, the murderer has been portrayed as a physically repulsive person. This projecting mechanism in folklore and in the popular imagination portrayed murderers as monsters and giants," he wrote in the *Federal Probation*[40] newsletter, a Bureau of Prisons publication that was issued three times a year. Banay unequivocally rejected the Lombroso "born criminal" approach, declaring it unfashionable and ridiculous.[41]

"Anybody jut-jawed, beady-eyed, and muscular enough to correspond to Lombroso's description gets snapped up by motion pictures or wrestling stadia before he can take to crime," he wrote, explaining that most people were more familiar with the criminal type than they realized. "He's a shy youngster with a slight physical defect: a nose that's too big, eyes of two different colors, crossed eyes, acne, a disfiguring birthmark, or a club foot," he wrote, offering the example of Bill, a former inmate of his.

Bill was born in a small town in upstate New York. He was white, with brown hair and eyes, and of average weight and height. His parents fought constantly, and his mother remarried when he was an infant. His stepfather was a cruel, gruff man who resented Bill's presence in his home, expressing his displeasure with his fists and belt. Nothing Bill could do was ever good enough for him. He vowed to leave home the minute he was old enough. Bill was a healthy kid, but when he was fifteen years old, he had a severe bout of chicken pox that left him fatigued for weeks, his skin blistered and red. The infection left his face pockmarked and pitted. He started looking for jobs, eager to save enough cash to move out, but his town was too small. People told him they weren't hiring. He needed to be in a big city, he thought, somewhere with lots of opportunities for a strong, capable teenager.

He scraped together funds to get him to New York City, where he applied to the Coast Guard—its recruitment posters were plastered all over the city's streets and its commercials played nightly on TV news.[42] "Vital to your country. Rewarding to yourself," the announcer declared. Bill's application was denied. He looked elsewhere, enquiring at restaurants and warehouses and stores. Also no. Finally, Bill went to the New York City Employment agency for help. He was puzzled; maybe he didn't understand how big cities work. "What am I doing wrong?" he asked. The administrator, a white man in a trim black suit, looked at him and sighed. "I'm going to give it to you straight," he told Bill. "No one's going to hire a man whose face would repulse customers."

Bill left the office feeling humiliated. Without a permanent position, he was forced to take on a bunch of odd jobs; they paid him in cash, but they paid very little. He was lucky if he could afford one meal a day, as well as the rent for the small cot in his boardinghouse. He tried to get his skin fixed, but the quotes he got from doctors far exceeded his income. But going home wasn't an option, not with his stepfather there. Frustrated and hungry, he began to steal groceries and clothing. Soon enough, his petty thefts escalated into armed robbery. New York police arrested him, and he was sentenced to ten to twenty years in prison.

"Nobody sees himself as he actually is in reality. Usually that's too painful," Banay explained.[43] "We can't accept the knowledge that we are ugly or repulsive." Plastic surgery paired with psychiatry was his preferred solution, addressing both the physical and psychological needs of offenders.

⌒

Thirty-year-old Richard Bloomenstein was one of the first resident cohorts to visit Sing Sing. He was a little starstruck that he was accepted into Lewin's program. In medical school, everyone had heard stories about Lewin's uncle, the renowned Dr. Jacques Maliniac, called by many "the originator of plastic surgery."[44] By extension, that gave Lewin a certain pedigree, Bloomenstein felt, in addition to his growing reputation. When Bloomenstein canvassed his peers about where to apply for training, Dr. Michael Lewin's name came up again and again. He's groundbreaking, one said. Well-respected, said another. Famously fastidious, warned another, erring on the side of overwhelming. "He's never satisfied!" huffed Dr. Morton Goldstein,[45] one of Bloomenstein's cohorts. "I often feel like a bug held pinned with drops under the crying of his dissecting microscope."

Bloomenstein's first day working with prison inmates was fraught. He'd been intrigued by the prospect. Conceptually, it made sense to him that surgery could improve behavior, and personally, he thrilled at the opportunity of operating in such a surprising location. Not to mention the numerous conditions he'd encounter—so many medical needs, so many challenges.[46] The morning he was scheduled to go, he scanned through that day's newspaper, the reality of just where he was going that day hit home, his eyes flitting from crime report to crime report. A local burglary. Two rapes. A murder. It seemed like every page was filled with people's misdeeds.

He was familiar with Ossining; his family owned a small farmhouse there, shared with his aunt and cousins. He'd spent many happy summers there as a kid, tumbling in the grass and eating sweets from the candy shop—but this trip was different.

Bloomenstein and the attending surgeon drove there in the afternoon. He thought they'd park outside the prison gates and walk in the entrance, but the senior attending surgeon breezed through the front gates, made a left, and pulled his car into a wide gravel lot. Exiting the car, they went on foot to the next set of gates, each checkpoint manned by armed guards. Looking up, Bloomenstein saw more guards standing at attention on the thirteen watchtowers[47] that ringed the prison like birthday candles on a cake. Five more guard posts

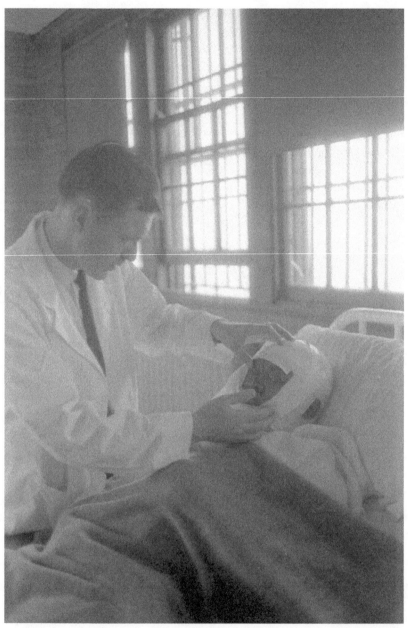

Inside Sing Sing Correctional Facility's hospital, a plastic surgery resident examines a convict's face-lift surgery, 1961. *Courtesy of McGovern Historical Center, Texas Medical Center Library*

flanked the river, and another oversaw the railroad tracks. Each station was armed with tear gas bombs, machine guns, and pistols.[48] He shivered, gripping his surgical bag.[49]

He relaxed when he got to the hospital. Inmates moved around in an orderly fashion, each man focused on the tasks at hand. The building was old but well-scrubbed, and he was surprised by how run-of-the-mill the place was, with its sterile surfaces and faded floor. An inmate nodded at him as they passed, and he took in the man's gray garb and polite smile; he wasn't starved or unkempt or aggressive! *I've alarmed myself for no reason*, he realized. Perhaps it was different in the cellblocks—he had no access to them—but as a medical building, the place was structurally sound.

"Your job is to interview and evaluate the preselected patients," the senior attendee informed him. A convict entered the clinic, a slender white man somewhere in his late forties, with a deeply wrinkled face. His nose deviated sharply to the right, with an additional bump on the bridge. "I'm here to get my nose and face fixed," he told them.

Bloomenstein instructed him to sit down and began the examination. He dug a small hand mirror out of his kit bag and passed it to the inmate. "Please hold it up to your face," he told him and walked behind the man. "For this type of surgery, what would happen is that we'd make an incision here, and another one here." He touched the corresponding parts of the face, first with his fingers and then again, this time with a small ink pen. "Ideally, the scars would sit in the natural lines of the face, but sometimes they'll be visible," he explained. He gently tugged back the loose skin on the man's face, shifting the folds to approximate what he might look like after a facelift and nose job. The man nodded approvingly.

"Remember, recovery from an operation like this is a process," Bloomenstein warned, explaining that he'd feel sore and tired after surgery and that it was imperative to stay hydrated and avoid unnecessary exertion while he healed. "And no blows to the face!" His goal was to manage the man's expectations and ensure that he understood that no surgical procedure had a definite outcome. Although he'd try to get the best possible result, it wasn't a guarantee. "There are real risks involved with surgery," he cautioned. "Are you still comfortable going ahead with this?" The man nodded; they were always willing to proceed.

Bloomenstein reached into his medical bag, fishing through the cotton wool, stethoscope, and thermometer till his hands settled on a small camera that he'd checked out from Montefiore's equipment room earlier that day. "Please sit still—and straight," he requested, thumbing the shutter open and adjusting the flash. It was important that the man sit upright, since he'd be supine in the operating theater, which would change the proportions of his face. Each type of plastic surgery required different pictures. For a nose job, he photographed a straight-on view, a close-up from the chin to the top of the head (to show the outline of the nose), and two lateral views. Later, he'd get the film developed and blown up, ready to pin around the operating theater as a reference point.

"We have some surgical restrictions," the attending surgeon informed him. For one, there was no anesthesiologist, and the doctors couldn't offer narcotics of any kind to the patients. Bloomenstein was shocked—that would be so painful! The visiting doctors often used antihistamines instead of opioids, settling for sedation rather than anesthetization, the attendee said. The prison hospital was accredited by the American College of Surgeons,[50] but Bloomenstein wasn't sure how it had passed inspection—the way the place ran seemed to defy accreditation.

All of the hospital's nursing assistants were convicts, but they'd been well trained in removing sutures, bandaging wounds, and related activities. "Sometimes we'll give the assistants a free nose job or tattoo removal as a motivational tool," his colleague told him. The main problem with the staffing was turnover; as men were released, new ones had to be trained.

As Bloomenstein became more comfortable at Sing Sing, his clinics got shorter. On a regular day, he'd operate or evaluate in the morning and then return to New York for an afternoon on the wards at Montefiore. Prison patients were different from civilians. Civilians complained a lot and often questioned his reasons for doing things. At Sing Sing, the men went out of their way to be agreeable and cooperative. Sure, the power dynamic was skewed, as sometimes they'd ask him for a letter of recommendation for their parole hearings (which he occasionally granted), but even so, they seemed more respectful and grateful for his help.

Surly or aggressive inmates were screened out early in the process. He also rejected men who expressed vague motivations for the surgery as well as men with needle tracks or obviously constricted pupils. Others were rejected because they couldn't seem to grasp what the process involved; some inmates requested scar removal when they had only a scratch—the procedure to get rid of it would create a greater scar! Sometimes he turned down needy cases, skittish about the lack of aftercare the man would receive. A big operation necessitated a lot of follow-up, sometimes even long-term monitoring, and most inmates wouldn't have medical coverage when they were paroled. Lewin understood

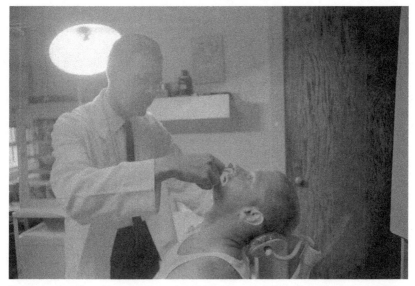

Plastic surgeon from Montefiore examines inmate's nose at Sing Sing Correctional Facility. *Image by Ted Russell. Courtesy of McGovern Historical Center, Texas Medical Center Library*

his resident's reluctance, but thought it was a shame—indicative of the bigger problem surrounding medical care in the world.

Bloomenstein sometimes wondered what crimes had landed his patients in Sing Sing, but he never asked. It's not my concern, he told his friends, who peppered him with questions about his experience. "I have no desire to know the details." Most of the work was fairly routine, he told them, mainly nose jobs, scar removals, tattoo removals, and bulking up recessive chins.[51] "Most were happy to look presentable again," he told them.

The operations at Sing Sing were a strangely quiet affair. Bloomenstein was used to the background hum and whine of Montefiore Medical Center, the beeping and buzzing machines and whatever music was burbling from the radio that day; during a long operation, you could always count on hearing the Beatles or the Supremes. Sing Sing didn't allow visitors to bring radios, so the only sounds during surgery were the slow breaths of the patient and the fleshy, slicing sounds of scalpels and sutures.

Bad reactions were rare, but they did occur. Some prisoners reacted poorly to sedation, bolting upright halfway through surgery in confusion and pain. When this happened, extra nursing assistants were summoned to secure the convict in place while more drugs were administered.

Bloomenstein was diligent about aftercare and regularly made the forty-minute drive on Saturday mornings to check on his patients' recovery. He liked making a day out of leaving New York, seeing it as an opportunity to picnic outside with his children and visit extended family. His wife and kids often would wait in the car in the prison's parking lot as he finished his rounds. It was business as usual for him, but for them, it was an eerie, unsettling experience. "What do we do if Daddy can't get out of prison?" his daughter apprehensively asked his wife. "There's nothing to worry about," she told her, keeping her face wide and bland, so the children couldn't see that she was also scared of the fortress-like encampment.

By the early 1960s, one or two plastic surgery procedures took place at Sing Sing each week.

# 4

# LIGHTS, CAMERA, VIOLINS!

## The Spectacle of Prison Surgery

Anyone tuning in to see the coronation of the Miss Universe 1959 on Saturday, July 24, would assume that twenty-two-year-old Akiko Kojima was perfectly comfortable in the spotlight. Kojima looked poised and professional, her back ramrod straight and her hands gently pressed to her sides as she stood next to the four finalists inside the Long Beach Memorial Auditorium in California. Her cerulean blue bathing suit showed every curve of her famous 37–23–38 frame.[1]

Earlier that night, she'd taken her turn down the runway alongside the other women, each clad in their regulation swimsuit. "Curvaceous contenders from every corner of the globe!" commented Ed Herlihy, the television reporter from Universal International. The TV cameras captured every turn of her heel and toss of her hair, every movement narrated by breathless broadcasters. "A rising beauty from the land of the rising sun," Herlihy announced.[2]

"Pretty packets of pulsating pulchritude's parading for the prize," joked the reporter from British Movietone. "Akiko Kojima from Japan. At 37–23–38 it adds up to a very nice figure. Bonsai!"

Kojima's hair gleamed under the stage spotlights as she calmly regarded the audience. Inside, she was quaking, battling to keep her nerves from showing on her face. Japan had never won a Miss Universe title—nor, in fact, had any Asian woman in all thirty-three years of the pageant's existence. There had never been a Black contestant.

On stage, she was sandwiched between Miss Norway and Miss England; both women were gorgeous, with their pale skin and light hair—their features so unlike hers. All the finalists came from highly privileged background; Miss USA, Terry Lynn Huntingdon, was a fifth-generation Californian and part of the Huntingdon dynasty! None of these women had ever had to struggle for anything!

How could a poor girl from Japan compete? Kojima could still remember the screams and the bangs—and even worse, the awful, loaded silence that occurred in the quiet after. . . . She'd been a little girl during the firebombing of Tokyo in World War II.[3] Her father died a few years later, and her mother struggled to put enough food on the table for Akiko and her three siblings. Her father's death had placed a strain on the whole family; how could she compete with these wealthy white girls? She continued smiling, following the advice of her pageant roommate, Miss Illinois: smile and think you're the best—and everyone else will too!

There was a pause, and the announcer slowly read the winners' names, in reverse order. Miss USA was second runner-up; Miss Norway was first runner-up. Then the trumpets rang out, and the plummy chorus of the eponymous "Miss Universe" theme song boomed from the speakers. "The way you walk, the way you talk, you take my breath away." One of the judges walked slowly behind the remaining women onstage.

Kojima stiffened as the judge's tuxedo tails brushed her lower back, and he tapped her on the shoulder. Her hands tightened into fists. Then her name was announced and her eyes teared up. She lowered her head, and the judge placed the Star of the Universe crown on her head, one thousand black pearls inlaid with gold and platinum and insured for $50,000.

"Oh my gosh!" she squealed, smiling as she straightened up. In one hand she grasped the four-foot trophy while a floor-length cloak was draped around her shoulders. "I am so very happy," she declared.

"The first Oriental to win!" reported the Saturday newspapers.[4] But Kojima didn't enjoy her win for long. Almost immediately, the rumor mill was at work, with columnists and commentators speculating that she'd cheated her way into a win. Had a plastic surgeon boosted her bust?[5] "Was beauty puffed by plastic?" asked the tabloids.[6] Tokyo plastic surgeon Dr. Toshizo Matsui alleged that Kojima had visited him for breast-boosting paraffin injections prior to her win.

Kojima vehemently denied his statement. "It just isn't true," she told the media.[7] The pageant officials backed her up; even if she'd had work done, there was nothing in the rules against it, they said.

Inside Dr. Michael Lewin's office at Montefiore Medical Center, his secretary deposited a fresh pile of envelopes on his desk. More mail from the penitentiaries, she remarked; one was postmarked from San Quentin prison in California, and another was stamped with the official seal of Pennsylvania's Department of Corrections. Lewin nodded his thanks and started in on the pile. It was easy enough to respond; each letter said basically the same thing, after all: some official had heard about his plastic surgery program at Sing Sing and wanted him to answer a few questions about its setup and so on.

"I feel like I'm getting a letter or a call every week about this," he told his uncle, Dr. Jacques Maliniac, during one of their monthly dinners in the Upper West Side. Still, it was flattering that so many officials were approaching plastic surgeons for help. Maliniac nodded his agreement. "It's a far cry from the attitudes of the early thirties and forties," he told Lewin. "I remember when our profession was considered quackish and disreputable!"

Lewin smiled in acknowledgment. During his residency, plastic surgery was considered the least respectable of all the medical fields, with trainee cardiologists and anesthesiologists at the top of the food chain. Despite the technical advances made during two world wars, "pandering to a patient's vanity" remained the common perception of plastic surgery. Operating for purely cosmetic purposes was viewed as distasteful, as if it somehow reneged on the surgeon's code.[8]

All those people, those organizations—they surely regret their behavior now, Maliniac continued, still bitter about his reception from New York's medical community, three decades after the fact. In 1931, the American Association of Oral and Plastic Surgeons had rejected his application. The organization accepted a maximum of forty members a year, and his work didn't make the grade, it informed him. His cosmetic surgery work—much of it on the war wounded—barred him from qualifying. It didn't help that the American Medical Association (AMA) guidelines stated that surgeons who performed elective cosmetic surgeries were unethical.[9] Without admittance to these societies, Maliniac and other plastic surgeons received little credit or respect from the medical community at large, and, due to the AMA's ban on medical advertising, struggled to find referrals.

In response, the cosmetic surgeons of that era had taken two routes toward authenticating their profession. Maliniac and Lewin had focused on gaining peer approval and recognition, writing lengthy research papers, publishing in journals, and petitioning the medical associations for inclusion. The second cohort of surgeons chose a showier, flashier path to success. Their goal was for public—rather than professional—approval. These surgeons took out full-page advertisements in newspapers and magazines detailing their "transformative!" services, some promising potential clients "Hollywood operations" that could restore youth "at any age."[10] They offered beauty salons a commission for referrals and accepted guest slots on radio shows, where they broadcast the magical nature of their scalpels to the nation.

Their existence infuriated Maliniac. He was trying to establish the skill and gravity required of his profession, and these so-called beauty surgeons were flipping that narrative, the exclamation points and bold lettering in their advertisments a mockery of everything he stood for. They sullied his work and made plastic surgery appear tawdry and cheap. He considered them all quacks and charlatans, he told Lewin.

Lewin disliked these surgeons' histrionics, but his antipathy was alleviated by a surprising recognition: the quacks had cheapened the value of his work in the 1930s and 1940s, but in many ways, they'd helped set the stage for his surgical work in criminal reform.

The newspaper coverage of plastic surgeon Dr. John Howard Crum said it all: "Why Beauty Treatments May Cure America's Crime";[11] "Miracle of Surgery Gives Ex-Convict New Start";[12] "Hardened Mugs May Emerge from Ether Resembling Great Screen Lovers;[13] "Operation on Face Changes Woman Slayer."[14]

Crum exemplified everything that enraged Maliniac about beauty doctoring. "He's just a showman," he grumbled to Lewin; in his opinion, Crum's work belittled their whole field.

Dr. John Howard Crum hailed from Cooks Mills, Illinois, and after a short stint in Chicago, he moved to New York, setting up shop on Fifth Avenue in Midtown Manhattan. The majority of Crum's plastic surgery experience stemmed from his time in the army patching up injured troops. Crum was vocal about the benefits that beauty delivered and, like many doctors of his time, strongly bought into the sociological theory that conflated people with "defective appearances" with an increased propensity for crime.

"A very large percentage of criminals have bad features," he told reporters. "I believe in all instances it was the factor that started them on their criminal careers. Every penal institution should give those about to be discharged the help of a cosmetic surgeon and a professional beautician."[15]

Crum wasn't the only New York cosmetic surgeon who held this view. "There is a definite place for rehabilitation of character through use of plastic surgery," wrote Dr. Maxwell Maltz in his popular science book, *New Faces, New Futures: Rebuilding Character with Plastic Surgery*:[16] "Judging human nature is still highly important, but unhappily we cling atavistically to this primitive arbitrary notions of deducing character which were popular amongst our antediluvian forefathers." Maltz reportedly had even offered his services—for free—to New York's Department of Correction, "If it would enable some man with a criminal record to forget his past, I would be honored," he told the Associated Press.[17]

Crum agreed with Maltz's opinion. He was adamant that cosmetic surgery could play a vital role in criminal reform, as well as provide "an economic necessity for thousands."[18]

And the self-described "showman" knew just how to prove it.

On March 17, 1932, on a brisk Manhattan afternoon, Dorothy Kilgallen, the eighteen-year-old special correspondent for the International News Service, marched under the wide, fluted columns that framed the entrance of the Hotel Pennsylvania on the corner of Seventh Avenue and Thirty-Third Street. Her dark brown hair swung as she walked, its tight curls framing her pale face. Inside, she joined the sea of polished leather brogues and dainty kitten heels click-clacking across the white marble floor of the hotel lobby, and turned to the right, making a beeline for the southeast ballroom. It was a popular attraction. A waft of scent and sound accompanied Kilgallen up and down the stairs, all the way to the high arched doors of the ballroom, which were flanked by fifteen uniformed policemen. They smiled politely as the guests entered, but their presence sent a clear message: disruption would not be tolerated.

Kilgallen smiled broadly at the officers, batting her sea blue eyes and flashing them her media credentials as she passed. Inside, she paused, startled by the somber surroundings. Thick black drapes swathed the stage in front of her.[19] Instead of the ballroom's usual bright array of freshly cut flowers and platters of finger foods, a few paltry pitchers of water dotted the room.

She spotted four musicians on the bandstand slightly to the left of the main stage, and her shoulders loosened a little—this, she understood. She watched as they warmed up for the event, the pianist stretching out his knuckles, one by one, while the cellist and the two violinists smoothed a final layer of rosin over their bows, strings plinking softly as they fine-tuned their instruments.

The crowd surged behind her, and Kilgallen quickly made her way to the front, claiming one of the reserved media seats near the front. The temperature

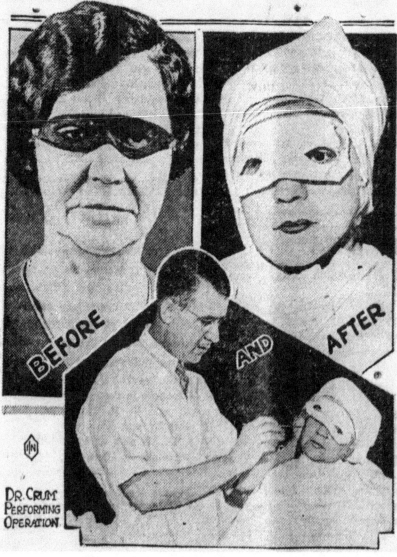

# Miracle of Surgery Gives Ex-Convict Fresh Start

\* \* \* \* \* \*

"Mystery Woman" Given New Face in Two Hours at Public Demonstration. Rogues' Galleries in Danger of Becoming Obsolete.

BEFORE

AND

AFTER

DR. CRUM
PERFORMING
OPERATION

Dr. John Howard Crum operates on mystery ex-convict inside the Hotel Pennsylvania, New York, 1932. *Blue Ribbon Books (1933)* rose as more and more people filled the space, the ballroom humming with their gentle chatter, laughter, and gossip. Almost one thousand people had packed into the space before the police officers decided it was at capacity and—despite protests from those still in line—swung the doors shut, barring the entrance with their bodies.

Ruth Maurer, vice president of the International Beauty Shop Owners Association, greeted the crowd, a small smile on her face. "Let me introduce you to the man who has done more for the fair sex than any other professional man in the United States. Dr. John Howard Crum!"[20]

The lights dimmed, and the room hushed in anticipation.[21] A spotlight turned on, its bright beam tightly focused to the left of the stage to capture Dr. Crum's entrance. The surgeon strode in from the wings, a tall, tidy man with broad shoulders, wide blue eyes, and thick brown hair that he parted to the left.[22] He was forty-five but looked younger, his smooth, wide forehead framing bushy brows that gave him a permanently thoughtful expression. His starched white surgical coat shone under the high beams that followed him across the stage. They stopped when he reached the sturdy enamel and nickel-plated chair that sat center stage.[23] It resembled something you might see at a dentist's office, Kilgallen thought. The headrest and seat were upholstered in a thick dark leather. A waist-high trolley, loaded with an assortment of polished silver tools, was parked beside it.

Dr. Crum scanned the ballroom, making a silent count of attendees in his head, then looked straight ahead and smiled at his audience. "Welcome," he said, the microphone bouncing his voice around the room, his low rumble reaching all the way to the rafters. "What you will see tonight is the triumph of surgery over circumstance," he proclaimed. "No longer do people need to be victims of their own experiences. . . . Those who serve their time can finally move on."

He gestured to his right, and two orderlies dressed in hospital scrubs escorted in a short woman, her eyes concealed behind a black domino mask. Hundreds of heads swiveled to take in her appearance. She wore a long black dress with white piping at the neckline and a delicate train of white buttons down the back. At first glance, she appeared slim, but a closer look revealed her body had that sort of shapeless quality achieved by women of a certain age. She walked with her head down and her shoulders hunched.

The orderlies assisted her into the chair and wrapped two white sheets tightly around her, covering her from the neck down. A smaller white sheet was wound around her hair and twisted at the nape of her neck into a tidy turban. The woman squeezed her eyes shut while this happened; all that was visible to the audience was a flutter of lashes under her mask and a pink slash for her lips.

Alice—not her real name—had just been released from prison after serving twenty years, Crum told the crowd.[24] Her crime was shocking. He paused to heighten the tension. She killed her husband! A disapproving murmur ran through the room, and chairs creaked as people shifted forward for a closer look at the murderess.

"But Alice served her time," Crum continued. "She paid her debt to society. Now, she's ready to start afresh, and make a new life for herself. She's older and wiser, and she's ready to make better choices. Isn't that so, Alice?"

His masked patient nodded.

"Thank you, Alice," he said and turned to face the room. Can any one of you argue with that? Doesn't everyone deserve a second chance?

The room stayed quiet.

Kilgallen scratched a note on her pad and leaned forward in her seat.

Crum frowned, pausing for effect, letting the light shine full on his face. Alice has not had that chance, he informed the room. She was poorly educated, and the world had changed dramatically since 1912. Twenty years ago, there were no refrigerators or radio stations or televisions. No jukeboxes!

The audience chuckled. Crum gave them a moment to laugh before he addressed them again, this time taking a more serious tone. "It has been difficult for Alice to assimilate," he explained. "She's eager to support herself, to get a job, and not be a burden to the state any longer. Before she was committed, she worked in beauty and had hoped to do so again, perhaps owning a small beauty shop—though she may have to work her way up to that. But that dream hasn't come to fruition.

"Do you know why that is?" Crum looked around the room, his arms wide. He pointed to Alice. "The answer is written on her face!"

He gently took hold of her chin, and lifted her face to the audience, his thumb tracing the contours of her face. Sometimes she was recognized and refused work. Other times, employers looked at her haggard appearance and decided she wasn't a good fit for a career in beauty. He lightly tugged her folded skin for emphasis. The powerful Klieg lights highlighted every flaw in her face, her litany of physical complaints starting at the drooping skin of her neck, rising to the deep grooves that ran between her nose and her lips and, finally, to the creases that crisscrossed her forehead like subway tracks.[25]

"She was turned away from every position, every salon," Crum continued. Every. Single. One. "She booked an appointment with me even though she had no money, no experience of plastic surgery, and no hope left." Many surgeons would have turned Alice away. But he believed that everyone deserved a second chance, a chance to reform—psychologically and physically.

Crum made eye contact with women in the first row. He knew that women understood the impact that their appearance has on their everyday life. "An aging and unattractive face will often have as disarming an effect on a woman's life as would some physical deformity," he explained in his popular book *The Making of a Beautiful Face*.[26] He shared these insights with the press. "When an employer has hundreds of women applying for a position, he will naturally single out the pretty one and give her the job. The less pleasing one will always have it harder. An ugly feature can warp a woman's life."[27] Feet shuffled and heads nodded in the crowd.

Crum sorrowfully shook his head. "Alice hoped for a miracle when she came into my office. Well, I'm no miracle worker, but I try and do His work. In return for participating in this event, I offered Alice the opportunity she'd been dreaming of—the removal of her lines of tragedy." He paused and the room broke into applause.

He nodded his thanks. "Alice, of course, was nervous about this," he continued. "Plastic surgery cannot, of course, eradicate the inward signs and scars from the heart, but the removal of the outward signs may do much to heal and restore her."[28] Fearful of being recognized, she wears a mask to protect her identity. "This is a serious operation, not a vaudeville act. Shall we get started?"

"The feelings of the age fearing women in the audience were probably one of relief, but to others, the first thought was, what a boon to criminals," wrote a United Press reporter sitting a few seats away from Kilgallen in an article published the following day. "Gangsters may now discard the old face and acquire a new one in less time than it takes to have a tooth extracted!"[29]

On the bandstand, the musicians began their set list, a repertoire of light dance-hall melodies, preselected by Crum. The opening notes of "Sweet and Lovely" thrummed through the ballroom. Some of the audience tapped their feet as the rhythmic jazz tune picked up tempo, others mouthing the words.

Kilgallen watched intently as Crum bent down and whispered into Alice's ear. He pulled back the wrap around her head to reveal the sides of her face. Kilgallen could see iodine lines inked up and down her jaw—where the surgeon would cut, she assumed.

Crum gestured to his assistant, who handed him a syringe. He held it up as he prepped it, the tip of the needle catching the light. He rolled up Alice's sleeve and slowly depressed the needle into her arm; the anesthetic ensured that she'd feel nothing during the procedure, he told the crowd. Alice would be hazily conscious throughout but would experience no pain. Kilgallen shuddered, rubbing her palms together.

The syringe was exchanged for a scalpel. Crum's sleeve dipped as he grasped the tool, briefly exposing the tattoo that twined around his forearm, a shaded line drawing of a snake wrapped around a staff, Kilgallen noted, a clear reference to the rod of Asclepius, the Greek god of medicine. The music rose expectantly as Crum's blade sliced up and down, and "Sweet and Lovely" transitioned into a rendition of "Goodnight Sweetheart" followed by "How Long Will It Last?" "An apt musical selection for this social work by scalpel," Kilgallen scribbled in her reporter's notebook.

The surgery continued. A slice here, an incision there, a fresh suture along Alice's hairline. Perspiration rolled down Crum's forehead. The metallic aroma of iron suffused the air, and bright red splashes pooled onto Alice's bright white wrappings. She didn't flinch. "Her small frame steeled to the test," wrote Kilgallen.[30]

The same couldn't be said for the tense-lipped spectators. Rapt and repulsed in equal measures by the smell and the sight of blood and bone, many faces bleached of color as time ticked on. Thirty minutes. Fifty minutes. Women fanned themselves with salts as the men shifted uneasily in their seats, nervously adjusting their collars. Conceptually, everyone here understood what was happening, but seeing this physical Cinderella process played out step by gruesome step in front of their eyes was a different matter. They'd known what was on the agenda tonight, but even so . . .

As the operation ticked into its second hour, it became too much for one observer who collapsed with a gentle fold of her knees and a drawn-out sigh. She was scooped up by two friends who exited the ballroom together. Three more women fainted and were ushered out.

Every few minutes, Crum paused to examine Alice's face, turning it this way and that. He picked up a pair of forceps and rolled them a few times between his thick thumbs before replacing them on the trolley and picking up a different pair. At one hour fifty-two minutes in, Alice let out a small sigh and slumped over in the chair, her head lolling to one side. The room rustled with chairs being pushed back, legs uncrossing as eyes unglazed.

Crum's assistant produced a small vial of ammonia, which Crum held under her nose, waving it slightly back and forth. The fumes snapped Alice out of her daze, and she sat up straight with a gasp. She visibly steeled herself, inhaling deeply. Then she shut her eyes. Crum administered another dose of Novocain, and the surgery continued.[31]

"Only once, when an anesthetic was injected with a hypodermic needle did she wince, and her mouth quivered, but that was the only sign of life she gave during the whole bizarre performance," wrote the United Press reporter.

At two hours, seven minutes, Crum was finally done. He placed his scalpels on the tray and peeled his gloves off. He turned to the audience, swinging the chair around to give everyone a full view of his Frankensteined Cinderella. Alice's head was swathed in bandages and a fresh white eye mask had replaced the domino mask covering her eyes. She blinked owlishly as she adjusted to the light.

Crum held a small hand mirror up to the audience, giving them a moment to take it in before passing it to Alice with a flourish. Her hands trembled as she raised it to her face. Gone were the deep grooves by her nose, her sagging chin, and the perennially angry furrows on her forehead. She tremulously raised a hand to her face, tracing the swollen skin with a finger. Her face had been replaced; she had a tight, defined chin and smooth plump cheeks framing her button nose. "How do you feel?"

"I feel fine," she said softly.[32]

"The metamorphosis was remarkable. In her place sat a smooth-faced agreeable-looking young woman," commented the United Press. "No one who had not seen the actual transformation gradually take place would believe it was the same woman." The applause was deafening.[33]

In the press interviews that followed this performance, Crum brushed off Kilgallen's concerns that criminals might benefit from plastic surgery or that Alice potentially might use her improved looks for criminal activity.

"I always take before and after photographs and make sure the appropriate authorities get them," Crum informed the pool of journalists. "And I refuse to work with men. I have been threatened on several occasions by criminals whom I have refused to help."[34] As for the theatrical nature of the event, well, it was intentionally "circusy," he informed them, so as to keep the audience engaged.

The reception to Crum's work was mixed. In Alabama, the *Montgomery Advertiser* was skeptical of Kilgallen's analysis. "She may be turned into a newer and better woman, but one cannot be operated on, and have their story told in the newspapers, and hope to go unidentified," the reporter commented.[35] "Somewhere in New York today there is a new woman . . . an individual woman who was somebody yesterday and is someone else today," reported the *Brooklyn Eagle.*[36]

Whether Crum's actions helped Alice start afresh and land a successful beauty career is unknown. Postoperatively, she was never seen or heard of again by Kilgallen or any other reporter . . . which may suggest Crum's work achieved the desired effect.

Michael Lewin was in Zurich when Alice's operation took place, but he'd made it to New York City by the time Dr. Crum's subsequent stunts occurred. In 1933, Crum staged a six-person live-action surgical extravaganza[37] followed by a Cinderella makeover of twenty-three-year-old Elsie Norman, an unemployed shopgirl, a year later—"she was so unprepossessing that I could see how people would be prejudiced." He performed an "ugly duckling" plastic surgery in 1936,[38] and in 1937, he raised the bar again by remodeling the "flat" noses of *three* Honduran siblings into a more aquiline shape live on stage.[39]

Crum's existence was an embarrassment to Lewin, but he had to admit—though never to his uncle—that his highly publicized exploits had laid the groundwork of criminal surgical reform with the general public.

Crum and his ilk's nonstop showboating unwittingly elevated the field of plastic surgery into the mainstream public consciousness. Not only did the average Joe now know what cosmetic surgery was and what it entailed (if a somewhat glamorized version), but the public also knew that they'd appreciate the chance to have some if possible.

The increasing demand for plastic surgery work caused the number of surgeons to balloon. In 1942, America and Canada had a joint total of 124 board-certified surgeons; by 1960 it grew to 400.[40]

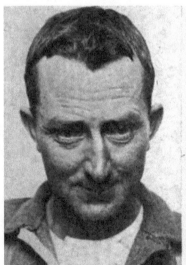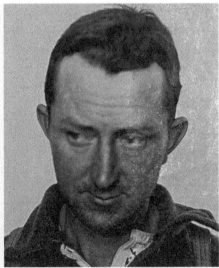

San Quentin inmate before and after plastic surgery of the nose. *The Laryngoscope, 1917.*

Lewin would have liked to forget all about his embarrassing predecessors, but to his mortification, they continued making newspaper headlines well into the late 1950s. At this point, both Crum and Maltz's careers had taken new and ludicrous turns. Crum's face was splashed across magazines promoting his donut reducing diet, "Dunk your pounds away!"[41] while Maltz had coined the term psycho-cybernetics, leading to a cultlike group to which he expounded on the benefits of visualization as a self-help tool. "It is still amazing to me how uncritical or unscrupulous some of our colleagues can be," Lewin wrote in his notebook.[42] He was disappointed with the general populace as well. "It shocks me how eagerly patients accept unvalidated approaches in their search for a fast fix."

Still, he tried to shake it off. Crum and Maltz might provide good sound bites for criminal reform, but Lewin was the one who was scientifically making that concept a reality. And he was doing it the right way, going through the official channels. He wasn't alone in this venture—across America, there were at least twenty-two prison plastic surgery clinics in operation, spanning from the gulf of Florida all the way to the Hawaii State Prison in Honolulu.[43] He wasn't even the only prison plastic surgeon in the state of New York; similar operations took place upstate at Auburn Prison and Clinton Prison in Dannemora.

Lewin knew he was making a difference at his hospital and in Sing Sing's medical wards; his work changed faces and lives and healed sick children and men, inside and out. What he did meant something, helped people put their lives back together. The file of thank-you notes in his office—some of them in crayon!—were proof that he *mattered.*

Even so, he was troubled. There was one big problem with his clinic at Sing Sing. He knew—well, felt—that without his surgical care and his residents' work, many of the inmates wouldn't have stayed clean when released—but he was very aware of how anecdotal his experience was.

He worked with a small sample size without any follow-up after they were paroled, Ricci being the one and only exception to date. "Once released, they are exceptionally mobile," he complained to a reporter from *Medical World News.*[44] Without a social worker or corrections official to follow up on the ex-cons' behavior—and report back to him—there was no easy way to keep tabs on their future endeavors.

Lewin had his own theories about how certain types of criminal acts seemed to relate to inmates' physical features. Some were obvious, of course. It was unsurprising that men with a string of robbery and assault charges might have a higher rate of broken noses and facial scars than inmates who committed check fraud. Lewin also noticed, admittedly among his small

selection pool, that men serving time
for petty crimes were more tattooed
than violent offenders—and significantly more concerned about having
their offensive inkings removed. But
this was all conjecture, he thought
despairingly. He had no hard data to
back any of this up.

Perhaps other plastic surgeons
had looked into this, he considered.
Maybe the answer was already out
there. He scoured medical journals
from across the world and asked his
secretary to track down every prison-
related medical report he found.
Stacks arrived in the mail, and he
scrolled through the footnotes to find
their source material and acquired
those as well. Peer-reviewed studies
were placed on top of his growing pile
of documents. His secretary sighed
but smiled as she lugged yet more
volumes into his crowded office.

At home, Berta smiled fondly at
him, shrugging in bemusement as
he settled into his favorite chair, a
thick leather affair by the fire, to read
his latest pile of mail. There was no
distracting her husband when he was
fixated on a problem![45] He scratched
notes in the margins of the most rel-

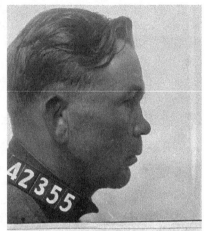

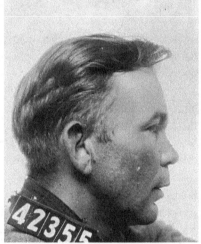

Before and after nose surgery, Album #17: San
Quentin Medical Department, 1913–1920, Dr.
Leo Stanley Collection. *Courtesy Anne T. Kent
California Room, Marin County Free Library*

evant works, squinting through his glasses to decipher every word.

One report published in 1949 covered a decade of plastic surgery inside the
Stateville penitentiary in Illinois.[46] Between 1937 and 1947, Dr. John F. Pick,
a plastic surgeon from Chicago, performed 663 elective cosmetic surgeries on
376 inmates, treating 556 "defects," which ranged from bulbous noses to facial
scars and drooping skin. The majority of the work was purely cosmetic.[47] Pick
reported that 76 percent of the inmate's disfigurements were acquired—through
violence, drug abuse, and poor self-care—with the rest congenital.

"Of those discharged after physical rehabilitation, only 1.7 percent became recidivists," Pick wrote. "There is a rather general agreement that physical appearance has something to do with an individual's behavior. I stand amazed at the obvious and often acute improvement in the individual's personality following surgery."

Pick became a regular attendee at the American Prison Association's annual conference.[48] "It is an old adage in science that anything new takes twenty years to become integrated into our methods of thinking," he told the assembled officials. "The next ten years may help to clarify much which is still unknown in this work . . . as concerns the application of plastic surgery to human behavior in general."

By the late 1950s, Pick had reworked the faces of more than two thousand inmates. Twenty years had passed since his estimate, but the adoption and scientific proof of the recidivism benefits of prison surgery remained elusive. Lewin was impressed by Pick's percentages and the number of patients treated, but he was frustrated that Pick wasn't more transparent about prisoner selection and what—if any—psychiatric and rehabilitative services were provided to inmates post-op.

He thumbed through a few more studies; most had smaller sample sizes than Dr. Pick, but they all appeared to follow the same trajectory, concluding that plastic surgery did indeed curb recidivism. However, these papers lacked the rigor he craved. "The manner in which these figures are reported makes it impossible to speculate on their reliability," he wrote in his journal.[49]

He had high hopes for a paper published earlier that year in the *British Medical Journal* titled "Use of Surgical Rehabilitation in Young Delinquents."[50] The author, Dr. D. A. Ogden, a medical officer at Her Majesty's Borstal Institution in Portland, England, explained that over the course of his years in the prison service, he'd noticed that hundreds of juveniles were showing up with facial and bodily disfigurements.

"A considerable number of these youths were afflicted with disabilities such as squints, crooked noses, internal nasal obstruction, limps, ugly scars, and other varied complaints. Many covered their resentment with an over-compensatory aggression," he wrote, speculating that many of their injuries could be attributed to parental neglect.[51]

Ogden arranged for fifty-five teenage volunteers to receive plastic surgery, theorizing that improving their appearance would improve their future behavior. He followed up with the youths every few months after their release. After two years of observation, 54.5 percent of the teens remained crime free compared to 34.5 percent of the delinquent population. Nose jobs, Ogden noted, seemed particularly effective, as only one of eighteen boys who'd had this procedure were reconvicted. "In one stroke, a source of chronic physical discomfort and of emotional embarrassment has been removed. In such cases, it is very difficult to tell where physical medical treatment ended and where psychiatric medical treatment started," he reported.

Another positive experimental outcome, Lewin thought, but once again, there had been no control group, no real scientific measure. If only Ogden had provided more data about how the boys were selected or the racial and economic breakdown of their home life once released. These were the details needed for a well-rounded picture of the success of the surgery. One's appearance did not exist in isolation. The lack of these details didn't invalidate Ogden's work, but his assertions carried less weight without them.

In the subsequent issue of the *British Medical Journal*, Dr. Allen Bartholomew, a prominent forensic criminologist and psychologist from Australia, rebutted Ogden's numbers. "As a piece of valuable research, it cannot be considered satisfactory as presented," Bartholomew wrote. "It is setting out clinical impressions in the guise of research work."[52] Stung, Ogden responded in kind in the next edition. "My conclusion is not drawn from inadequate work that lacks the necessary degree of methodological sophistication as Dr. Bartholomew suggests; it is a direct observation. I remain convinced there is a crying need for further development of the use of remedial surgery in delinquency and believe the best proof of the pudding will lie in the further eating thereof."[53] Lewin chuckled as he read Ogden's aggrieved counter. The British did have a way with words sometimes—"best proof of the pudding" was priceless!

In August, the new Miss Universe, Akiko Kojima, was in the headlines again. *Parade* magazine polled all the Miss Universe contestants about whether beauty contests should be judged by men or by women. "Give me a man judge every time," Miss USA told the reporter. Miss Georgia, Miss Maine, Miss Florida, and Miss Missouri nodded in assent.

However, Miss Poland disagreed with the Americans' summation. "Men are the children of passion. Women are the children of calculation," she explained. "It is best to judge without passion and only on the facts." As the reigning Miss Universe, Kojima's answer held the most weight. Her statement was definitive. "In Japan, where I come from, both everyone and everything are judged by men. I am not about to make any exception of beauty."[54]

Lewin had reached an impasse with his prison surgery research. Every report he'd collated suffered from the same issues: a lack of controls, consistent checkups, or any real investigation or analysis into how an individual's race and economic circumstances might have influenced his or her recidivism rate. They mirrored the exact same problems he faced at Sing Sing!

"We share a common weakness with all other programs, namely lack of social follow up. We have no hard data about the effectiveness of our program," he wrote.[55] It gnawed away at him. He thumbed through the studies again, scanning the text to find some hidden proof or point of logic that he'd overlooked. His surgical training had drummed into him the importance of documentation and replicable research, and he tried to drill the ethos into his residents—even his children! It was untenable that his prison surgical work could continue to take place without confirmation of its long-term success rate.

What was he missing?

His research was clear on one thing: for now, at least, the Western world was in favor of prison plastic surgery, with projects similar to Sing Sing's taking place across the United States, Canada, and the United Kingdom. The New York Department of Corrections was a big supporter as well—it felt like every time he turned on the television or picked up the *New York Times,* there was State Corrections Commissioner Paul McGinnis, shoulders raised almost to his ears in his boxy gray suit, voluminously praising the practice. Plastic surgery is a useful reform tool, McGinnis noted in a widely circulated report highlighting a new survey, which found that 6 to 8 percent of New York's inmates blamed their crimes on their physical appearances.[56] "It is a new approach to an old problem," McGinnis told reporters.[57]

With so many people in authority backing the prison plastic surgery programs, Lewin felt certain they'd support an in-depth research project to conclusively prove or disprove the long-term benefits of this treatment. How could they not? Hopefully it would validate the very treatment they praised.

He scheduled an appointment with Warden Denno to explain his proposal. "I'm requesting permission to run a full research trial," he said, pitching his concept to Denno. His tentative plan was to oversee a large-scale scientific study on Sing Sing's inmate population that would potentially prove his thesis about plastic surgery as a long-term recidivism treatment for inmate rehabilitation.

Denno refused. The prison didn't have the budget to fund a project of that scale, he said. End of story.

That wasn't good enough for Lewin. He wasn't ready to let the idea go.

# 5

# THE RIKERS ISLAND EXPERIMENT

## a.k.a. the Surgical and Social Rehabilitation of Adult Offenders

Surgeon at Prison Helps Remove Scars That Foster Crime—
*New York Times*, 1963[1]

Prisoner's Life Scarred by Crime and Confidence—*Raleigh Times*, 1963[2]

In late 1963, Douglas Lipton, a newly appointed junior researcher at the New York Department of Correction, was handed a strange assignment. "I want you to go to Montefiore Hospital," his boss, Sol Chaneles, told him. "There's a plastic surgeon there who wants to talk to the department."

Twenty-seven-year-old Lipton was intrigued. What did the plastic surgeon want with the department? Lipton knew nothing about the field, other than what he saw on movie posters and magazine commercials; it helped people who'd been wounded in war or auto accidents, and it was beloved by the vain, those unsatisfied with what they'd been given and sought to cheat nature. Still, it seemed like an exciting space, and anything that changed the humdrum of his day was welcome. Too many hours sitting at his desk and his thoughts would turn sorrowfully to his father, who'd passed a few months back. He'd barely seen him in the years leading up to his death; he'd been so busy working on his doctoral dissertation (provisionally titled "The Conforming Boy in the Deviant Family"), teaching criminology classes at Vanderbilt University in Nashville, and spending time with his wife, twenty-three-year-old Carol.[3]

Then his mother called; his father had a heart attack—his fourth in as many years. Lipton packed a bag and booked a flight. "Whatever gets me to New York the quickest," he told the ticket agent. His father looked smaller than he remembered and so pale, even against the starched white hospital sheets. He stood by his bed, holding his wrinkled hand, and drank in the contours of his face, committing them to memory. His father died that night. He was fifty-three years old. Everything went a little blurry after that. There was a funeral to organize, relatives to contact, and his mother to comfort. He'd known his father had ongoing health issues, but he hadn't realized the severity. Now he was gone. He felt guilt, regret, sorrow—so many emotions.

While sorting out his father's affairs, he tried to plan his next steps. He had intended to move to New Hampshire for a position as an assistant professor, but now he was reluctant to leave his mother. She was healthy, but now she was on her own in New Jersey, living in a house that seemed far too big for one person. Besides, he'd missed the hustle and bustle of New York City. It was home in a way that Nashville or New Hampshire never would be.

He'd tried—unsuccessfully—to move back to New York before, but his lack of experience had been a barrier: he was turned down by New York University and City College of New York. This time around, he was determined to get a position. He reached out to Sol Chaneles, head of the sociology department at City College, who turned down his earlier application. Chaneles hired him as a criminology professor, with extra classes held at the Police Science College. He was happy to be back in his home city, but he missed being challenged at work. At Vanderbilt, he'd been immersed in research, and he wanted that sense of discovery and investigation, the rush of a project coming together.

Chaneles made him an offer: Chaneles had been headhunted to run the department of correction's new research unit and was looking for staff; how did Lipton feel about becoming the first official research associate for the Department of Correction in New York City? He could teach classes at City College on the side, if he wanted to. Lipton happily agreed; it was more money, and the chance to dig into research again.

So far, the work hadn't proved as exciting as he'd hoped. He'd been handed some partially completed projects to continue, one that assessed the connections between addiction and criminal behavior and another that measured the impact of computer training on juvenile recidivism, but he wanted a project he could own. Lewin's invitation was exciting, and Lipton was curious about what they would discuss during their meeting. And, as the most junior member on the team, he didn't have a choice.

By 1963, Montefiore Medical Center had grown into a sprawling institution in the Bronx, its twenty-four buildings enfolding more and more of the neighboring brick blocks as it expanded its medical offerings. Lipton had been born in the Bronx and spent the first fourteen years of his life in a small house on Macombs Road, less than three miles south of the hospital. He hadn't been back in more than a decade, and it felt strange to walk his old haunts as an adult. Had that park always been so small? Was his favorite deli still there?

Lewin's private office was in the back of a small building to the left of the main hospital. From the outside, it looked like a repurposed family home, with a small awning at the entrance and ivy trailing up the trellis windows on either side of the door. Inside, Lipton noticed the lovingly retrofitted interior, the original furnishings stripped out and replaced with large wooden desks, polished typewriters, and black rotary phones. Gilt-framed certificates and awards hung on every available bit of wall space. It felt cramped but comfortable, like the hospital had forced an office into a residential home.[4]

Dr. Michael Lewin stood when Lipton entered and shook his hand with a firm, cool grip. He sat back down and gestured Lipton to a leather chair across the desk from him.

Lipton appraised the famous surgeon; he was smartly dressed in a full suit and tie despite the heat of the day, and his hair, although receding, was still thick, though silver peppered his brown strands. Lewin appraised Lipton right back, liking the inquisitive look in the younger man's eye and his air of self-confidence. His suit was cheap, but he wore it well, and his tie was expertly knotted. He'd heard Lipton's polite address to his secretary when he entered; being respectful to others, no matter their position, was a characteristic Lewin valued highly.

He cleared his throat, hoping his first impression was correct. "Let me get straight to the point," he said to Lipton. "I'm sure you're wondering why I requested this meeting." Lipton nodded, and Lewin pursed his lips as he decided how to introduce his request. Perhaps by contextualizing the problem, drawing from one of his unpublished papers.[5] "Literature is replete with characters whose antisocial behavior is determined in large part by some physical defect," he said, briefly summarizing the "ugly" tropes so common in popular culture, from Victor Hugo's Quasimodo to the wart-covered Wicked Witch of the East in *The Wonderful Wizard of Oz*, and then recapping his work at Sing Sing.

"Not all situations are as clear-cut or dramatic," he continued; the surgeries differed in intensity, but even so, each operation was a concerted attempt to help inmates reclaim their identity. To allow them to match their outsides to how they felt on the inside. "I've seen inmates transform from surly, violent cons to model citizens," he explained. This wasn't about beautification; it was about *transformation*. Surgery made a real difference to someone's life. Lipton's eyes narrowed in thought. The surgeon's story sounded like a fairy tale, with Lewin playing the role of the fairy godfather. It seemed too good to be true. Would fixing a nose or a chin really change someone's behavior? This wasn't at all what he'd expected—had his boss sent him to humor the old surgeon as a joke?

These surgeries are *already* taking place in correctional facilities across America, Lewin continued—he estimated that around 2,500 or more occurred inside prisons annually.

Lipton raised an eyebrow and Lewin leaned forward in his chair. "I'm not joking," he informed him, ticking off the programs on his fingers. "They're happening at Huntsville prison in Texas, at San Quentin in California, at Stateville penitentiary just south of Chicago, at the Western Pennsylvania State Correctional Institution, in Ohio, Michigan, North Carolina, Minnesota, Oregon, Utah, Georgia," stopping when he ran out of fingers and breath. Lipton smiled, convinced.

"However, there's one problem," Lewin added. The recidivism benefits of his surgical work—and all other prison programs—was mostly anecdotal. Sing Sing's warden had refused his request for a study. There was no conclusive proof that prison plastic surgery affected recidivism. "They've been measured by subjective yardsticks," he told him.

Lipton grasped the problem immediately. Getting the right kind of data was key here, and there simply wasn't enough of it. Without that, no real statistical analysis could happen. He might not know much about the world of beauty—the closest he got to that was his wife's assortment of scented glass bottles and nickel-plated plastic tubes—but numbers he understood. What Lewin was getting at was a logic problem—did A plus B equal C—but within the parameters of beauty.

He glanced at the surgeon again with new respect. The man was a conundrum. His knowledge and verbosity of literature was a rare find in a medical man, as was his passionate interest in research. He clearly cared deeply about the inmates he'd worked with; it was surprising, really, considering how much other work he must have. To be that dedicated to the people that society had discarded—it was awe inspiring.

Living with physical defects is a major obstacle in life adjustment, Lewin continued. "What is the effectiveness of surgical treatment alone or in conjunction with vocational counseling and treatment?"[6]

Now that was research thinking! Lipton nodded his agreement, his mind buzzing with possibilities. There were so many ways to design a study like this. "We'd need to quantify this, get some hard scientific data on the effect of surgery on inmate reform," he told Lewin, plans bubbling away in his brain. There was a dramatic quality to the notion that by changing someone's face, you freed them of a handicap. He'd need a control group, some variables . . . did the specific type of plastic surgery count as a variable? He needed to do some research!

Lewin was pleased with his enthusiasm. "Plastic surgery is not a cure-all," he told Lipton. "But I'm convinced from the success we have that it can be of great benefit." He looked seriously at Lipton. "Be aware, this may be a controversial study," he told him. "Many people have uninformed views on what a plastic surgeon does and whether inmates should benefit from their work."

Lipton nodded. He could handle it, he said; he was used to ruffling feathers—already, it was a hallmark of his short career.[7] He'd been the only sixteen-year-old freshman at Vanderbilt University, too young to drink, smoke, or attend most social gatherings.[8] He'd enrolled in premed but quickly switched to sociology, finding what was inside people's heads more interesting than their bodies. Post college he'd spent three years in the service teaching war gaming to army cadets and officers—all far older than he—before returning to school for his master's.

"As long as you understand what you're getting into," Lewin said and held out his hand.

In Lower Manhattan, Corrections Commissioner Anna Kross was busy fielding a fresh avalanche of horrors from the city's jails. A twenty-seven-year-old junkie had died in his cell, apparently from severe withdrawal, and his lawyer wanted her to affirm that a situation like this would "never happen again."[9] She wished she could make that promise; she didn't see that happening till addicts were viewed as sick people rather than criminals, according to the law. *They should be in hospital beds, not cellblocks*, she thought.

She picked up the next report. There had been more escape attempts on Rikers Island, with inmates braving the cold East River to get to freedom. The body of William Brooks, a sixteen-year-old fugitive from Rikers juvenile institution, had just washed up near Queens.[10] There was a case of diphtheria at the Woman's House of Detention.[11] These were only the most pressing issues—they didn't include the never-ending reports of rape and violence inside New York City's jails.

With every report, Kross's eyebrows rose above her owlish glasses. "We have a real problem," she informed Mayor Robert Wagner. "Places like this are about to explode." She sounded like a broken record, she knew; she'd told him over and over again that the city's correctional facilities needed a serious over-haul. "Only a realistically enlarged budget could lead directly to more adequate implementation of the rehabilitation program underway," she wrote to Wagner via interdepartmental mail.[12]

His response was noncommittal, as usual. Overcrowding and sanitation is-sues at the Women's House of Detention, a bastille-like structure in Greenwich Village, were especially severe, and the medical care inmates received was shameful. Kross had pulled out all the stops: she'd written to Wagner, called him, and even begged him *in person* for the $16 million needed to build a new women's facility on Rikers Island.[13] Although Wagner agreed that it was a con-cern, her allotment for medical care never rose significantly—hence the assort-ment of deplorable doctors on her payroll.[14]

If only I could fire the lot of them, she thought wistfully, but that was out of the question. The jails were understaffed as it was—a problem that was not unique to New York City. A survey in the March 1963 issue of the *American Journal of Correction*[15] reported that there were a total of 137 full-time doctors and 95 full-time psychiatrists serving 133 state and federal penal institutions across forty-three states. Sixty-three institutions lacked even one full-time doc-tor! It was outrageous, Kross thought.

Still, just because Kross was enmeshed in a no-win staffing situation didn't mean that she was prepared to praise the jail's medical team. When the *New York Times* reached out to her for comment about the rumored low-quality care, she was frank. Our medical services are "bizarre and obscure," she told the re-porter, her tone clipped and angry.[16] There is no such thing as twenty-four-hour care, she revealed; the department just didn't have the money. The Department of Correction already paid its medical staff well below the going rate for their work. "The only physicians that can be hired at current rates are those too old for active office practice, those with unfortunate personalities, and those mental or physically handicapped," she continued.

The reporter nodded sympathetically, his hand dashing across his pad to capture every word she said. A choice phrase or so from Commissioner Kross could always be counted on to sell newspapers. Kross eyed the reporter's hand and shrugged internally. He was going to print every single word she'd said, which would irk some officials. But that was how the game was played. Whereas her entreaties were ignored, the media and any frenzy it stirred up was harder to brush off.

She'd resisted meeting with reporters when she'd first taken the mantle of commissioner, stung by their response to her appointment: "Anna Kross Clipped, to Be Figurehead Only," read one headline.[17] "Kross wants city to foot the bill to attend a penology conference in Geneva," sniped the *Daily News*.[18] Was it that hard to imagine a woman in charge? She knew it wasn't personal; they were just trying to sell papers, but their mean-spirited attitude was frustrating. Even female reporters got their jabs in; Texas reporter Elizabeth Carpenter described Kross as "the doughty queen of her own domain" and "a squat shapeless plain little woman."[19]

Kross was the second woman in city history to be appointed corrections commissioner and didn't all five-foot-two of her know it?[20] Katherine Bement Davis had preceded her in 1914. Davis took charge six years before women— white women, that is[21]—got the vote, and Kross often wondered what her tenure had been like, a mere sixteen years after a Virginia court had decided that, under the law, a woman was not "a person," having no legal existence save from her husband or guardian.[22]

But Kross had grown cannier over the years, realizing that it was better to embrace the press than run from it. Treat reporters well and give them some choice quotes, and they'd happily devote pages to furthering her causes.

The *Times* story created a public uproar. Citizens wrote letters and op-eds and waved placards in front of city hall, demanding that serious changes be made. It wasn't right that inmates were subjected to such substandard care.

There was turmoil inside the department as well. Doors were slammed and heated words exchanged. "She's caused a complete breakdown in the morale of personnel," Dr. Joseph Glass, the attorney for the Physicians and Dentist Association of the Department of Correction told the *New York Times*. "As representative for the association, I demand a public apology." He deemed Kross's comments "irresponsible." Kross disagreed. "If someone feels aggrieved there are adequate channels for redress," she told the reporter.[23] Basic medical care was not a luxury.

Nor was treating inmates like human beings. That was how you got people to reform, she believed: by recognizing their humanity, their individualism, not by treating them as a faceless evil group.

She did her best to make their jail stays more tolerable; this year, one focus was design, and she'd ordered the walls of the Rikers Island reception and classification center repainted in bright turquoise, lemon yellow, light blues, and warm tan, with inmate artwork hung in the hallways.[24] People interact with their environment, and appearances can make a difference, she knew. In her days on the bench, she'd added similar touches to her courtroom with rose etched doorknobs, crystal water glasses, and colorful drapes at the windows.[25]

Her new classification system was a step in the right direction; rather than loosely assigning inmates into groups by age or criminal history, she developed a week-long orientation and diagnostic procedure for new admissions, which involved interviews with social workers, vocational counselors, health care workers, and school representatives. They funneled new arrivals into appropriate rehabilitative treatments, with an emphasis on group psychotherapy. Correct classification was the engine that drove effective treatments, she believed.

"Experts should make the decision on the best course to pursue with each prisoner, to give him an incentive for success in his return to the community," she wrote.[26]

But despite Kross's best attempts at reform, during the last decade New York's jail and prison population had swelled almost 50 percent—a problem she attributed to the intersection of economic disparities, racism, addiction, and the New York Police Department's vengeful but not unsurprising hard-line response to the spike in crime-related officer deaths.[27]

On weekends in Harlem, drunks throw empty liquor bottles in street which is a dangerous condition. This occurs mainly around the Manhattanville and Gen Grant projects.—anonymous male, letter to Mayor Robert Wagner, 1961[28]

The early 1960s were a pivotal time of change in New York City, with the celebration of America's first spacecraft flight, the introduction of Barbie's boyfriend Ken, and the invention of electric toothbrushes.[29] But this excitement was tempered by the spate of airplane hijackings, the growing concerns about the possibility of nuclear war, and the mounting number of troops sent to Vietnam.[30]

Still, young people swarmed the bars and nightclubs of Manhattan and Harlem most nights, the dance floors filled with men and women dressed in drainpipe jeans, capri pants, and boxy shift dresses. They jived along to *Billboard* Hot 100 hits. At any given time, revelers were likely to hear "The Monster Mash" by Bobby Pickett and the Crypt Keepers or "He's a Rebel" by the Crystals blasting the air. They danced, drank, and laughed, but a hysteria to their humor hinted at the precarious nature of their play in a city on edge.[31]

On August 28, 1963, in the middle of a long sticky summer, the "Career Girls Murders" shocked Manhattan.[32] Two white roommates, a twenty-three-year-old schoolteacher and a twenty-one-year-old *Newsweek* researcher, were brutally murdered in their Upper East Side apartment. Each woman was stabbed more than sixty times with three different knives. Both victims were recent transplants who had headed to the big city to further their careers. Their deaths suggested that all those small-town concerns about big-city dangers were real. No arrests were made; their killer remained at large.

It was hard for New Yorkers to dismiss such tragedies. They might dance joyously to "the graveyard smash," but behind that happy-go-lucky facade, the reality was that civilians wanted their monsters firmly locked up behind bars.

The push for more policing didn't help Kross's cause. She wanted to rehabilitate her inmates, not throw away the key. Bigger changes were needed, Kross decided. It was vital to treat the root causes of offenses, not just punishing them—the city's social welfare departments had to step up. Reducing the city's crime rate was more complex than simply scaring people into good behavior, no matter what the higher-ups said.

She knew that Mayor Wagner meant well, but he was the son of a U.S. senator, albeit a progressive socialist one. He had no idea what it was like to grow up in poverty, day in and day out, to sift through garbage cans hoping to find a threadbare blanket or a stale slice of bread for the day's meal, to never know quite when your next meal would be, let alone to plan for your future. She did.

In 1894, when Kross was three years old, her family emigrated to New York from Russia. She'd seen firsthand how unfairly America's promised land of opportunity had played out for her parents. Her father worked as a buttonhole maker and barely had been able to afford their tiny tenement apartment deep in the slums on the Lower East Side of Manhattan. The stench of horse manure and sewage filled their four boxy walls, and the roaches and rats that infested them seemed endless. In winter, she huddled over street grates to warm her frozen limbs. The squalor motivated her to seek out every opportunity; throughout high school she worked in a suspender factory during the evening and taught English to new immigrants on weekday mornings and weekends. Somehow, she excelled in school and was awarded a full scholarship to New York University law school. She skipped her graduation ceremony due to the cost of a dress.[33]

Kross was the only kid in her tenement who went to college. Year after year, she saw kids she'd grown up with get into trouble with the law: petty theft, loitering, vandalism. They were bored, they were broke, and they were angry—with little education, they didn't see any way out of the slums. Her heart went out to them, and she started volunteering at the local jails, doing what she could to ease people's pain. They'd been set up to fail by an unjust system; had things gone differently, perhaps she would have been behind bars.

"Youth is no better than the soil it grows in," she was fond of saying; she disliked people being punished for the "crime" of poverty.[34] She was a strong believer in criminologist William Bonger's theory, which named poverty and deprivation as the basic cause of crime. Bonger preached that "crime was a direct result of a capitalistic system of private property and mass production."[35] As a judge, she'd done her best to even out this dichotomy, beginning with the basic principles of parity. In her court, all defendants were provided with free day care—she didn't want a woman getting sentenced because she was afraid to leave her three-year-old alone at home.

Ideally, she'd prefer not to sentence the majority of the women that came before her; in her opinion, around 90 percent of the women and teenage girls in prison should never have been arrested to being with. Her approach to law was contrary; early in her career, she famously insisted that the clients of prostitutes, as well as the women, be charged with solicitation. "Prostitutes don't belong in prison; they're social accidents," she informed Mayor Wagner. Providing these women with medical and psychiatric treatment would be far more effective in reforming them, she urged to no avail.

Kross was adamant that the best way to lift people out of poverty—the by-product being a decrease in recidivism—was education. Giving them marketable skills was just common sense, she thought, but it was a radical change from the way correctional care was carried out in America, which had focused on punitive sanctions for the last thirty years. She'd had some success implementing a raft of new programs—at the Women's House of Detention, there was a waiting list to get into the beauty school, and on Rikers Island, jobs in the prison bakery and machine shop were highly contested. There was even an experimental drama workshop designed to help inmates access their emotions. Youths at the Adolescent Jail on Rikers could sign up for an intense work-training program—essentially, a cram course in work skills and training, behavioral adjustments, and real-world socialization—developed to aid in their reassimilation upon release. There had been a sharp drop in re-offenses from youths who participated in that program.

Kross was pleased her programs were producing results, but she wanted to go bigger. She wanted more data about the effectiveness of her programs—and, ideally, to utilize penal research from across the world. "The general attitude to prisoners was lock them up and forget them," she wrote in an interdepartmental newsletter. Not on her watch.

The day after his meeting with Dr. Michael Lewin, Douglas Lipton awoke early and headed straight for the office. The sun was still creeping its way over the

Manhattan skyline, gradually fanning away the night chill when he pulled his car into the lot for the 134th Street docks.[36]

He blinked at his steering wheel. He felt tired. All night, he'd been turning Lewin's proposal over and over in his head, trying to think of the best strategy. He was still mulling this over when a loud honk—the ferry horn!—pulled him from his reverie. He half-ran toward the water, smiling breathlessly at the guards as he boarded the *Greenwich Village*, the 245-ton steamboat that ferried riders to Rikers Island.[37] This was the only entry point to the jail for inmates, officers, and janitors alike. There had been talk of building a bridge, but nothing had come of it so far. Onboard, Lipton stared at the tumultuous gray waters of the East River as he planned his day's schedule in his mind—he'd need to consult with his boss, write up a plan of action, maybe draft an outline to a bigger proposal. . . .

When the boat pulled into the dock, Lipton was first in line to disembark, hotfooting it up the hill to his desk inside the warden's house;[38] when Commissioner Kross created the department of research and planning a year prior, half of the space had been converted into a research facility.

He typed feverishly as he drafted an outline of their proposed study, the keys clacking as he tried to clarify his thoughts on paper. He scanned the page, sighed, and pulled out a new sheet. It was helpful to see the concept written down; it made it more real somehow. His first draft ran more than twenty pages. He skimmed it critically—it needed a lot more work, but he felt that the basic elements were there. At least, he hoped they were. Another week or so of work and he'd be ready to show it to people. He'd need approval from the Department of Correction higher-ups, specifically New York Corrections Commissioner Anna Kross, to get the project off the ground.

*What would Commissioner Kross think of his inmate beautification scheme?* he wondered. It made sense, once Lewin had explained it, but it felt like a hard sell. Still, he'd dealt with this type of problem before—the summer before he started his graduate studies at Vanderbilt, he'd taken a summer job at the University of Western Kentucky to teach basic criminological theory to freshman and sophomores. His expertise on the subject matter coupled with his track record of military war-gaming elicited another offer, this time from the police commissioner of Bowling Green, Kentucky. "We'd like to offer you the position of Bowling Green's chief of police," they told the startled twenty-six-year-old. "This would be a temporary appointment. . . . We're hoping you'll revitalize our systems, shake them up a bit, so to speak."

Bemused, Lipton agreed—when would an offer like this come along again? The station was hostile at first—who did this kid think he was, displacing their sixty-something-year-old police chief like this?—but the staff soon warmed up when he replaced their rusted revolvers with sleek new handguns and developed a free college program for officers. He brought in FBI marksmen to run their unit's weapons training. They were sad to see him leave.

It had been a wild ride of a summer! Surely, if he could handle rural Kentucky, he could make a case for his project in forward-thinking New York. He was hopeful about Kross's reaction. Although he didn't know her personally, her reputation as a staunch advocate for criminal justice reform and love of innovative solutions preceded her. The word on the prison grapevine was that she was a different type of commissioner. For some officers, this was a good thing; for others, Kross was a disruptor they could do without.

When Lipton's proposal landed on Kross's desk inside the New York criminal and supreme courthouse in Lower Manhattan, she was immediately struck by the title page—"The Surgical and Social Rehabilitation of Adult Offenders." That was . . . unusual, she thought, a little uneasy. She was old enough to remember the height of the eugenics movement of the early twentieth century, when the idea that criminality was hereditary and that certain physical features identified criminals held sway with the general public.

This so-called criminal appearance took a very white Eurocentric approach to "goodness," which placed targets primarily on immigrants and Black, brown, and Asian folk.[39] The eugenics banner was upheld by many of the country's major universities: Stanford, Yale, Howard, plus 370 other colleges offered courses on the topic—eugenics wasn't so much a trend as a nationwide gospel.[40] There were some outliers, even then, to that school of thought—in 1919, Harvard University rocked America when it vociferously rejected a $60,000 bequest from Dr. J. Ewing Mears, a surgeon from Philadelphia. Mears's endowment was contingent on the founding of a eugenics course, "notably relating to the treatment of the defective and criminal classes by surgical procedures."

Harvard's refusal was doubly surprising, as the university seemed to embrace eugenic philosophy, since the president of Harvard and many of its faculty were strong proponents of this belief. For years, Harvard sent a full breakdown of the race and background of their students to the eugenics record office in Cold Spring Harbor, New York.[41] "We did not deem it right to pledge to teach somewhat permanently that the treatment of defective and criminal classes by surgical procedure was a sound doctrine," its statement said.[42]

In 1963, eugenics had long been debunked, but Kross reasoned there might be a kernel of truth to the concept, floating somewhere along the lines of how one's appearance might affect his or her behavior from a societal rather than a naturalistic point of view. She was troubled by the racist and classist overtones inherent in assessing a person's physical attractiveness—the poor had less access to health care thus were more likely to be scarred and lesioned from a lack of treatment rather than heredity.

The previous summer, a research paper by Erik Kozeny, a German psychologist, again muddied these waters, creating a stir in corrections. Kozeny, using the 1939 Nebraskan penitentiary study as the basis for his experiment, assembled a collection of 730 mug shots sourced from the Austrian federal police. He then divided the photographs into sixteen binders, each binder representing a different crime. He morphed the images in each binder together, noting the measurements of each composite picture, including the space between the eyes and the skull shape. He asked members of the public to match the composite photographs to their crimes. He found a statistically significant correlation between the physical features of offenders and their respective category of crime,[43] stirring up the old debate that criminality *was* an inherited trait.

Kross was disappointed by Kozeny's conclusions; it was hardly rocket science that muscular men were more prone to violence or that slender, athletic men were cat burglars. Their body type might have influenced the type of trouble they got in, but it was a ridiculous generalization for the entire population. Physical appearance *did* play a role in stereotypes, she knew.

Not too long ago, an earnest young man from New York's state employment agency had informed her that the agency struggled to find work for many law-abiding white job seekers due to facial disfigurements. In 1962, they placed only 450 of their 840 disfigured applicants. Even then, most of these jobs were of the menial back-of-the-house type—the kind that have no advancement prospects, he added. Life was difficult for "facially ugly" New Yorkers—and that was without the added burden of a criminal record. It was exceedingly unfair, and Kross hated unfairness.

In a perfect world, she'd change people's biases and rid the city of these discriminatory practices. Psychological studies showed that an individual's beauty bias *could* be changed; however, the process of doing so at scale would take decades, if not centuries, and those being retrained had to *want* to shift their attitudes, unconscious or otherwise. That time line was too long for Kross. She drummed her fingers on the desk. Lipton's proposal had potential, she thought. And Rikers Island inmates would make ideal test subjects for his plastic surgery program.

The island—and its unfortunate residents—were ripe for a study.[44] Less than one square mile wide, the jail complex was smaller than Central Park but larger than San Francisco's infamous Alcatraz. Opened in 1932, it lay in the center of the East River, halfway between the Bronx and Queens, with a full view of

LaGuardia's runways on a clear day. Originally 100 acres wide, the island had quadrupled in size to meet demand—truckload after truckload of sanitary waste landfill had extended its borders to 413 acres. On hot days, the stench of rotting garbage wafted through the jail.

Due to its vast expanse, a huge proportion of New York's prison population was first processed on Rikers Island, shipped across the water, and absorbed into one of the squat red brick buildings and concrete cellblocks that dotted the isle. This city-within-a-city was a wretched place, cramped, noisy, and ringed with razor-ribboned wire. The island's twenty-year-old tree nursery provided some respite from the shackles of jail life, an enterprise Kross had thrown her support behind. She hoped the fifteen thousand leafy London plane trees[45] would provide the men with some respite from their surroundings. The island's many jails, which included an adolescent division, a classification center, and a workhouse, originally was intended for a population of four thousand but had stretched to hold some nine thousand men and adolescents, the overcrowding meaning that inmates were regularly doubled up, with two or three to a cell.[46] The numbers had doubled, but housing accommodations had not caught up— there were 18 percent more beds now on Rikers than a decade ago.[47]

Many saw the walls of Rikers time and time again; their re-offenses ranging from murder and assault to byzantine changes in the law,[48] parole violations, or defaulting on a fine. Nationwide, the country's jails and prisons had similar problems—but no one had solved the "revolving door" of crime so far despite the funds the government was pouring into recidivism research.

Perhaps Douglas Lipton's experiment would be the one to make a difference, Kross thought. It was possible that plastic surgery could impact prisoners' behavior—and how others responded to them—when they were paroled, potentially leveling the playing field for once. It was time to challenge the beauty bias, she decided, flipping through the pages again. This type of discrimination had to end. Every morning as she climbed the steps to her courthouse, she took a moment to glance up at Thomas Jefferson's quote carved in three-foot letters on the granite exterior: "Equal and exact justice to all men of whatever state or persuasion." It was time the city lived up to its word.

Granted, Lipton's experiment was different, but different thinking was clearly what New York needed right now.

⌒⌒

With Kross's backing, Lipton spent some time tweaking the project proposal, getting it ready to submit to the Department of Health, Education, and Welfare in Washington for funding. There were some inherent difficulties with using Rikers Island as the setting for the study rather than a state prison. For one, the jail had significant turnover, and inmates needed to be there long enough to go through the psychological tests and analysis needed to qualify. Second, there was a large educational element involved with the work. Lipton assumed that, like him, most inmates would know little about the mechanics of plastic surgery.

For informed consent, they needed to fully understand the projected outcomes, time commitments, aftercare, and have realistic expectations about what was and wasn't possible. *Would they even be interested in this?* he wondered. He knew that facelifts and breast enlargement surgeries were popular with women, judging by his wife's magazines and television newscasts, but would male inmates care in the same way? It was hard to imagine. None of his friends or colleagues had ever had any work done—at least, he didn't think they had. Surely he'd have noticed if Martin was suddenly sporting a new nose or if James had had ab implants—if that was even something that people did.

"You also need to think about how the correctional staff will fit into this plan," Sol Chaneles urged him. "Trust me on this, their education needs to be addressed as well." Lipton frowned at his boss and looked down at his notes. The Surgical and Social Rehabilitation of Adult Offenders study, or SSR, as he'd started calling it, didn't call for the island's correctional officers to actually *do* anything, save escort the inmates to and from their appointments with the research staff.

Chaneles smiled at his confusion. "Talk to Wally," he said.

The Department of Correction's research division was so new—barely a year old—and understaffed that Chaneles had forged partnerships with outside agencies. It was a necessity, as he lacked the manpower to do everything in-house.[49] But along with the extra paperwork and communication challenges, he also benefitted from the combined wisdom of externally related agencies. For one of his current initiatives, researching the benefits of education as a community integration tool for juvenile delinquents, he'd partnered with psychologist Wallace Mandell from the research wing of the Staten Island Mental Health Society and the nonprofit American Foundation.[50] It was likely that Lipton would be working with these agencies on the SSR project.

He headed to Staten Island to see Wallace "Wally" Mandell. Mandell got straight to the point. "There's a lot of back and forth with the institutional staff," he told Lipton. "The jail's officers have made a lot of things very difficult for us. They've 'forgotten' to inform us when a few of our adolescents were paroled, and we've waited for hours for them to bring in an inmate for our scheduled time . . . and they never arrive."[51] Lipton pursed his lips. That sounded frustrating. "It's often impossible to get anything done," Mandell continued. "I've raised these concerns many times—Sol understands—however, the guards' behavior never changes."

Lipton fidgeted in his chair. He knew Mandell was telling the truth, but it was *his* truth. It made sense that the Rikers officers might act up if they felt that extra work was being unfairly added to their schedules. Getting an inmate out of his cell and across the island might not take that much time, but someone would have to cover his station, someone else would have to check the inmate out of one logbook to the next—all the fussy bureaucracy that made a corrections facility tick.

But Mandell was an outsider. He didn't work on Rikers Island, and he didn't really know the *ways* of the island. He'd likely learned correctional protocol through a series of mishaps—and those small mishaps were precisely how dangerous incidents started. No wonder the officers thought he was clueless and didn't prioritize his requests, Lipton thought.

But Lipton wasn't like that—he was an insider. He saw the guards every day—on the dock, at the gates, at reception, in the staff dining room—they knew him in a way that they didn't know Mandell. They'd seen him in every single one of his suits, they'd searched his beat-up car in the lot, and they nodded their heads to him in the hallways. He wasn't exactly *friends* with any of them—most of the guards had high school educations and the concept of high-level research with controls and scientific standards didn't make sense to them—but they didn't mess with him like they did Mandell. "I appreciate the warning, Wally, but I think I'll be fine." Lipton gave the psychologist a big smile—for the SSR study to work the way he'd envisioned, he needed to play nicely with all the agencies involved. Getting along was vital to the project's success.

But first things first: without funding, the project wouldn't get off the ground. Kross had given him the green light, but her budget was empty—he needed Washington to sign off on his idea, or it was toast. He'd never applied for a grant before and hadn't realized how much paperwork was involved.

For the next two months, he developed his proposal further, holding biweekly consults with Lewin, Chaneles, and Mandell. To run the rigorous experiment that Lewin suggested—which Lipton backed wholeheartedly—he needed a watertight outline that answered every question a grant assessor might have. Lewin was emphatic that the study have a number of variables, but he wasn't sure what that looked like.

"Well, we obviously have one group that has plastic surgery and a control group who doesn't," Lipton said.

"That's a little cold-blooded, don't you think?" Lewin demurred. It seemed unfair to get an inmate's hopes up with a selection interview and multiple physical and psychological tests without providing them their desired treatments.

"It's necessary," Lipton told him. Without a control the study would be as unscientific as all the others that existed.

Lewin frowned, two lines converging into a deep $V$ above his eyes.

"You can always offer them treatment at a much later date," Mandell interjected. "We won't tell them that or put it in the proposal, but once the work is completed, there is no reason that can't happen."

Lewin dipped his head in reluctant agreement.

They hashed out the other variables. Should they provide relationship advice and surgery? Married inmates tended to have better recidivism rates than single ones.[52] Housing help? Housing insecurity was a major factor in recidivism rates.[53] After much debate, they settled on the basic outline of the program.

Inmates accepted into the trial would be randomly divided into four groups, each with a different variable. One would receive plastic surgery and social and vocational care, another group would receive only plastic surgery, the third group would receive only social and vocational care, and the final would be a control group that received no treatment or additional services.

Lewin and his team of surgeons would assess the inmates for eligibility at the jail. Those who were approved *and* assigned to the plastic surgery group would be scheduled for their chosen surgeries at Montefiore Hospital once paroled. It seemed foolproof enough, Lipton hoped; they'd gone over their plan so many times that he was anxious to get started.

That is, of course, if Lipton got the grant—the struggle of researchers since the beginning of time. Fingers crossed, he mailed his application to the attention

**The Rikers Island Surgical and Social Rehabilitation Project for Adult Offenders Groupings**

Group 1: plastic surgery and social and vocational services
Group 2: plastic surgery
Group 3: social and vocational services
Group 4: no treatment (control)

of Mary Elizabeth Switzer, the director of the Vocational Rehabilitation Administration (VRA) in Washington, D.C. The VRA was a freestanding division of the Department of Health, Education, and Welfare. Switzer's team focused on preparing mentally and physically challenged Americans to enter the workforce, and the organization invested heavily in correctional research.

He hoped she approved the application. His proposal was turning out to be one of those love-it or hate-it ideas—during dinner parties, whenever his project came up, opinions veered firmly into two camps. One cohort understood what he was doing and why, whereas the other camp took a more negative view. "Is it fair for convicts to profit from their jail time?" they argued. "Will criminals use this free surgery to evade the law and cause more trouble?"

There was real justification to such concerns, so he couldn't flat-out refute them. Their apprehension had precedent, after all, the most notorious being the real-life exploits of the infamous Chicago gangster John Dillinger.

Throughout 1933 and into early January 1934, John Herbert Dillinger terrorized bankers and policemen across America's Midwest.[54] Thirty-year-old Dillinger and his crew—known by the feds as the "Dillinger gang"—went on a spree of

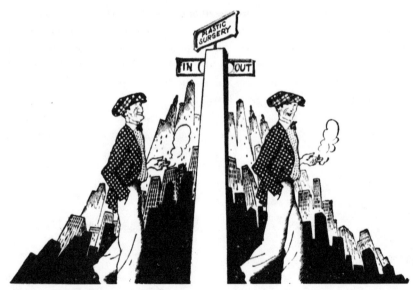

A criminal transforming through plastic surgery. *"Underworld Takes up Plastic Surgery,"* Hartford Courant Sun, *July 8, 1926*

high-stakes heists, successfully robbing twenty-four banks and four police stations. There was a finesse to his felonies that hadn't been seen before; Dillinger elevated bank robbing from a snatch and grab to a carefully orchestrated event. He viewed it as a team event, with a getaway driver idling outside in a nondescript Ford coupe, a lookout, a safe-cracking expert, and more. His gang wore bulletproof vests, toted machine guns, and kept a fully stocked medical kit in their getaway car. After a year of taunting the cops, in January 1934, he was captured in Indiana. Six weeks later, he held the jail deputies hostage with a wooden gun he'd carved in his cell and escaped.[55]

A national manhunt ensued. In absentia, he'd been indicted by the local grand jury, and the Federal Bureau of Investigation threw all of its considerable resources into finding him. To evade detention, Dillinger paid a visit to Chicago plastic surgeon Dr. James Probasco, demanding the man provide him with a new face.

The surgeon tightened his jaw, lifted his cheeks, and excised a small oval of skin from his chin, the infamous cleft that had been splashed across wanted posters. Dillinger complemented his new look with a pair of shell-rimmed spectacles and dyed his hair, eyebrows, and newly grown mustache dark brown. To finish his reinvention, he winced, lifted his left palm, and methodically shredded the tips of his fingers with a razor blade.[56] He repeated this on his right hand. Without fingerprints, they'd never catch him, he reasoned. Even if he somehow got in trouble with the law again, nothing about him would connect him to his previous identity. Dillinger was wrong. Shortly after his surgery, a tip from the bureau's nationwide network of informants placed him at his Chicago hideaway. Dillinger was killed in a shootout.[57]

"Our agents had no trouble recognizing him," FBI director John Edgar Hoover told the press. "There were two strong characteristics he couldn't remove. He had a very queer yellow eye and a crooked mouth. The men spotted him in a moment."[58]

His fingerprints didn't foil them, either; enlarged photographs displayed a recognizable pattern of whorls and phalanges with a small white blotch in the center. Hoover framed Dillinger's prints and hung them in his anteroom above a glass exhibit case of relics from the bureau's big catches. The photographs were physical proof of how ineffectual his feature-obscuring surgery had been. There was one way that he could have successfully concealed his prints, Hoover acknowledged—but only if Dillinger had been brave enough to bathe his palms in nitric acid.[59]

To avoid criminal copycats, the FBI issued a stern warning to the medical community at large: surgeons who abetted criminals would feel the full force of the law. Their licenses would be revoked, and they would serve a minimum two-year prison sentence.[60] Plastic surgeons touted their support for the FBI's hard line—they didn't want their practices curtailed or viewed with suspicion. It had taken long enough for them to gain acceptance as it was.

"No new weapons should be allowed to fall into the hands of outlaws," commented Dr. Jacques Maliniac, Lewin's uncle, in the 1935 winter edition of the *Journal of Criminal Law and Criminology*. "Every precaution should be taken to prevent the diversion of a reputable branch of medicine to the service of the lawless."[61]

Despite Dillinger's premature death, Hoover's warning, and Maliniac's grim pronouncements, Dillinger's surgery inspired a number of felons. The newspapers gleefully embraced this narrative. "Plastic Surgery Has Become Fad for Criminals," hooted the *Tonawanda Evening News*.[62] "Plastic Surgery Used by Criminals," sneered the *Los Angeles Evening Post Record*.[63] "Facelifting for Criminals Now Fine Art," revealed the *News Journal*.[64]

Reporters wrote story after story about criminal plastic surgery subterfuge and penned lengthy, hand-wringing editorials. Criminals are using surgery to hide from the law, they warned; or, as in the case of first-generation Californian Fred Korematsu, undergoing plastic surgery to evade the Japanese internment camps.[65]

A raft of Hollywood studios embraced this trope, further drawing the connection that plastic surgery abetted criminals. In the movie *Another Face*, released in 1935, a gangster receives plastic surgery to hide from the cops. His looks are so transformed by the scalpel that he parlays them into a career in Hollywood. In 1936, there was *The Man Who Lived Twice*,[66] in which a mobster escaped his past through surgery, giving up his criminal ways after his face was transformed. In *Mississippi Gambler* (1941), a remodeled fugitive starts a new life as a plantation owner. There were many others in the same vein.

Sometimes, these movies explored the power of plastic surgery as a criminal reform tool. In the 1938 movie *A Woman's Face*, Ingrid Bergman starred as a criminal kingpin who reformed her behavior once she was given a new look. In 1941, Joan Crawford played a scarred ingenue in a movie of the same name. Her character's criminal behavior was due to a lifetime of social rejection. By the end of the film, she morphed into an upstanding citizen, thanks to plastic surgery giving her an appearance of which she could be proud.

⌒⌒

The public's fascination with the transformative and redemptive nature of plastic surgery grew stronger each year, and more and more programs popped up

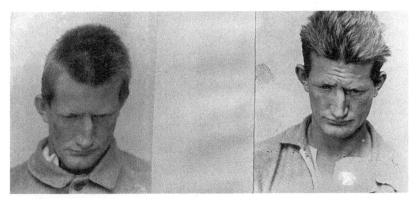

Before and after nose surgery, San Quentin. *Courtesy Anne T. Kent California Room, Marin County Free Library*

in prisons. However, the excitement surrounding its potential for reform went hand in hand with fears about being misled and anger about such an opportunity being offered to criminals rather than law-abiding and low-income folk.

The sheer novelty of this practice was irresistible to journalists, who used their headlines to hammer this point home. "Gaol's Facial Cures," disclosed the *Sydney Morning Herald*[67] in 1960. "Convicts Receive Plastic Surgery for Improvement Inside and Out," detailed the *Santa Cruz Sentinel* in 1961.[68] "Is Ugliness the Root of Crime?" queried the *Miami News* in 1962.[69]

Lipton was uneasy with the tone the papers had taken. So far, it had been relatively clear sailing, but he knew that, inevitably, there would be some hiccups as his research progressed. He didn't want his work derailed—it would be such a waste of the months spent immersing himself in plastic surgery and its history within a prison population. There was still so much he didn't know, and within those answers lay, potentially, the key to cutting recidivism rates. If—and he knew was still an if until he had that data in hand—beautifying surgery, like face-lifts and nose jobs could be proven to cut crime, there was so much that could be done with that information!

Dr. Michael Lewin was pleased with Lipton's enthusiasm but cautioned him not to get carried away. "Our operations are not one-size-fits-all," he apprised him. Every patient responded differently to treatment. "A patient's race often informs their outcomes," he explained—Black people were more prone to keloids after surgery, so a scar removal procedure might result in a scar that was double or triple the size of the original. "That's obviously not our desired outcome." As approximately 50 percent of New York's state and federal inmates were Black, a subject's race would be a relevant concern to the experiment.

Then the reply arrived from Washington, D.C. Lipton slit open the slim white envelope nervously; in his experience, thin envelopes were more likely to be form rejections. He scanned the sheet of paper, then reread it more slowly. It was a yes! He'd been approved! The Vocational Rehabilitation Administration had awarded the SSR project a federal grant of $240,000, enough to fund his study for a few years, effective July 1, 1964.

A few days after Lewin and Lipton announced their funding, Pastor James Keller highlighted New York's criminal plastic surgery programs in "3 Minutes a Day," his nationally syndicated column. "The fact that physical factors can incite to crime is a pointed reminder of the intimate relations in God's plan between body and soul," he wrote. "Help your fellow man in any way you can to satisfy his legitimate bodily needs. This will be a step towards reducing human misery which will prepare man for his ultimate destiny of heaven. Grant O heavenly father that I may see all men as Your children and serve their best interests."[70]

The pastor ended his column with a passage from Romans 15:1—"Now the strong ought to bear the infirmities of the weak, and not to please ourselves."

# 6

# JAIL HOUSE PSYCH OUT

Prisoners to Get Plastic Surgery—*New York Times*, 1964[1]

Of Children and Convicts—public affairs pamphlet distributed by Montefiore Hospital and Medical Center, 1963[2]

Twenty-seven-year-old Fred Marshall didn't like his cell. His was a common enough complaint on Rikers Island; the cramped spaces were notoriously sewage ridden and infested with rodents and bugs. Confinement was harder for Marshall than his bunkmate; Marshall weighed 280 pounds and stood six-foot-one in bare feet. His nine-foot-by-four-foot room was so narrow he could barely stretch his arms out. But he was lucky, in some ways, he knew, to be sharing his space with only one other person. Down the hall, cells the same size as his were crammed three to a room.[3]

"The number of prisoners in jails has reached an all-time high," Commissioner Kross told the press. "We shouldn't treat cattle the way we have to house our inmates."[4] In 1964, more than 121,234 new inmates trudged through the city's jails, the majority of them incarcerated for petty crimes or addiction-related problems.[5] The overcrowding was so bad on Rikers Island that Kross regretfully ordered the tree nursery bulldozed to make space for new cellblocks. The gymnasium was converted into a 250-bed dormitory, and hours at the carpentry workshop, machine shop, and sewing shop were cut to allow men to bunk there at night.

"No doubt you have heard the noise of the pile drivers, bulldozers and jack-hammers all over the institution," wrote Warden Henry Noble in the *Rikers Review*, the inmate's quarterly newspaper. "We are in the midst of a construction project to enlarge the institution, providing better facilities for our rehabilitation program . . . and help[ing] considerably in morale."[6]

The warden's announcement didn't improve Fred Marshall's frame of mind. He wasn't looking forward to better, bigger cellblocks, and, despite his relatively large cell, he didn't feel very lucky. This was his fourth cycle through the jail; his rap sheet included assault, theft, and drug possession. He had a six-month sentence ahead of him; a man he'd tried to rob had fought back, and he'd gotten cornered by the cops. He knew what was in store for him here: plates of mush for dinner, jabs in the yard, and written warnings from racist officers for not jumping or kowtowing as they wanted—rebukes for the crime of existing in a Black body. Another half a year of his life wasted behind bars, half a year in which he'd get older and heavier while his hopes grew smaller.

"Talking about morale, a man's appearance has a great deal to do with it," continued Warden Noble. "It appears to me that the clothing we provide could look a good deal better if it was worn properly and taken care of properly."

*What great advice*, Marshall thought sourly. As if a pressed shirt would somehow make him presentable! His bulk had grown over the last few years—he'd always been large, or "big boned," as a kindlier person might say, but now he was enormous. He'd catch a glimpse of his appearance in the cloudy tin mirror above the sink or the stainless steel mirrors in the corridors between the cell blocks and shudder and look away. At least there weren't many mirrors in the big house. All he could see was excess flesh, and it disgusted and depressed him. When he eventually got sprung, what was his life going to look like? What was *he* going to look like?

New York City wasn't a good place for a big Black man. Often, his mere presence was viewed as a threat, some combination of his skin color and his size, he supposed. It didn't matter how much he smiled; it seemed as if most people made up their minds about him within ten seconds of seeing him. He couldn't change his Blackness or his height, but maybe if he was slimmer, things would be better. He sadly pressed one of his stomach rolls between his thumb and forefinger and pinched till it hurt.

He'd been heavy for as long as he could remember. When he was small, his baby fat had been cute, but by middle school, it had turned to pudge. Kids had teased him, teachers had dismissed him, even his own mother seemed to prefer his slimmer brothers to him! He'd tried dieting, but there was rarely fresh food in the house, and smaller servings of bread and potatoes only made him hungrier. He grew larger and larger till he couldn't shop in the kid's section anymore, and soon, he'd outgrown the adult department—his Mom had to buy his pants at places like Rochester Big and Tall Men's Clothing or Sig Klein's Fat Men's Shop[7] or, more likely, their Goodwill equivalent. He'd been embarrassed by his shapeless threads but had no alternatives; his father rarely worked, and his Mom supported their household on welfare checks and running cash-in-hand errands for their neighbors.

Somehow, she always managed to put food on the table each day, mostly fatty, starchy carbohydrates, with the occasional side of meat—which was rumored to be horse meat.[8] Not that he ever asked her. Dinner time was always a tense event, with his mother glowering at his father or berating him for blowing their rent money on whiskey and horses, and his father's responses alternating between charming or snarling, depending on that day's die roll. Marshall stuffed his mouth with bread rolls, so he didn't have to engage.

Maybe that's how this started, he thought, his thighs rubbing uncomfortably together as he walked around the rec room. He glanced at the mess of flyers gathered on a table near the door; there was one about Operation Alphabet, a college Shakespeare course for illiterate inmates—"Tell your friends!" it implored—the latest edition of the inmates' paper, the *Rikers Review*, a flyer announcing the new books in the prison library, and so on. His eyes flicked down again, his eyes blinking as he scanned one particular page: "Interested in Free Plastic Surgery?" it said in bold lettering. Marshall paused then picked up the sheet of paper.

Now that they had the official stamp of approval—and funding—from the U.S. government, Lewin and Lipton were quick to put their plan into action.

"I hope that enough inmates sign up," Lipton told Lewin. The jail population could be remarkably challenging sometimes, and it was hard to predict how inmates would respond to their offer. "I'm sure we'll get the numbers needed," said Lewin. In his experience at Sing Sing prison, inmates tended to be enthusiastic about free plastic surgery. Surely jailed inmates would feel the same?

Lipton hoped he was right. The inmates on Rikers Island were different than the inmates he'd encountered in west Kentucky; they seemed more jaded, harder, and more dismissive of authority. Lewin might feel positive about this, but the surgeon had worked with a prison population with long sentences. In New York City, sentences averaged around nine months, and most of the men were focused on their immediate future rather than any long-term gains.

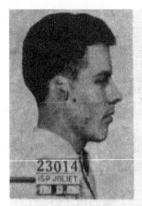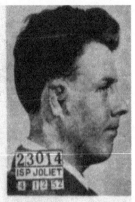

These official photos from Joliet Prison show how
ear surgery bettered this prisoner's appearance.

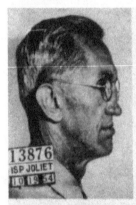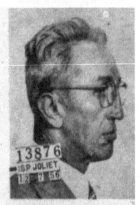

This man's problem was a badly battered nose—
but see (photo at right) how surgery helped him.

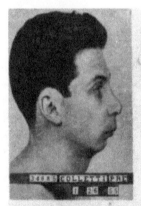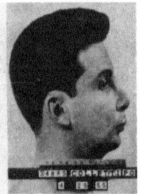

The commonest facial deformity at Stateville is
a receding chin. This one was improved in 88 days.

Before and after plastic surgery mug shots of convicts in Joliet
Prison, 1957. *American Weekly, July 1957. Inmate mug shots/
Illinois Department of Correction/Illinois State Archives*

"I think we need to do more," he told Lewin. To gauge interest, he passed out posters and flyers to the correction officers, asking them to distribute them throughout the island's jails. Tear-off slips were attached, which inmates could fill out and submit in a sealed box placed below the poster.

He ran a couple of informational sessions for the convicts and convinced Lewin to ferry in from the Bronx to answer any medical questions that arose. Around twenty inmates piled into their first session. Half came out of boredom, happy to do anything that broke their daily tedium. They slouched low in their chairs, joking around with their friends. Lipton eyed them suspiciously but began his presentation, which was interrupted every few minutes by a crude comment or laugh. Time wasters, he thought. But some attendees seemed intrigued, their eyes focused on the speaker.

"Now, do you have any questions?"

"Can you make my penis bigger?" called out a young Hispanic guy near the back.[9] His friends snickered.

Lewin's brow furrowed. "Excuse me?"

"My penis—y'know, me hog, my salami, my—"

"Yes, of course," replied Lewin. "No, that is not an operation we will be providing. Any more questions?"

"Will it hurt?" asked an inmate near the front, a middle-aged white man with a crooked nose.

"The operation in of itself will not be a painful experience," Lewin assured. "However, it's likely that you will feel some discomfort after the procedure and may be sore and tender. Depending on the specifics of the type of surgery performed, patients should also expect skin ecchymosis—sorry, bruising—for a number of weeks."

"But will I feel it?" the inmate repeated. This time, Lipton replied, "You won't feel the operation at all," he said, looking to Lewin for confirmation. "For the actual work, you will be fully anesthetized."

"The criteria to enter the study is small," he told the assembled convicts. "We're looking for inmates aged twenty-one to fifty years old, and, at the time of their admission to our study, who have more than thirty days left on their sentences. Once approved, the requirements are to attend follow-up interviews at six months and then again a year out and to keep in touch with our staff."

Meeting adjourned, the men filed out, jostling, joking, and grumbling. "That went well, I think," Lipton said to Lewin, pleased that a few of the questions had been related.

"I was happy with their responses," Lewin replied. "I think we can safely assume there's interest." Lipton chewed his lip. He hoped the surgeon was right.

He tried to keep himself distracted during the next few weeks as flyers and boxes were distributed in each jail block. That was easier to do so than expected; the 1964 Olympics were in full swing in Tokyo, Japan—and, for the first time, were telecast internationally—meaning New Yorkers could watch the games live, rather than with a twenty-hour delay as the tapes flew across the Pacific.

People crowded around televisions in bars or at home to enjoy the athletes' feats. They marveled when Ken Sitzberger, his toned physique ripped straight from a high school biology book, won a gold medal in springboard diving for the United States. They gasped as Fred Hansen pole-vaulted himself into the air, his sinewy forearms straining as he twisted himself up and over, clearing 16.7 feet to claim another gold for America.

The American Olympians brought home a total of twenty-six gold medals, but they also returned with the promise of equality and unity between the races. In photographs taken at the events, the U.S. gold medalists, Black *and* white, linked arms and grinned at the camera in a show of solidarity. Their camaraderie and beaming smiles were broadcast nationwide and printed in magazines and newspapers, serving as a beacon of hope to millions of Black and brown Americans. Black athletes have equal footing with their white teammates, the pictures implied, which were taken three months after Title VII of the 1964 Civil Rights Act was enacted, making employment discrimination on the basis of race, color, religion, gender, or nationality illegal, along with the desegregation of schools, public pools, restaurants, hairdressers, and other establishments.

However, the Civil Rights Act only covered certain attributes. Fred Marshall's skin color was protected from discrimination under the law, but his physical appearance was not—protections covering a person's height, weight, hair color, or personal beauty were noticeably absent from the act.

After what felt like an interminably long amount of time, the correctional officers delivered the application boxes to Lipton's office. He opened them nervously, tipping a pile of crumpled papers onto his desk. He smoothed each one out, trashing those that were illegible or covered in crude comments and drawings. He sorted through the pile, numbering each application on his notepad. It felt like he had been counting for hours, but it was still light when he finished. He looked at his pad, frowning, and counted the applications again.

He shook his head in confusion. It was a great outcome—the more participants the better in any scientific study. But the response was more than he or Lewin could have imagined: 1,424 inmates had applied for plastic surgery.

At the Staten Island Mental Health Society, Wallace Mandell was thrilled to hear about the volume of applicants. Not only would this be good for the study, but it would be great publicity for the project. The kind of publicity that could lead to bigger grants and greater prestige for his center. Having a big profile was an important factor in his field for allocating funding. Having 1,424 inmates apply on their first recruitment round demonstrated a huge interest in their work. The Surgical and Social Rehabilitation of Adult Offenders project had just gotten a lot more exciting.

"Cosmetic surgery is an attractive subject for publicity purposes," Mandell wrote in an interdepartmental report. "It has a perpetual fascination for the public, and we are committed to looking for projects which could win allegiance and develop the image of jails as being involved in exciting programs."

He repeated his comments to Anna Kross when he visited her Manhattan office.[10] She smiled thinly at him. "This study is a risk," she told Mandell. "I don't

## City Prisoners to Receive Plastic Surgery; Three-Year Study to Test Its Social Value

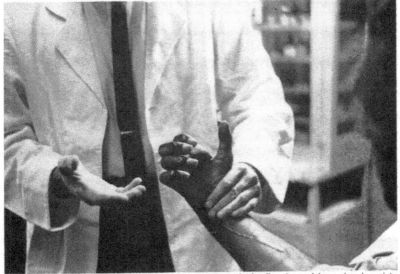

**SURGERY CAN MAKE IT WORK:** Mutilated, disabled hands are a major handicap to regaining a place in society. Plastic surgery makes crippled hands usable and thus can broaden job opportunities for prisoners.

News article in *Montefiore Tempo,* Montefiore's in-house newsletter, in spring 1965. *Courtesy of the Archives at Montefiore Medical Center*

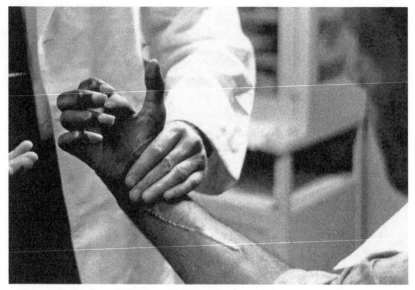

Detail from news article in *Montefiore Tempo. Courtesy of the Archives at Montefiore Medical Center*

want to think about what happens if something goes wrong. . . . If their surgery doesn't work, or if they're unhappy with the outcomes, or, worst case scenario, there's a surgical accident."

She looked thoughtful. She was pleased that there was more research happening on Rikers, but with actual surgery involved, the consequences seemed greater for the inmates—and for herself.

During the eleven years of her administration, Kross had earned herself the unhappy distinction of being the only commissioner—ever—facing three major simultaneous investigations.[11] She'd been taken to court by disgruntled officers she'd fired, she had been accused of being a bleeding heart, and she had been called "shameful" by the state legislature. Two years later, a New York Grand Jury investigated claims that she wasn't performing well. "We do not think Anna Kross is a good administrator," they wrote, blasting her for not reforming the medical care of inmates.[12] The grand jury had summoned her four times. All charges had been dismissed, but even Mayor Wagner, her biggest supporter, had told the media that "Perhaps in all matters she has not used the best judgment." Her critics poked at other things: the suspicious money losses on Rikers[13] and the arrest of a prison cook who had moonlighted as a drug smuggler.[14]

Kross had plowed on, trying to shrug off the barrage of outside complaints. She got no small sense of satisfaction that the inmates, at least, seemed to appreciate her efforts. In the latest *Rikers Review*, the convict editor, Sumner Waddell, had praised her in an article titled "Her Cross Is Heavy": "This is a tribute to a woman who stands like a tall oak tree in the valley of society where fear and hate walk hand in hand with bigoted giants," wrote Waddell. "Her devotion to use her talents to make this institution better along all facets, confuses and frustrates some. . . . Once a program is proposed her fights become relentless for its approval, not accepting one or several rebuffs as being final."[15]

Anna Kross had higher-level support as well. In March she'd attended a gala ceremony hosted by the Women's National Press Club in Washington, D.C., thrown to celebrate the inaugural Eleanor Roosevelt Memorial Award. She'd worn a string of pearls along with one of her favorite dresses, a long black number with crocheted sleeves, her hair turned up in a chic chignon (forgoing her usual hat, for once[16]). President Lyndon Johnson and First Lady Ladybird Johnson arrived at the Statler Hilton Hotel at 9:20 p.m.,[17] having dined earlier that night. Once they'd posed for the necessary press photos, shaken hands, and kissed cheeks, they made their way into the gala, where the president got down to business.

"For establishing the first public school to be held in a prison, for her initiative and her courage in bringing about major reforms in New York City's penal system, and for her success in bringing a woman's heart and a woman's insight to bear on the darkest social problems, the first Eleanor Roosevelt Golden Candlestick Award is presented to Judge Anna M. Kross," he announced. Kross blushed as he handed her a weighty golden candlestick that stood almost three feet tall. What would her parents think of her now, she wondered, their little mushka applauded as she received an award from the president of the United States! She beamed as she looked around the room, warmed by the friendly faces of her well-heeled supporters. It felt good to have her contributions valued.

Like always, that feeling didn't last long. Back in New York, the complaints started up immediately—the continued spate of avoidable addict deaths in the jails,[18] a guard's suicide inside the men's house of detention.[19] The mayor was on her back—he was being pressured by *his* higher-ups, most notably by Paul McGinnis, New York State's Corrections Commissioner, and New York's Governor, Norman Rockefeller, who was pushing for cities to rehabilitate their inmates—fast.

Two years earlier, during the 1962 legislative season, Governor Rockefeller signed the first major prison reform bill in the state, offering discretionary reductions of the maximum term of an indeterminate sentence.[20] Additionally, Rockefeller wanted all inmates to have access to counselors and psychiatrists, a position Kross believed in but hadn't the resources to achieve. She had fifteen psychiatrists and six psychologists total to treat all inmates, which averaged one professional for every 560 men, clearly an inadequate number. Still, it was a big improvement on the *three* mental health professionals she found on the payroll when she became commissioner in 1954.

Across America, the numbers were far worse, with an average of one psychiatrist for every 4,400 inmates held in state and federal penitentiaries. They were all woefully below the guidelines of the American Correctional Association's *Manual of Suggested Standards for a State Correctional System*, which stressed that there should be one psychologist, minimum, for every five hundred inmates.[21] On the other hand, the inmate-to-staff ratio for corrections officers averaged one officer per seven inmates.[22]

Still, psychologists aside, Kross had made other significant changes; the medical and mental health care at the jails now fell under the city's Department of Health and Community Mental Health Board instead of the Department of Correction, a helpful consolidation, she felt. It also increased the quality of care; doctors were less reticent about working for the health board than the jails. Despite all of her changes, it was never enough. There was so much more to do. That's why she'd petitioned—and won—an extension of her term in office; technically, she should have retired in July, when she turned seventy-two years old.[23] The idea was to have the maximum impact possible while she held power. But she was tired of the fighting, of all the back and forth, and the interminable meetings that filled her schedule. Kross was beginning to feel indifferent about the plastic surgery project. It was one thing to back something you believed in, but there were unassailably frivolous elements to the study.

"Listen to me," Kross said fiercely to Mandell. "There are a lot of departments at play here—the Department of Labor, the Bureau of Prisons, the Board of Education. . . . I don't have time to do all your hand-holding. I need to know you're in control of this. That problems will be handled."

Mandell swallowed. "I understand," he told her. "We are following every recommended protocol."

Lipton's excitement about the number of applicants soon turned to panic as he realized the huge amount of work it would be to process such an enormous group. For starters, Dr. Michael Lewin and his residents needed to screen each applicant for suitability, which meant numerous trips to the jail and back-to-back physical examinations. Most exams took place in the newly opened Reception and Classification Center,[24] a $10 million three-story building designed to be more inviting than the other cellblocks. Its seven-by-ten-foot one-person cells were twice as big as Fred Marshall's cell and painted pastel green or light beige. They were outfitted with "non-sag" beds and included a table with built-in stool, a washbasin, and a mirror.

In a small white room inside Rikers Reception and Classification Center, just off the main intake hall, Lewin examined inmates, one after the other. Each assessment took a minimum of thirty minutes during which he checked their medical histories to ensure they had no contraindicating problems, unknown or otherwise. Then the real assessment began: confirming whether there was a real need for surgery and to what degree, as well as whether their requested outcome was achievable. Inmates were scored by two metrics: severity and prognosis. Severity levels were classed as minimal (one), moderate (two), marked (three), or gross (four). Then he scored them from one to four (one being poor and four being excellent) as to the likely outcome of the operation. He looked for a minimum score of two on each axis. Applicants with minor issues or potentially unwelcome outcomes were rejected.

The inmates were an eclectic bunch. One man swaggered in and pointed to a thimble-sized mark tattooed between his finger and thumb. "I'm desperate to have this off," he told Lewin, who smiled and noted the mark on his pad, along with the ten other tattoos—all much larger and more obvious—that covered the man's chest and arms. Denied. There was a guy who wanted his nose "fixed" when his nose was perfectly straight and well sized. Another man complained about his large "flappy" ears. "I look like taxicab coming around Forty-Second Street with its doors wide open," he told him.[25]

Then there was Dennis Jordan, a white man of medium build and height who wanted *all* of his features remodeled. He told Lewin that he disliked his oversized nose, his concave forehead, his receding chin. He hated his appearance so much that he tried to avoid people in general. At Rikers, he was serving time for theft; his particular modus operandi was casing funeral parlors and stealing the belongings of the bereaved during the service. "I want to look like Kirk Douglas," he told Lewin. "Well, I can't assure you of that, but I can assure you of an improvement," Lewin told him. Jordan nodded reluctantly. "Okay," he said. Inmates who cleared the medical screen were then shunted in Lipton's direction to undergo interviews and psychological testing. It was imperative that anyone who had surgery was mentally equipped to handle the aftercare and healing process.

Lipton had more flexibility than Lewin regarding the timing of the interviews, as he was based on Rikers Island. The officers fetched his inmates for him, lining them up in the hallway outside his door. He kept the door ajar; he'd never been hurt by an inmate, but it wasn't unknown for a situation to escalate. Every year hundreds of corrections officers and support staff were injured in the nation's jails and prisons.[26]

He looked down at his pad and noted that he had six evaluations scheduled that day. He was interviewing men as fast as he could, and Chaneles was pitching in, but the number of inmates didn't seem to be decreasing. He sighed. Who knew you could have too much of a good thing?

There was a knock on his door, and he looked up, and still farther up, to see the full length of the man entering; this was Fred Marshall from the Men's House of Correction, according to his case file. Marshall loomed over him, his large frame filling the small room.

"Sit down, please," Lipton said, gesturing to the chair opposite him. Marshall adjusted his bulk and sat, crossing his legs with surprising grace.

Lipton smiled in welcome as he gave the man a once-over. Marshall's face was round, and his expression was open. His teeth were very white, and his eyelashes were girlishly long. He glanced down at his file again; the man was twenty-seven years old, a year younger than he was. In another life, perhaps, they could have been friends.

"Hello Fred," Lipton said. "Thank you for coming today. Now, please tell me about the reasons why you're here. I see from your file that Mike—I mean, Dr. Lewin—says here that you've asked for liposuction of your flanks."

"Flanks?"

"Fat removal from your stomach," Lipton clarified.

"Yup."

"OK. Now, tell me, how are you feeling about your body at present?"

"I hate it," Marshall said, a grimace on his face. "I told the doc to cut it off." He rubbed a hand across his belly, emphasizing the flesh straining through the thin fabric of his prison scrubs.

"Have you always felt that way?"

Marshall shrugged. Some of this used to be muscle—kind of—he explained. He'd been a boxer in high school for a little while. People had told him he'd be good at it, that he was the right size for a boxer, but he didn't practice enough to be any good at it. He didn't like the feel of his fist hitting the punch bag.

Lipton dipped his head sympathetically as he flipped through the rest of the case notes. Fred Marshall was born in Detroit, the second youngest of four boys. His parents split up when he was seven years old, and his file indicated that both of his guardians had alcohol and gambling problems.[27]

"Did you like school?" "Not really," Marshall admitted. It didn't come naturally to him, not like the other kids. When he looked at books, the words would get all jumbled up in his brain. There was no money for a tutor. The other kids teased him about his weight. He dreaded going to school. Frustrated, he looked for a way to kick back. He didn't want to drink—that was what his deadbeat dad did—instead, he tried heroin one weekend with some of his friends. He liked the feeling of his body softening and his mind going blank as the narcotic spun through his nervous system. After multiple warnings about his bad behavior from teachers, he was expelled in his third term.

After that, he had a lot of free time, so horse on the weekends with his pals became dope during the week on his own. He lost himself in that hazy void, all of his feelings suspended in a comforting fog. But smack cost money, and he didn't have much. He pawned most of his possessions—and some of his ma's—but the money didn't last long. He began thieving to fund his habit, petty easy-to-pocket stuff that he quickly sold. His days blurred into a mockery of the official workday: steal, sell, meet his dealer, shoot up, and repeat. He wasn't a good thief; he was too slow, too clumsy, and he got caught easily. Arrests stacked up. He felt stuck. "That's when I joined the army," he told Lipton—he'd hoped that the stringent service would break him out of his destructive cycle.

Lipton blinked. He hadn't expected that. He thumbed open Marshall's file again to check, yes, there it was, in black and white type. Two years of service in the army—drug free, he assumed—followed by a dishonorable discharge.

"I was clean, real clean for a long time, and then I ran into an old friend," Marshall admitted. He thought he'd have just one hit, but. . . . After he was dismissed, he moved to New York, hoping for a fresh start. He got hired as a hospital orderly, but then he messed it up. He was back to square one and his old tricks—and then back in jail. But Lipton's flyer had given him hope when he thought he was done with that emotion forever. Something had clicked when he'd read that missive—a strange and unexpected opportunity had come his way, and he didn't want to lose it.

"I just want it gone," he told Lipton, a pleading expression on his face. "I want to get a job. . . . I want to meet a girl. . . . Please help me."

Lipton nodded. "Thank you for your time." If Marshall passed the subsequent psychological tests, he was in.

On Rikers Island behind a dilapidated wooden desk a few feet from where Lipton sat, Sol Chaneles, the director of research and planning for the Department of Corrections, was having a bad day. The thirty-eight-year-old was feeling increasingly skeptical about his position in the correctional hierarchy.

Two years earlier, Anna Kross had summoned him to her mahogany-walled office inside Manhattan's Center courthouse. At the time, he'd been happily ensconced as a research professor inside City College's sociology department, his days a mix of teaching and research projects. He was wrapping up his latest project, a Ford Foundation–funded[28] investigation into goal setting for juvenile delinquents when she called.

"Your work caught my attention," Kross told him. She liked his study design, and how it factored in community and educational achievements. "I have a proposition for you."

Kross offered him the position of director for her brand-new penal research department. This job is an opportunity to affect things on a wider scale, she promised him. "In this position, you can make a real difference in how we run this city, potentially influencing policy." Chaneles was flattered by her regard and intrigued by her invitation. He often felt like his worked existed in an academic silo, rarely making it into the hands of people who might make use of it—an issue that almost *all* researchers suffered. Developing a research department from within the correctional department—on Rikers Island itself, no less—offered the possibility of bridging that gap.

Then she told him the pay: $13,100 per year, considerably less than he presently earned. "This is just the starting salary," Kross told him. "We'll review it in our next budget revision and it will go up accordingly, adjusting for your experience and efforts." Chaneles frowned. He didn't like the sound of that, but the directorship had so much promise that he allowed Kross to sweet-talk him into a temporary pay cut. It would be for just a little while, till the department realigned its budget. He couldn't let something like *money* stand in the way of making such a big impact. His wife wasn't thrilled that he'd be traveling to the jail every day, but she was used to his eccentricities.

Kross was pleased when Chaneles accepted her offer; she enjoyed being surrounded by a focused, motivated team. She had high hopes for her new department—once she had the data, she could start to make some real scientific-based changes. Chaneles already held clout within the criminal justice community, but his new appointment significantly boosted his profile. Top-tier journals solicited his papers and invited him to submit op-eds. Organizations across the United States booked him for their conferences, eager to discuss his methodologies.[29]

"An experimental attitude towards innovation is essential," he told the National Council of Crime and Delinquency in Washington, D.C. "If new goals, plans and insights are to function effectively within the Department of Correction, public ignorance must be reduced." The audience was rapt.

Chaneles was gratified by the positive response from professionals *and* the press. It helped ease his transition; instead of a warm, bright office in the heart of the city, he now suffered the indignity of having his trunk searched daily, before enduring a rocky boat ride to Rikers Island and a seat in a cold, drafty office. The isle's dank, cloying smell irritated his nose.

There was never any quiet; the sirens, squawks, and shouts were a daily distraction from his research books. He never knew when he'd be called to fill in—when the entire medical staff quit in March 1964, citing poor pay and an impossible workload, Chaneles was conscripted into helping out in the classification center. He didn't blame the nurses and doctors and orderlies for resigning; Rikers inmates totaled thirty-one thousand clinic visits a month, an untenable number for such a small team.[30]

When Douglas Lipton agreed to join him, Chaneles breathed a sigh of relief. He liked the younger man's go-getting attitude, and having someone to delegate to lessened his to-do pile. His wife, however, remained annoyed about his reduction in salary: "They should pay you what you're worth!" He agreed. "Soon," he told her; the commissioner had promised him she'd increase it. He laid out the expected salary terms with respect to his work experience and management responsibilities in a report to Kross marked "confidential: for discussion only."[31]

"The training program is conceived, at the outset, of a high-quality graduate program. Hence salaries should reflect, ideally, conditions of numeration to be found in the best graduate schools." He proposed $22,000 a year as project director.

Despite his detailed brief and Kross's assurances, after the next budgetary meeting, his salary remained the same. Crestfallen, Chaneles sat at his desk, feeling belittled and unappreciated. Commissioner Kross hadn't taken a pay cut to take her job, had she? Why was it one rule for her and another rule for him?

He appealed to her in writing. "Since the beginning of the division, the scope has, as you know, increased many times, and concomitantly my responsibilities as its director," he wrote. "The current salary level for research directors engaged in comparable programs is $20,000. I therefore respectfully request that immediate attention be given to a salary increase."

Kross refused, reiterating that Chaneles's department had her full support and that she'd be happy to increase his pay when the mayor allocated her more funds, which she believed would be soon, she added. *She* was paid $20,000, she reminded him, and her pay also hadn't increased.[32] I believe that your research work may change the correctional world as we know it, she told him.

The budget crisis in New York City's Department of Corrections and its ballooning convict population mirrored the widespread crisis in which the city was mired. In 1964, more than eight million people crowded New York City's five boroughs.[33] The Bronx alone held 1,450,000 residents—more people than San Jose, Nashville, and Austin combined.[34] It was home to people from every walk of life: psychiatrists in their gilt-plated Upper West Side apartments, models in their East Village lofts, smooth-talking salesman, rough-and-tumble plumbers, immigrants in tired, shabby tenements, pockmarked addicts curled on stoops or splayed out in basement alleyways, senators locked away behind high wrought-iron gates, weary-looking shop girls crammed two to three a room. . . . Turn any street corner and you'd hear a jumble of accents, car honks, and alarms sweeping down the avenues and curling around the condos. The city buzzed at all times of the day, running on a pulsing, nervous energy that made it feel almost alive. But there was never enough work or money to keep its denizens fed.

The city's many problems crystallized for Chaneles as he strolled the many halls of the New York World's Fair, which spanned almost the full 646 acres of Flushing Meadows Corona Park in Queens. He goggled at the ingenious gadgets displayed: a picture telephone that allowed users to *view* their callers, an animatronic Abraham Lincoln, and men in jetpacks zooming precariously around the halls.[35] "Every day brought word of marvels to come," he told a reporter from *The National Geographic*. For him, the fair's tagline, "Man's Achievement on a Shrinking Globe in an Expanding Universe," encapsulated the flip side to these technological marvels.

"For problem youths, none of this makes sense," he explained. "There's a terrifying need for people who can operate data processing machines, but to apply for the necessary training you need to have at least a high school education." The technology divide was impacting the class divide, displacing skilled and unskilled workers alike.

"A lot of dishwashing is done with machines now. Why should people take time to show you how to do it when you might not work out?" an administrator at New York's state employment agency told the same reporter. Accordingly, unemployment numbers were going up in line with the increasing number of inmates at Rikers, who'd turned to crime through desperation, boredom, or sheer opportunity.

Chaneles knew that the statewide spike in crime had resulted in huge sums of money pouring into correctional and social welfare at both state and federal levels, much of it earmarked for research. What wasn't apparent was how it was being spent; in New York City, the cash seemed to go into a black box. And it wasn't like those dollars were being put to good use elsewhere; week after week he wrote Kross memos about the substandard condition of Rikers' ramshackle facilities and its dangerous staffing shortages.

Kross acknowledged the problems and shared her own frustrations with Chaneles, always with the assurance that she'd requested more funds for his department. "We value you highly," she told him. Chaneles was unmoved. He'd been flattered the first time but not anymore. It might not be personal, but knowing that didn't make it any easier to survive in the city on his now-meager wages. His former colleagues were pulling in almost 40 percent more money than he was and using their disposable income to enjoy all the culture and luxuries that New York offered. They were enjoying their forties, while he, with all his vaunted experience, was eking by—he'd taken a part-time evening shift at the Staten Island Mental Health Society just to cover his household expenses. There was never a hint of this in his interactions with the press; in public he was a suave, confident proponent of Lipton's plastic surgery study.

"It's a completely new move in prisoner rehabilitation," he told the *Sydney Morning Herald*.[36] "It helps those already burdened with other social, economic, and psychological limitations."

"Tattoos and scars are an added problem for a prisoner. . . . [They lower] a prisoner's motivation and his chance of making good," he told the *Gazette and Daily*.[37]

But in his day-to-day life on Rikers, Chaneles started checking out, tired of the constant pushback about being paid what he was worth. The work would still get done, he knew; Lipton was a solid, reliable worker with a young man's energy. Let him take the lead. Chaneles would sign off on Lipton's work, but he didn't have the energy—or desire—to direct the SSR project. He was going to work his mandated hours, nothing more. Chaneles redirected his energy into a personal passion: children's books. He loved watching kids' faces light up as he told them stories, and, with grandkids on the horizon, he wanted a head start. He'd been noodling with the idea of a Christmas picture book in which Santa switched up his traditional outfit for a new look.[38]

With Chaneles taking a backseat, Lipton's other commitments left him scant time to handle the growing SSR caseload. He'd overcome his surprise at how eagerly the inmates shared their darkest stories—the tragic floodgates that opened in the small interview room. They treated it like a confessional, with Lipton their priest and savior. One story blurred into another; so many of the men had grown up in poverty, surviving racial and nationalistic discrimination, mistreatment or abuse by their parents, and poor performance in school—if they hadn't dropped out entirely. Subsequently, many formed unhealthy attachments to drugs and alcohol. Some tales were generational—their broken lives a repetition of their parents' own troubled upbringing.

He wanted to devote every applicant the time he deserved, but it was growing increasingly evident that he couldn't do it alone. It would take him months—
possibly years!—to make it through the pile of applications working alone—
meaning the study wouldn't get underway for a long while. He needed help.

Unlike Chaneles, Lipton wasn't restricted by the meager budget provided by
the Department of Corrections. He had $240,000 from the Vocational Reha-
bilitation Administration to draw on. The grant document specifically allotted
funding for manpower, as well as for leasing new office space to home any new
hires. He began by canvassing the sociology and psychology departments of
New York's colleges, asking the program administrators to notify their graduate
students of this opportunity.

Twenty-eight-year-old Richard Kurtzberg, Dick to his friends, was his first
hire for $8,000 a year. Kurtzberg was halfway through his PhD in school psy-
chology at New York University, a private university in the heart of Greenwich
Village, and had never worked with inmates before. He was green but eager, and
he took some of the pressure off Lipton. It wasn't enough.

Then the careers department at Hunter College, a public university in Lenox
Hill in the Bronx, with approximately 50 percent students of color, called.[39] "I
have someone I think would be perfect for you."

On the cracked sidewalk of 64 University Place, outside a redbrick office
building situated just off Union Square between Park and Tenth Street in
Lower Manhattan, twenty-nine-year-old Norman Cavior took a deep breath.
He smoothed the pleats on his blue guayabera shirt—a fashion he'd picked up
while stationed in Panama—pushed back his shoulders, and nervously pressed
the buzzer. *Bzzzzztttt. Bzzzzztttt.*

Cavior pasted a smile on his face, ready to respond. He wanted to make a
good first impression—he really needed this job. A few months back, inside
a small hall just off the Grand Concourse in the Bronx, he'd slipped a ring
onto Helene's finger. In front of seventy-five witnesses, he'd vowed to love
and cherish her for the rest of his life. Cavior and Helene were Bronx kids,
growing up barely a mile from one another, but they'd met only a year ago—in
Madison, of all places!—when Cavior was hired as a researcher by the University of Wisconsin, where Helene just so happened to be taking classes. It was
a whirlwind romance.

Cavior wore a yarmulke for the ceremony, which was presided by a rabbi—
Helene's family was Jewish, and his mother-in-law insisted—and spent the

whole time looking dreamily at Helene, who looked even more beautiful than usual. His best man, a Jewish guy he'd known since he was five, had to prod him to move, he was so starstruck. His choice of best man had been the one burr on the otherwise perfect day; his best friend was a mixed-race Black man, and Helene's mother had objected. Apparently, it wasn't his race that bothered her, but that he wasn't Jewish. Reluctantly, Cavior rescinded his best man invite; his pal shrugged, smiled, and said he understood, but Cavior still felt bad.

The couple spent two months in Wisconsin's winter, but hated the subzero temperatures so much so that Cavior quit his job and they decamped back to New York. Helene was hired by a local elementary school, and Cavior picked up his studies at Hunter College. But Helene's meager salary couldn't support them both. Cavior, the only child of a single mother, had grown up on welfare. Most nights, his mother got home late, her fingers chapped and torn from her work operating a sewing machine in a sweatshop. His mother raised him to be self-sufficient and to abhor debt, and the mounting household expenses bothered him. This job was a lifeline.

Cavior liked Lipton—"call me Doug!"—immediately. The man had an affable, no-nonsense demeanor, and his energy for the project was infectious. He found himself genuinely interested in the concept behind the experiment. Cavior never really considered the effect of personal appearance on criminal behavior, but he could see why it would be valuable to explore. Many of the kids he'd grown up with—mainly the Jewish ones and Italians—had their noses slimmed and straightened by surgeons. They proudly showed him before-and-after sketches when he went round to hang out.

Lipton was impressed by Cavior's sincerity and that he'd some experience with inmates. As an undergrad, Cavior had volunteered at the drug rehabilitation clinic on North Brother Island, a twenty-two-acre plot halfway between Rikers Island and the South Bronx. Most patients were part of a pipeline of addicts sourced from the neighboring jail. Lipton hired him on the spot with a starting salary of $6,000 a year. He hoped his team's lack of experience—for both Kurtzberg and Cavior, this was their first full-time psychology job—would be balanced by their desire to develop something important—and to put in the long hours necessary to achieve this.

Cavior was thrilled to be hired. That evening in his small Queens apartment, he poured two small tumblers of dark rum and raised his glass to Helene. They weren't big drinkers, but it felt good to mark the moment.

His new office was a thirty-minute drive from home—if traffic was light. Traffic was *never* light. After two weeks of sitting in his beat-up car, drumming his hands impatiently on the dashboard as he inched up Grand Central Parkway, he'd had enough. He bought a used two-cylinder BMW 600 motorcycle, which shaved his commute in half, and used the extra time to wolf down Helene's bacon and eggs as he scanned the day's headlines.

He liked Richard Kurtzberg—the man was a little serious and uptight, but he was reliable and honest and respectful. They worked well together. Kurtzberg had had a more luxurious upbringing than Cavior, but his parents were high school dropouts who'd clawed their way up. Richard was the second person in his family to go to college. The pair quickly established roles that best suited their skills; Kurtzberg crunched the data, and Cavior took the lead in the psychological assessments. There was a lot riding on their analysis—if they approved inmates with unrealistic expectations or ulterior motives, they might jeopardize the study.

Once a week or so, the pair received an inspirational update or memo from Dr. Lewin, written on Montefiore Hospital notepaper. "The inmate with a visible disfigurement is handicapped; not only does he have the disadvantages of a criminal history but he carries with him a visual stigma which constantly reminds him and those that deal with him of the fact that he is different," Lewin wrote.

Kurtzberg and Cavior split their time between their Union Square office and Rikers Island, generally heading uptown in the afternoon to ferry over, then decamping to their assigned testing rooms inside the intake building. The surgical screens had whittled down the number of volunteers, but with the application boxes redistributed among the jails, the numbers were going up again. There was never enough time in the day! To standardize testing, all inmates were shepherded through a variety of psychological tests.

Cavior liked to start with the Tennessee Self-Concept Scale: one hundred word-association questions designed to measure the inmate's personal identity and social identity, including how he felt about his appearance. He followed this with the Sacks Sentence Completion Test, which followed a similar trajectory but delved a little deeper into how the subject felt about himself and his surroundings.

The next test, the Minnesota Multiphasic Personality Inventory (MMPI), was held in a large conference room with twenty or so men testing simultaneously. Cavior and Kurtzberg took turns proctoring these two-hour sessions, restating over and over that the men needed to answer *all* of the 566 seemingly random questions. The MMPI measured personality traits such as depression, paranoia, schizophrenia, and flightiness, and inmates who exhibited unusually strong psychopathology results would be eliminated from the study.

**Sample questions from the Minnesota Multiphasic Personality Inventory**
*Answer true or false or omit if unsure.*

*False/True. I am an important person.*
*False/True. It would be better if almost all laws were thrown away.*
*False/True. My family does not like the work I have chosen.*
*False/True. I have not lived the right kind of life.*
*False/True. I like to read newspaper articles on crime.*
*False/True. I do not always tell the truth.*
*False/True. Evil spirits possess me at times.*

The few inmates who received inconclusive results were given the Rorschach Theme Apperception Test and reinterviewed. Cavior quickly realized that many of the prisoners had requested plastic surgery for the "wrong" reasons. Some wanted to change their identity, in the vein of John Dillinger. These he quickly excluded.

It was harder to turn down the men who genuinely believed that plastic surgery would dramatically improve their lives, those who felt that a new nose or chin or ears would transform them from pupa to butterfly. The problem was that these men wanted surgery *too* badly. That level of intensity meant that they were too dangerous to be allowed in the study. People with strong fixations on their body parts were known to react poorly to treatment—disappointment was inevitable for these men, Lewin explained to the psychologists. Even if he turned them into doppelgängers of Sean Connery's Bond, they'd still find things to complain about.

Still, it pained Cavior to shuffle this group into his discard pile. They'd been brave enough to share their deepest insecurities, and he'd viewed enough troll-like faces to know that they really *would* benefit from the scalpel. Living with their looks would be hard for anyone to handle. Kurtzberg didn't seem to be as torn up as he was, but then Kurtzberg had always been tall and athletic—he'd played high school football!

Cavior hadn't been tall *or* athletic. He'd been a shy, fat teenager, carrying forty-odd excess pounds. He'd looked soft and round, with a small double chin and flabby arms. His size made him awkward around girls. He'd felt trapped in his slow, cumbersome body. He'd transformed in the army; he'd signed up at eighteen and was promptly shipped off to Panama. On the cusp of Central and South America, with a daily temperature of 83 degrees, he trimmed down, tanned, and discovered salsa dancing. His newfound confidence made him popular with women—girls love to dance, he realized—which had helped him woo

Helene. He'd broken out of his shell, but he knew that not everyone did. Once stuck in a cycle of self-loathing, he understood why some people acted out.

Cavior found that the team's final test, the Goodenough-Harris Drawing Test (colloquially known as the "Draw a Person" test) offered the most intriguing insight into inmate's psyches. "We use this to get a rough estimate of intelligence," Kurtzberg explained to him. "The drawings are used to analyze the subject's unconscious image of himself." The test design was straightforward—applicants were handed a paper and pencil and asked to quickly sketch a person—any person, any gender—on the sheet.[40]

Coby Harris, a white twenty-six-year-old heroin addict on his fourth cycle through Rikers, scrawled a blond white woman who looked to be in her late twenties or thirties across his paper. He dressed her in a collared shirt and knee-length skirt. "Now, please draw a person of the opposite sex," Cavior instructed—the Draw a Person test was a two-parter. Harris glanced up at him, his bulbous nose shining under the fluorescent lights. He grasped his pencil and, with a look of concentration on his face, squished in a drawing of a slim man with buzzed dark hair, protruding ears, and a tense expression behind his sketch of a woman. The man wore a suit and tie and was about one third of the woman's size.

"It portrays a frightened, tense, and constricted young man," Cavior noted in Harris's case file. However, Harris impressed him during their one-on-one interview. At first, when questioned about the roots of his addiction, Harris tapped his nose.

"I blame my big honker," he answered. Cavior nodded, his face expressionless. Harris paused, biting his lip. "Maybe there are other reasons . . . my lack of education . . . hanging out with the wrong people," he backtracked. "My honker isn't the only problem." Pleased by his self-awareness and ability to think rationally, Cavior added him to the "yes" pile.

⌒⌒

**For Immediate Release**
U.S. Department of Health, Education, and Welfare[41]

Plastic surgeons at Montefiore Hospital in the Bronx, New York, will remove tattoos and scars from a group of prisoners in the hope that this will help prevent them from returning to a life of crime. Miss Mary E. Switzer, U.S. Commissioner of Vocational Rehabilitation, said, "We are hopeful that this project will contribute to one phase of a solution to the great problem of crime and criminal acts in our society."

Cavior and Kurtzberg's inexperience showed in little ways—their naivety with inmates, the way they phrased their questions, and other small details, none of which were an issue alone, but together, they added up to a headache for Lipton. He thought about expanding his team—perhaps someone to oversee the two would solve this—but found a surprising shortage of experienced applicants. He rang Wallace Mandell for recruitment advice.

"It's hard to attract professionals because of the low status of these jobs in the community," Mandell told him; he couldn't even staff *his* part of the research project as he'd like. "My team is making all kinds of fumbles," Mandell sighed. "People have found their questions a source of concern, if not resentment."

"Mmm hmm." It helped, a little, Lipton thought, to hear that everyone struggled with this, but it didn't fix his issue. Time would change this, Lipton reasoned, and positive media attention about the project would help attract more skilled employees. If his staff needed a bit more managing in the interim, so be it.

The applicants who passed the physical and psychological screens were admitted to the study and then randomly assigned to one of its four groups: plastic surgery only, plastic surgery and services, services only, or the control group that received no surgery and no services.

Cavior and Kurtzberg acted as liaisons among New York's social services, employment bureau, welfare departments, Montefiore Hospital, and the inmates. The next step was facilitating the inmates' exit interviews, which would take place a few days before they were released with a bologna sandwich and 25 cents (an unofficial tradition of supplying ex-cons with something to eat and money for a telephone call or subway token[42]).

Every subject in the study save the control group was required to have one final meeting with SSR staff before being released. Group three—which had been assigned to social and vocational services only—would be informed that plastic surgery would not be available to them. The team would also finalize the hospital appointments for groups one and two, as well as any social or welfare meetings.

That didn't happen.

Lipton was furious. "Please explain to me what happened here?" he asked, brandishing a sheet of paper that listed all of their approved subjects. He tapped three names. All three men had been cleared for treatment and assigned to the plastic surgery and services group. All three has been released without an interview, and hence had no scheduled time for their surgeries.

Cavior and Kurtzberg looked at one another warily and half-shrugged.

"Was this not the plan we agreed upon, the plan we established in meeting after meeting? Well?"

Lipton frowned. "Talk to me. What am I missing here?"

Kurtzberg pursed his lips. "It's . . . been difficult communicating with the officers on the island," he said delicately. "They have . . . that has . . . it's been challenging."

Lipton looked at him expectantly.

Guard turnover has been a real problem, Kurtzberg explained. Every time he'd established rapport and processes with one guard, he'd leave. He and Cavior had to start all over again with new officers. They were rarely informed when an officer was reassigned, which created an information gap with his replacement. Sometimes, after a bit of sweet-talking, the officer manning the reception desk might grudgingly tell them that officer so-and-so now worked a different shift or that he'd been transferred to another jail, but it was never straightforward. And that was just on the officer side!

One the inmate side, before they could conduct any interviews, they had to find the block in which each of their inmates were housed then send a list of names to the related warden's office the night before they were scheduled to meet. The following day, the guards would hold back the requested men from their work assignments, and then a security officer would collect them and take them to the intake center. The jail could spare only one guard to transport these men, meaning the entire transportation process took around thirty minutes, which cut the scheduled sessions short.

On a few occasions, they waited forty-five minutes to an hour, and no one turned up. They tried searching for them, only to be turned back at the main desk, since their clearance didn't extend to other parts of the building. Even when this process went smoothly, at any given test session, the inmates themselves might revolt, a ringleader announcing that the tests were stupid or boring and that they didn't want to take them anymore. He gathered five to ten men with him as he left the testing room.

"There's more," chimed in Cavior. "Some fellows get out early or transferred to another institution, and the corrections staff aren't flagging that for us. That's why we're losing subjects."

"That's not good, not good at all," Lipton said.

Cavior and Kurtzberg looked dejected, but Lipton didn't have time to hold their hands.

He flipped through the list of names, checking the release dates. The next men scheduled for release were a twenty-six-year-old addict and a thirty-one-year-old burglar. "Where are we with these men? Please tell me some good news."

"They are . . . we have . . . ah, we expect their exit to go smoothly," said Kurtzberg, recovering his composure. The addict had been cleared for rhinoplasty by Dr. Lewin and was scheduled to meet with him at Montefiore Hospital two days after his release, he explained. He's very eager to have the surgery and scored very highly in terms of motivation. He's single and thinks this will help him attract women.

"Good, good. Thank you, Richard," said Lipton, some of the tension easing from his shoulders. There were so many unknowns here—how the cosmetic work would turn out, how the men would react, how their communities would respond to their new appearances—but his team had to get the work done, first, for them to get to those questions.

"And the other one?"

"The second subject is set to be released the day after and is scheduled for surgery four days later," said Cavior. "His operation is a more complex procedure as he wants his facial scars removed."

"Drug scars?"

Cavior shook his head. "They're from a nasty car accident he got into a few years back. He's been prepped for what to expect and has received his appointment date."

"Good, good. Thanks Norm. I'm glad something's going right with this. Let me know how it goes."

The following week, he got a call from Cavior. Neither of the released men had showed up for their appointments, and the team hadn't been able to reach them by phone.

The team was in crisis. If the inmates failed to attend, their whole study and all their work, was for naught.

# 7

# BEAUTY BEHIND BARS

Texas Penitentiary Lets Inmates Put on a New Face before
Leaving—*Dallas Morning News*, 1965[1]

Plastic Surgeons Fight Crime with the Scalpel—*Democrat
and Chronicle*, 1965[2]

Dock Jobs Sold for $1,000 Each. Kickbacks to Loan Sharks—
*New York Daily News*, 1965[3]

The mood inside Montefiore Hospital's auditorium was somber. Lewin had summoned everyone involved with the SSR project to the Bronx for an emergency meeting. Kurtzberg and Cavior trekked uptown to attend, the Rikers Island team ferried in, and Wallace Mandell and his associates drove in from Staten Island. Surgical residents in starched white coats sat next to the social workers in their rolled-up shirtsleeves and the sociologists and psychologists in their work-casual wear, Norman Cavior's guayabera shirt providing the only pop of color in the auditorium.

Michael Lewin paced up and down, inhaling deeply on his pipe. "I need to understand what is going on here," he said, gesturing to Lipton and his team. "What is going *wrong* here? How can we fix this?"

Cavior opened his mouth and then closed it. He didn't have a good answer. He looked around the room, taking in the tense, anxious faces. Was this really going to end before it had even begun?

"One issue we've found is the delay," ventured Lipton. He blamed his staff—a little unfairly, he knew—but he was responsible for them. "The period of time between an inmate's release from the jail and their admission to the hospital is problematic."

"Go on," Lewin said, taking a seat.

"If we could get them into the hospital the same day that they're released, that would help tremendously," Lipton replied. "That's a big pain point—once they're in their community again, what was pressing inside the jail lessens. For many, a waiting period of even a few days is enough to deter the subjects from their original desire."

"I agree," said Chaneles, raising his voice so it would carry. "The holdup is at the Montefiore end."

"Noted, and thank you for your comments," Lewin said. He looked around the room, observing the discomfited expressions of his surgeons. "Well? How do we address this? Can any of you add something to this discussion?"

"There's a city-wide shortage of beds," piped up one surgeon. "That's the real problem."

"We can't just let them cut the line," argued another surgeon. "They're criminals. Why should they get bumped ahead of honest, hard-working men and women who've been patiently waiting their turn?"

Lewin frowned. He'd expected that some people might feel this way, but he didn't like to hear it from his own residents. But this wasn't the time to reeducate them.

"Nonetheless," he said, ignoring the comment, "What's clear is that we all need to reevaluate how this works."

Chaneles stood up. "It's simple," he said. "Inmates should be seen as soon as they leave the jail. They feel like they're being let down again."

Lipton nodded his agreement. For many offenders, the decision to commit to surgery had been difficult, and their general disillusionment with the "system" led them to view the admission waiting period as a reason to exempt themselves.

"I can't see how that will work," objected a surgeon. "We don't have hospital beds open like that. They need to come on their scheduled date, or they'll get turned away."

"The longer they wait, the less likely they'll be to attend," argued Lipton.

"But no one has attended."

"My point exactly."

Lewin steepled his hands in thought.

A copy of the *New York Herald Tribune* lay on the table in front of him, folded to page three, where the headline, "Surgery Tested on Twisted Lives," glared at him.[4] Next to it lay the *Rochester Democrat and Chronicle*, where the article had been reprinted with the headline "Surgeon's Scalpels Fight Crime."[5] The reporter's write-up about their fledgling program was mostly positive— he'd met the man in his private apartment and felt like they'd built a rapport— but it also mentioned that their first two subjects had failed to show up. So far, the reception to the article had been positive, but it was easy to visualize public sentiment turning against them.

"What about the social workers?" asked Lewin. "Can we utilize them more? Perhaps send them to the inmate's lodgings and personally escort them to their appointments?"

Lipton looked at Mandell, who oversaw this portion of the project.

"Ye-es," he said slowly. "We don't have the resources to do that for a long period of time, but for a period, it's possible, especially if we contract out."

Lipton smiled, as he sighed inwardly. It was amazing how quickly that grant money was disappearing.

"I don't think we have a choice at this point," Lewin said grimly, and everyone there nodded in assent, all hoping this small change would be enough to turn the project around.

"One more thing," said Chaneles, standing up again. "I have an announcement. As everyone's present, I'd like to inform all of you all that the next few weeks will be my last as the director of research for New York's Department of Correction. I've handed in my notice, effective next month, on February 18."

Dear Miss Kaufman,

Thank you for your letter. With regard to your comments about equal rights for negroes there should never be any question about people "earning" basic legal rights, guaranteed to all by the constitution of the United States. We all have a duty to ensure that citizen rights are not abrogated regardless of race, religion or national origin. I appreciate this chance to explain these matters to you.

Sincerely yours,

Robert F. Wagner, mayor[6]

Kross was saddened that Chaneles was leaving, but she had bigger things to worry about. The systemic biases that underscored New York's criminal justice system ran deep, and her fight against them drew rancor from within her department. Officers whispered about her judgment and grumbled about her directives. They didn't want the department's racial and gender biases dismantled. Last year, after a three-year court battle, female police officers were finally allowed to sit for the New York Police Department's sergeant's exam. It was an outrage it had taken so long, but the post of corrections commissioner held little sway over the police commissioner.

Changes in her own administration were poorly received. In January she'd promoted Captain James A. Thomas, a gruff, well-liked World War II veteran, to warden of the Men's House of Detention on Rikers Island. Thomas had been on the force since 1946 and went by "Big Daddy" or "Kingfish" to his subordinates; he was tough but fair and handled himself well around troublesome inmates.[7] Born in 1914, he heralded from Hawkinsville, Alabama, a poor scrubby town that grew out of the blood and tears and lashes of Black slaves. Thomas grew up in poverty, with dire warnings to get home early; lynchings were an unhappy occurrence in his neighborhood.

Kross's promotion caused a stir—many in the administration disliked the idea that a Black man had attained such an important position. They questioned her judgment and made digs about Thomas's experience. Kross raged against the pushback—Thomas was smart, qualified, and popular—but she had battles on so many fronts that, as a concession, she made his title provisional, naming him acting warden instead.[8] This didn't help—instead, it made her unpopular with officers of both mindsets.

Thomas took the news stoically. "Don't you preach to me about trust until you've grown up a Negro in the Twenties," he told *Penthouse Magazine*.[9] "You don't satisfy anyone in this job. Trying to do anything in this place is like hitting a giant pillow: you hit it, there's no effect. You're sitting on a powder keg and if you push it too far, it's going to blow the hell up."

Kross hated that she was forced into making the call, but she needed her staff to back her—her biggest concern was that the officers would stop following their orders. She'd have no recourse but to fire them, but if the department ground to a halt, chaos would ensue. The SSR plastic surgery project was just *one* of her rehabilitative ventures, and every project depended on officer compliance to run smoothly.

⌒⌒

Her relationship with President Lyndon Johnson and Ladybird Johnson helped. After he'd honored her with the Eleanor Roosevelt Candlestick Award last year, they'd developed a friendly rapport. The First Lady in particular was especially charmed by Kross's forward-thinking reforms and her refreshingly brutal honesty about the state of the world. Whenever Kross was in Washington, D.C., or the presidential couple visited New York, they made it a point to carve out time for a chat over coffee or a dinner meeting.

Kross was happy to dine with the First Couple. They were pleasant company, and the added benefit of their attention helped keep her officers in line. They might grumble, but with the president in her corner, they couldn't rebel outright, at least for now. President Johnson respected Kross's insight and knowledge of the criminal justice system and used some of their conversations to shape his address to Congress in January.

"Crime has become a malignant enemy in America's midst," he told Congress.[10] "We must identify and eliminate the causes of criminal activity whether they lie in the environment around us or deep in the nature of individual men." He smiled at the assembled senators and members of the house as he unveiled his plan; he was doubling down on education as a way to curb crime across the nation.[11]

"Jobs filled by high school graduates rose by 40 percent in the last ten years. Jobs for those with less schooling decreased by nearly 10 percent," he said. "We can measure the cost in even starker terms. We now spend about $450 a year per child in our public schools. But we spend $1,800 a year to keep a delinquent youth in a detention home, $2,500 a year for a family on relief, $3,500 a year for a criminal in state prison. I hope 1965 will be regarded as the year when this country began a thorough, intelligent and effective war against crime."

President Johnson's rhetoric was persuasive, and numerous senators nodded in agreement when he proposed a $4.1 billion education budget for the next fiscal year, plus an added $1.5 billion to cover his new schemes. "This is a small price to pay for developing our nation's most priceless resource."

The president hammered home his belief that the crime problem was best attacked by developing and testing experimental methods in subsequent sessions with Congress. "Crime will not wait while we pull it up by the roots. We must arrest and reverse the trend toward lawlessness," he told them. "The first offender's initial contact with our correctional system is often a turning point in his life. We should consider how we can best ensure that his first contact will be his last."[12]

Kross was pleased with Johnson's public backing of correctional research, but his speech intensified her pressure to get results. Fast.

She offered Chaneles's directorship to Lipton, which he accepted with pleasure; the promotion came with more power and responsibility, as well as salary bump to $14,000—$900 more than Chaneles had earned. Kross also made an executive decision to appoint Wallace Mandell as the SSR project head—he wasn't a corrections employee, but with so much of the next stage of the study taking place outside the jail, it made sense to have the collaborating agencies more involved.

At Montefiore Hospital, administrator Ronald Milch penned a letter to the Vocational Rehabilitation Administration to notify them of the personnel changes, a reporting requirement for federal grants.[13]

By the end of March 1965, more than 9,150 inmates had been physically screened, each surgeon screening around sixty inmates a day. Of those, 7,300 were approved for surgery and passed on to the psychology team. Cavior and Kurtzberg kept careful notes about each interviewee, holding regular discovery sessions to avoid any surprises.

In general, inmates who applied for plastic surgery had greater mental health and behavioral problems than the general inmate population. "This suggests to us that the real or imaginary handicap of a physical defect was an aggravating factor," Kurtzberg wrote in his preliminary report. Additionally, their ethnicity seemed to be causal to their cosmetic requests: 74 percent of inmates requesting heroin track removal was Black, whereas 65 percent of nose jobs were requested by white prisoners. Puerto Ricans requested 44 percent of all tattoo removals. The numbers didn't make sense to the pair. Tracks can be more conspicuous on dark skin, Lewin explained, marked with underlying thromboses and usually on the forearm. They are distinctive scars, instantly recognizable to law enforcement, employers, and other addicts. "The cured addict feels that the eradication of this stigma is essential," he said, hastening to add that this didn't mean that Black inmates were heavier drug users.

Even so, the high confluence was curious. Kurtzberg and Cavior dove into the data. Their main focus was on the benefits that cosmetic surgery could provide, but on a granular level, those benefits intersected with the inmate's personal privileges. The relevance of their economic status and background had to be analyzed.

Around half of all new admissions to Rikers Island were Black, despite accounting for 23 percent of Manhattan residents, a statistic that was mirrored through the state's prisons.[14] It was not surprising, really, when they thought about it; entrenched racism and the media's constant narrative about Black criminals had undoubtedly swayed the police. A recent report from the FBI depicted Black men and Black neighborhoods as a training ground for violent criminals, and crime also skewed higher in urban cities. Overall, white men clocked more arrests each year, but Black men were arrested more for the "serious" crimes, including murder, rape, and aggravated assault.[15] No question, minorities started at a disadvantage in society.

Surprisingly, Kurtzberg found that Puerto Rican inmates statistically had the most handicaps. Overall, this group had the least "natural cultural identification" with New York City and achieved the lowest levels of education when compared to their Black and white counterparts. Education also played a role in a former offender's likelihood of compliance with the SSR project. So far, the more educated inmates had failed to attend their appointments, either at Montefiore or with their social care team. "This may reflect the more cautious attitude toward new experimental programs of those with more education," noted Lewin.

By now, one or two subjects were trickling into the hospital each week. The ex-cons who most consistently showed up were those with glaring facial scars and battered noses. The more visible the issue, it seemed, the stronger the drive to get it fixed.

They analyzed the data of 473 consecutive admissions to Rikers Island to get a better understanding of the prevalence of disfigurement. Their sample included 375 adults comprised of 176 Black, 104 white, and 95 "Puerto Rican" men[16] and 98 adolescents. They found that 47 percent of the adults and 28 percent of the youths exhibited one or more "significant" deformity. They did not include an addict's needle scars and tracks in this assessment. "They comprised primarily of nose, ears, chin, and traumatic nasal deformities," Kurtzberg wrote in their report. "White subjects showed a significantly higher incidence of deformity than the Negroes." Despite the large number of admissions with fixable physical issues, only 6 percent of the adult inmates in this data pool applied for free plastic surgery. Even accounting for those lost to parole or transfer, it was a smaller number than expected.[17]

Two days after Fred Marshall was released from Rikers Island, he was visited by a social worker who escorted him to Montefiore Hospital for his treatment. He looked different in his everyday clothes. He walked a little taller and his shirt draped his bulk in a flattering manner, quite different than his prison scrubs.

TABLE I

Incidence of Physical Deformity[1] Among 375 Consecutive Adult Admissions to the

New York City Correctional Institution for Men:

| | Addicts | | | | | | Non-Addicts | | | | | | |
|---|---|---|---|---|---|---|---|---|---|---|---|---|---|
| | Negro | | Puerto Rican | | White | | Negro | | Puerto Rican | | White | | Total | |
| Deformity | No. | % | No. | % | No. | % | No. | % | No. | % | No. | % | No. | % |
| No Sign. Deformity | 87 | 75% | 26 | 33% | 11 | 25% | 41 | 68% | 11 | 65% | 24 | 40% | 200 | 53% |
| Facial Scars | 5 | 4% | 3 | 4% | 1 | 2% | 5 | 8% | 1 | 6% | 0 | 0% | 15 | 4% |
| Other facial[2] Deformities | 9 | 8% | 9 | 12% | 11 | 25% | 4 | 7% | 1 | 6% | 9 | 15% | 43 | 11% |
| Tattoos | 10 | 9% | 39 | 50% | 19 | 43% | 4 | 7% | 4 | 24% | 20 | 33% | 96 | 26% |
| Body Deform | 4 | 4% | 1 | 1% | 2 | 4% | 5 | 8% | 0 | 0% | 7 | 12% | 19 | 5% |
| Hand Deform | 1 | 1% | 0 | 0% | 0 | 0% | 1 | 2% | 0 | 0% | 0 | 0% | 2 | 1% |
| TOTALS | 116 | 101% | 78 | 100% | 44 | 99% | 60 | 100% | 17 | 101% | 60 | 100% | 375 | 100% |

1.
In cases where a person had multiple deformities his primary (most severe) deformity was used for classification. Needle tracks were not considered as a deformity for this table.

2.
Comprised primarily of developmental deformities of the nose, ears, and chin, and traumatic nasal deformities.

Incidences of physical deformity at the New York City Correctional Center for Men, Rikers Island. *Wallace Mandell, Michael Lewin, Richard Kurtzberg, Marvin Shuster, and Howard Safar,* The Surgical and Social Rehabilitation of Adult Offenders *(1967)*

Lewin greeted him in one of the surgical prep rooms. He wanted to check in with Marshall about the procedure and confirm he was still eager to proceed. "I'm ready for this," he told Lewin. "I did what you wanted, doc. Make me a new man!" He jiggled his body for proof; the surgical team had requested he lose twenty pounds before the operation, and he'd shed most of it. He held out his arms for Lewin to see; they were covered in needle tracks, but there were no fresh marks. He was drug free.

"That's great, Fred," Lewin said, genuinely pleased with his attitude. Excising that much skin was going to be a difficult operation and would leave pink raised scars on Marshall's body, crisscrossing his stomach and sides. Thankfully, Marshall seemed to be in the right frame of mind to accept them.

Lewin had chosen to operate on the first batch of inmate admissions himself, assisted by his residents. With inmates still gun-shy about participating, he felt he had the best chance of reassuring them about their surgery. Going forward, he'd take on the role of attending physician, in a supervisory capacity, with one of his residents leading the operation. So far, he'd slimmed down the nose of a fraudulent bookkeeper, removed the heroin tracks from a wannabe artist, and pinned back the ears of a renowned burglar.

Once Marshall had signed the necessary forms, a white-smocked nurse, her hair tied back under a crisp white cap, handed him a hospital gown and left the room while he changed. "Thank you, ma'am." When she reentered, she bade him lie on the gurney and methodically cleansed and shaved his chest and groin area. "This is just to prep you for the doctors," she told him before wheeling him to the operating theater. The overhead lights were dazzling, and he felt a needle slide into his arm before everything faded.

His operation took around four hours. Lewin painstakingly sliced him from hip to hip, the transverse incision a few inches south of his navel. He vacuumed out Marshall's excess fat through a small canula and tightened his abdominal muscles with a neat row of stitches. The excess tissue and skin was trimmed away, and he closed his incisions with a few tidy lines of butterfly stitches. Marshall never stirred. Lewin had erred on the side of caution with his sedation; it was hard to gauge the tolerance of former addicts, and he didn't want any surprises in the middle of his surgery. He assessed Marshall's prone body. His skin apron was gone, but his emotional scars—and his new physical scars—would be permanent reminders of the procedure.

Marshall startled when he woke up in his hospital bed, his body trapped beneath a tightly tucked sheet. For a moment, he panicked, thinking he was back on Rikers. But his sheet—and his surroundings—were far too clean to be the jail, and his shoulders released as it all came back to him. His whole body ached, like he'd been run over by a truck. Even his arms and legs were tender—and the doc hadn't even touched those! He tried to sit up straight and gasped; it felt like he was being pulled apart. He relaxed back onto his pillow. He lifted his sheet for a peek but couldn't tell if the surgery had been a success because swathes of white bandages encased his torso, with a small drain running underneath one piece of gauze.

It hurt. He hadn't expected it to hurt so much. "Nurse! Nurse!" he bellowed. "I need painkillers. Bring me some painkillers!"

A different nurse appeared, a frown creasing her forehead. "There's no need to shout," she said.

"*I hurt!*"

She looked at his chart. "Your nerves should still be numb from the surgeons' anesthetic," she informed him. I can give you some medication in a couple of hours. The sensations should have returned by then.[18]

"You're not listening to me," he growled, gritting his teeth in pain. "@#*!!! bitch!"

The nurse sniffed and walked away. She'd been warned that ex-cons would be on the ward and that they'd try to wheedle extra drugs. She refused to be made a fool of.

"Come back!" He knocked over his bedside table in disgust, its arrangements of papers, pens, and cardboard somethings scattering across the floor.

A different nurse finally brought him medication an hour later, once they'd ascertained that his size and prior addictions meant that the anesthetic had worn off faster than usual.

Through his recovery, Marshall was a grumpy and demanding patient. He summoned nurses in the middle of the night, asking for snacks or drinks. He bullied the other patients into conversation, despite their obvious discomfort, and took control of the television remote.[19]

He behaved around Lewin, but that was it. Everyone on the ward breathed easier when he was discharged. He was still swollen, but now that he could see how much less of him there was, he was relieved—and grateful. "I've signed up for those drug detox programs," he told Lewin, as he left. "I want to stay clean."

Another problem was bubbling up inside the city's jails: the rising number of female inmates. Overall crime rates had doubled 50 percent from 1935, but, historically, women made up a small fraction of that population. In 1964, 11,273 women, all first-timers, were sentenced to a week or more in the Women's House of Detention, around a 35 percent increase since 1960.[20]

Crime was up overall that year, with 1,504 rapes (a 17.8 percent rise from 1963), 14,831 felonious assaults, 26,284 stolen cars, and a 16 percent increase in murder despite the 26,885 cops who patrolled the city.[21] Mayor Wagner wanted answers, but Commissioner Kross couldn't find an obvious instigating event for the spike.

Some on the force claimed that the Equal Pay Act of 1963 had made women more "uppity," leading to the increase in female offenders, a backward opinion Kross refused to entertain. "The women's liberation movement has triggered a crime wave like the world has never seen before," the chief of the Los Angeles Police Department told the papers.[22]

Women also received short shrift on the victim front. "I wonder if our snowballing crimes of passion might not be traceable, at least in part, to schoolgirls who look like tarts," wrote ABC radio host Paul Harvey in a letter to FBI director Edgar Hoover. Harvey invited Hoover to comment on his newest column, "Do Short Skirts Invite Trouble?" The director's response, via his assistant, was also short. "Don't ask for trouble. Dress sensibly. Provocative clothing may attract the attention of a potential sex criminal."[23]

It was a damned if you do, damned if you don't situation. The messaging for women constantly contradicted itself. Wear this dress, be taken seriously. Buy those heels, you're a working gal. American women, almost from the moment they were born, were bombarded with advertisements about how to look and dress to be viewed as a "proper" woman, the subtext being that to be a proper woman, one also had to be beautiful and desirable. There was an insidious side to this fetishization, the emphasis being that an improved appearance absolved or subsumed personality defects.

Revlon cosmetics, which launched in 1932, was an extreme offender. Vice president William Mandel doubled down on the transformative power of makeup. Ads proclaimed that one could "Pat on a whole new face in seconds!" or "Reflect this lovely radiance, always." His favorite quote, lifted from the playwright Jean Cocteau, summed up Revlon's philosophy: "If there is a defect on the soul, it cannot be corrected on the face; but if there is a defect on the face and one corrects it, it can correct a soul," he told reporters.[24]

It was disingenuous to pretend that appearances didn't matter, Kross knew. Take the bail system, she thought; she'd been seriously troubled by its vagaries since she'd entered the criminal justice space. On paper it seemed to make sense: a bond to ensure that people returned for judgment without forcing them to reside in a cell, should they be innocent. The reality, however, was a set of standards that benefited the wealthy and penalized the poor.[25] Kross highlighted this injustice in her annual reports. "Men, women, and adolescents, the majority of whom are too poor to pay bail must remain amongst criminal associations, for weeks, months and often longer," she complained. There was evidence that this greatly affected the outcome of their cases.

"The man who is jailed is less likely to get equal treatment in court," reported criminologist LaMar Taylor Empey. "He may be unwashed and unkempt. His appearance under guard further destroys his image and is far different than if he presented himself neatly dressed and more self-confident." Empey's research reflected the appearance bias at work in the courtroom; the presentation of the offender greatly affected the judge's verdict. "The irony is that this outcome does not seem to be rationally based on the accumulation of evidence relative to the offense, but whether he can raise bail," he commented.[26]

Kross never paid much attention to her own appearance. She proudly told people that she had *never* capitalized on her femininity and that she only wore new dresses because her daughters bought them for her. She found the whole beauty industry confusing.[27] It was so unnecessary. Still, she recognized that beauty *was* an industry and one that had a lower barrier of entry for women than many office jobs.

She considered this as she turned her attention to the Women's House of Detention, a medieval twelve-story turreted fort full of dark, narrow cells and hallways, situated two miles from her courthouse. It looked more like a badly designed public housing project than a holding facility; it served double time as a detention and assessment center, the only jail for women in the five boroughs. The "House of D," as it was known colloquially, had such a poor reputation that a woman once asked a judge to charge her with a felony instead of a misdemeanor—accepting the correspondingly longer sentence—just so she could serve her time elsewhere.[28]

That was not an acceptable state of affairs to Kross, who believed that jail should provide a respite to women, a place to learn new skills and reform their lives.[29] She tackled this a couple of ways, starting with the aesthetics. Constrained by the building's dimensions, she couldn't enlarge the cells, but she could make them more comfortable. The bars were painted a pastel pink. Each cell was outfitted with two cots, a washbasin and toilet, and a number of shelves and hooks. Each woman received one pair of black oxfords with Cuban heels,

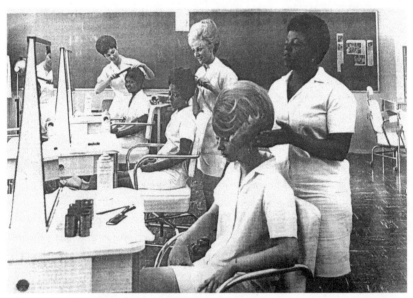

The cosmetology program at California Institute for Women teaches inmates skills they can use to acquire jobs after release (California Department of Correction and Rehabilitation file photo, circa 1970s). *Courtesy California Department of Correction and Rehabilitation*

two pairs of ankle socks, three cotton dresses, two cotton slips, two panties, and a few brassieres.[30] The pink bars entertained the inmates. "Ain't we the fancy schmancies? Pink prison bars," they laughingly told reporters.

Then there was the education side. Before Kross took over, the Women's House of Detention had no extracurriculars. The entire education budget was allotted to the men's jails. In 1956 she opened a beauty culture program, which taught the inmates how to press, wash, and wax hair. Over the years, Kross had equipped it with the latest tools and products and offered inmates the chance to sit for their cosmetology license.

The jail also offered courses in typing, sewing (in which inmates were taught to make items of clothing from scratch), knitting classes, laundry classes, and culinary classes. Equipped with these skills, Kross hoped they'd be better able to forge a life for themselves on the outside. Without education, their choices were limited. Kross rejected the conception that a woman's role was at home. Perhaps that premise works if you're wealthy, she told reporters, but if you're impoverished it's ridiculous to suggest that you don't contribute.

To be sure, criminal history could make it challenging for inmates to find work, but she wanted her officers to understand that offenders' problems didn't start when they entered the correctional system. The bigger issue was that the inmates tended to come from marginalized, impoverished communities and were poorly educated.

For once, the wardens welcomed the new programs. For them, the schooling had a twofold benefit; in addition to work skills, it improved the offenders' demeanor. "Even those with a poor self-image who mutilate themselves, use makeup," Warden Gloria McFarland told Kross. Women received a weekly free treatment in the beauty shop for "morale building" and the jail held an annual fashion show to boost their self-confidence. But Kross's system suffered from some built-in flaws. Most women averaged ninety days in the jail before being released into the community or shipped to a prison upstate. That meant that they rarely completed the one thousand hours of training required for the state cosmetology license.[31] In 1964, only twenty inmates had been able to certify with the state.

Despite being fed, clothed, and educated, many inmates and staff pushed back against the quality of care received. "Ninety-five percent read under a sixth-grade level," charged one officer; in his opinion, the women attended classes to relieve boredom, not to learn. For forty-four-year-old inmate Molly Sands, serving her latest stretch for prostitution, the worst part of her stay was the clothes. "Every time I look down at myself, I think I'm less than nothing," she told a visiting writer; her bra was far too small and her cleavage spilled out over the top and sides.[32] "What's the use of going on with this life anyways when you were born to be an ugly duck like me?"

For once, the SSR team felt like they were making good progress. By mid-May, seventeen ex-cons had successfully had their operations, and groups one and three had been successfully matched with the social and vocational services they required, mostly a mix of employment help, rehab clinic referrals, and housing services. The project was behind schedule—the initial plan had predicted that seventy inmates would have received surgery by now—but considering the challenges up to this point, they felt pretty good about where they were.

News of their progress had leaked to the media and was gossiped about from coast to coast. In San Francisco, Dick Nolan, a prominent gossip columnist, dedicated his column in the *San Francisco Examiner* to the premise of criminal reform surgery. "Pretty is as pretty does, my dearies. One thing pretty may do is get people out of the clink and keep them out," he wrote. "If Cyrano made the pokey today the penologists would cut his nose off. With a handsome new face, he would start each day with a song. . . . We just don't know whether it really works."[33]

To be sure, Rikers Island as a whole was still a shit show. In January, two of the prison's full-time physicians died within weeks of each other, both of natural causes. No replacements were available. A skeleton staff with limited field experience was placed in charge of all medical care on the island. "After 4 p.m., we have to rely on nonlicensed physicians," Rikers chief medical officer complained to Kross. "Coverage continues to be perilous."[34]

Then word arrived from Washington, D.C. The Vocational Rehabilitation Administration was concerned about the viability of the study due to the project's personnel changes. The organization already invested $240,000 into the experiment—the cost of ninety brand new cars—and wanted to ensure it was being utilized correctly. Representatives would be making a trip to New York to investigate. Please expect them shortly.

Lipton fretted about their imminent arrival. What would their delegation make of it all? Even with the new regime, ex-cons still cancelled or absconded from their appointments with alarming frequency. Research studies had been cancelled for less.

He prepped his team for the visit; they were all to be on their best behavior and express a positive outlook. Transparency was fine, but negativity was not.

He didn't want to hear any gloomy comments while they were here. He polished his shoes and wore his best suit to greet them.

The delegates met him at his office on Rikers Island, and he gave them his most charming smile before he briefed them on their triumphs so far.

"Why are you experiencing such a large turnover?"

The change of staff has been disruptive, Lipton admitted, and that handicapped the first few months of the study. However, he now had a dedicated, loyal team and they've progressed much further.

He walked them around the reception and classification center, pointing out the rooms they used for screening, and where they held the psychological tests. "Note the bright colors and modern feel of the place," he said proudly; the center had been designed for maximum exposure to sunlight and fresh air. "Our Corrections Commissioner has a forward-thinking approach towards incarceration." They nodded and scribbled on their pads. He wished he could see what they were writing down.

"What are the issues surrounding their discharge?"

"Ah, well, there have been various problems that were not initially anticipated. For one, the narcotic patient offers a difficult recovery problem because of the need to administer opiates postoperatively. However, we are the first study of this kind to have a control group."

"Can you explain why female inmates have not been included in your study?"

"That's not intentional," Lipton replied. He'd posted the project's particulars in the women's jail but had so little interest that including them wasn't statistically viable. "I'm not sure why," he said. "We wanted to include them."

"Hmm," said a delegate, scrawling something on his pad.

"The few who showed interest were provided with plastic surgery on release," he said quickly, hoping that admission would please them. But yes, he conceded, his data did not contain any information regarding the surgical treatment of female offenders.

The delegates asked that question again during their meeting with Michael Lewin and Anna Kross. "It is surprising," Lewin told them, with his usual transparency. In his private practice, 90 percent of his patients were women. "They tend to care more about their appearance than men, likely due to social conditioning. I would say that number is true for all elective surgeries in New York City." Kross smiled and changed the subject. Later she vented her frustration to the team. "This is unacceptable," she said. "Women make up 50 percent of the world." She didn't like being blindsided.

Back at their Union Square office, the team discussed the visit. They'd made a good impression—they hoped. The delegates expressed genuine interest in their work. Still, they were all surprised that the committee had raised the point about women. For years, female offenders had received radically different treatment than men—they had fewer amenities and freedoms and less opportunity for growth. As men made up around 90 percent of all prison inmates, most correctional research focused almost exclusively on men. Women were absent from the majority of federal and state recidivism programs.

Kross was extremely displeased. Throughout history, much of women's perceived value in society had been relative to their appearance. The more attractive a woman, the higher her dowry. In the 1960s, that translated into a higher salary and, if lucky, a higher society husband. Her own daughters were beautiful *and* smart, one a clinical psychologist and the other a children's psychiatrist. But even they agonized over what to wear on a date and what outfit would make the best impression at work. Every woman inherently understood the socioeconomic boost of being beautiful in all situations.

More and more women sought cosmetic surgery's promise of physical perfection. This was a global phenomenon. In Tokyo, one in twenty nightclub hostesses underwent nose slimming surgery.[35] In Oklahoma, surgeons were deluged with requests for ear pinning surgery, caused by the ponytail trend.[36] In Minneapolis, face-lifts were de rigueur as older women competed with college graduates for jobs.[37] In Brazil, the importance of one's appearance was so highly regarded that in the late 1950s the country launched a "beauty is not just for the rich" program, offering free cosmetic surgery to its citizens. The tagline: *The poor have the right to be beautiful.*[38]

Given all of this, it seemed especially strange to Kross that there were so few interested females in the Women's House of Detention. It was almost suspicious. She asked her wardens to report. "It's hard," Warden Mary Lindsay told her. She'd place the requested fliers around the jail and had personally approached individual inmates about the program.[39] For example, take Toni, who's on a ninety-day stretch for soliciting, she explained. In her opinion, Toni, a slight Puerto Rican woman with curly dark hair and a sprinkle of freckles across her nose,[40] would have been considered a very pretty girl if not for the deeply gouged needle marks that tracked up her neck and down her arms—the unmistakable stamp of a junkie. "I offered her the surgery, and she refused. She said, 'Why bother? I'll just be putting them back again.'"

Warden Lindsay had no success with Agatha, either, also incarcerated for prostitution. "She's fat and ugly and has a large birthmark covering her face!"

Agatha's clients tended to be bums or bulls (street slang for cops)—and Lindsay assumed she'd be pleased by the chance to have the stain on her face removed. But Agatha just shrugged and walked away. "If only somebody had waved a magic wand when she was younger," Lindsay sighed. In her opinion, Agatha was past saving.

There were a few outliers, she admitted. Edna, an addict also in for soliciting, had eagerly welcomed her offer. She wanted the scarred, puffy skin over her left eyebrow smoothed out. Edna took pride in her appearance; unlike most addicts, she'd never injected into her legs, which were slim and scar free. She enjoyed showing them off in a short blue dress, reveling in the appreciative stares. Edna was a decade older than the average prostitute but had kept her clientele interested by maintaining her face and figure; she kept her needle tracks strictly on the inside of her left forearm. Edna liked working the streets—it made her feel independent, she said; it was a point of personal pride that she'd never claimed welfare. She was excited about getting her facial scar removed. She'd scheduled her Montefiore visit as early as possible. My guess is that she wants the surgery to attract more johns, Lindsay noted—bettering herself, sure, but not exactly what Commissioner Kross had in mind.

Even so, Lindsay believed Kross had picked up on something important with the SSR study. "There really is a need for surgery on women," she said; in her experience, law enforcement generally tried to avoid jailing pretty young offenders. Instead of a jail sentence, they connected them with social workers and welfare staff. The opposite was also true. "When they're not kind, it's because she's so unattractive that they don't feel protective," Lindsay remarked. "When they do go to prison it's because they're incorrigible and not very good looking." Lindsay's observations fueled Kross's desire for the surgery project to succeed—and for it to include women. The burdens society places on its women are not going to change, she insisted.[41]

Around the United States, new plastic surgery programs had sprung up. They were sprinkled across the states in no particular order: in Kansas, in Connecticut, in Iowa. Nonetheless, approximately 95 percent of all prisoner beautification surgeries were performed exclusively on men. There were no published studies—even among the less rigorously reported ones that Lewin disapproved of—about the recidivism benefits of surgery on female inmates. It seemed very strange, Kross thought, especially accounting for the growing body of research that suggested 70 percent of female inmates suffered from low self-esteem and a poor self-image compared to 40 percent of men.

One of the few prisons that focused on improving women's physical appearances lay forty miles north of Manhattan in Bedford Hills.[42] Since 1961, plastic surgeons from the University of Rochester had trekked to the 264-acre West-field State Farm for Women. They treated the women's various complaints,[43] straightening their noses, removing their tattoos, and clearing their acne to the tune of fifty-some operations a year. Early that year, popular author Kathrin Perutz visited Westfield State Farm to research her next book and conversed with inmates and staff. "The major problem is public acceptance of the parolee," Superintendent Lillian Fish told her. "Few places want to hire her." The surgeries helped with the women's "cosmetic imperfections," which had a knock-on effect with their job prospects.

Fish had strict rules about what makeup was appropriate: eyeshadow and mascara were a no-no, as they could appear "trashy," but lipstick and hair styling (natural colors only) were approved. "We want them to go out of here looking like ladies." Westfield ran a cosmetology course similar to the one at the Women's House of Detention, but here inmates had the unfortunate luxury of time to complete and earn their licenses. At least, in theory. During Perutz's visit, she was especially taken with Sylvia, a young, heavily pregnant Black woman she met in the prison's beauty shop.

Sylvia was a natural cosmetologist and loved spending time in the salon. She specialized in styling, waxing, and trimming weaves and was in such demand that she had to be booked a week or more out. She'd excelled in the salon's school, breezing through the theory tests, and passed the state cosmetology exam in the top percentile. However, the state refused to issue her license, she told Perutz. She had multiple felonies on her record, and New York allowed a maximum of one felony for licensing purposes. She continued working at the salon; it was her favorite place in the prison. "There's still hope," she told Perutz. "Maybe the law will change? They're working on it."

Kross was glad to learn that women's needs were at the forefront of Westfield's reform strategy but disappointed that most correctional facilities failed to take the needs of their female inmates into consideration overall.

In Washington, D.C., the delegates from the Vocational Rehabilitation Administration began the long task of sorting through their New York field notes. Once assembled, they conferred over the results. They had noticed how nervous Lipton, Cavior, and Kurtzberg had been, but Anna Kross's calm confidence and Dr. Michael Lewin's gravitas had impressed them.

Overall, their findings were positive. There was a clear need for surgical work for inmates. In their short time on Rikers Island, they'd personally seen many men who could have used beautification. Having a control was a nice touch and helped validate the study. But they were concerned about the project's day-to-day administration—staff turnover had thrown a wrench in the project, and they weren't convinced that it would be a one-off. The SSR researchers earned significantly less than researchers employed by private corporations or universities; who could say they wouldn't be lured away? They sent their report to the Vocational Rehabilitation Administration's commissioner, Mary Elizabeth Switzer.

Despite the aforementioned setbacks, Switzer was excited by the SSR's progress and green-lighted its continuation, with a warning to increase the frequency of their reports. She'd funded eighteen inmate rehabilitation projects including the SSR, and she was patiently waiting for them all—well, at least a *few* of them, hopefully—to reap results.

The fact that some of the SSR subjects, albeit a small number, had completed step one of the process would make her pleas for continued funding more substantive. It was one more piece of ammunition for President Johnson, who needed to show Congress that his reform plans were actionable.

The future of corrections and policing was a hot topic on the president's agenda at the eighty-ninth Congress. He'd run on a campaign of rehabilitation

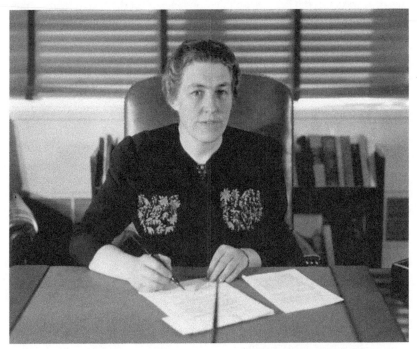

Portrait of Mary E. Switzer. *Courtesy Schlesinger Library, Radcliffe Institute, Harvard University*

and reshaping America, and he wanted to make good on his promises. So far he'd passed the Prisoner Rehabilitation Act of 1965, which made broad provisions for numerous prison programs, including halfway houses, granting inmates leave for emergency purposes, and community work furloughs.[44] He also made prisoners eligible for Pell grants under the Higher Education Act of 1965[45] and authorized the secretary of labor, under the ManPower Training Act, to run an experimental two-year training program for inmates that transitioned into employment on release.

With a smile on his face, President Johnson praised Congress for their foresight in peacefully passing these acts. It was just the kind of crime-probing "blue ribbon panel" he'd called for in his State of the Union address. Better care and treatment for prisoners went hand in hand with his widespread social welfare projects; he passed subsidies to allow low-income renters to enter the property ladder and developed Medicare and Medicaid to care for the elderly and the poor.[46]

Switzer deeply appreciated having such a welfare-minded president, but that didn't mean she wasn't going to push him for more. Inmates didn't have anyone else in their corner. Once imprisoned, inmates were permanently disadvantaged. It was even tougher for disabled prisoners. "At the time of parole, they face the double handicaps of disability and a prison record," she announced to Congress,[47] emphasizing her department's accomplishments. We've achieved so much with a paltry $900,000, she told them, listing some of the projects in play. In Dobbs Ferry, New York, a psychologist had set up a day care service for delinquent teens; a team in Atlanta was producing movie shorts showcasing the struggles of disabled offenders; and in Los Angeles, researchers were doing a deep dive into the recidivism rates of alcoholic inmates.[48]

"We have a variety of approaches," Switzer continued. "An area that's more dramatic is the people who get into trouble because of some disfigurement, which gets them off to the wrong start." She gave a brief overview of the Surgical and Social Rehabilitation of Adult Offenders project. As she suspected, her audience was enthralled with the Hollywood-esque nature of the work. "This was one of the first dramatic pieces of intelligence that caused us to go and do something about it," she said.

"Let me say we believe strongly in this program. We believe this study is very important for the improvement and general stepping up of the whole professional area of work in the field of public offenders," Joseph Clark, the Pennsylvania senator, announced in support. Switzer's passionate rhetoric swayed the room. They approved the Correctional Rehabilitation Study Act of 1965, which increased the Vocational Rehabilitation Administration's research budget.

Not every senator was as enthused as Clark about Switzer's plans. "While I know this program is needed, this program of prevention is like solving the floods in New Orleans by damming up the Mississippi," said Sam Gibbons, Florida's Democratic representative, in a separate session. Gibbons was famously contrarian; he'd voted against the 1964 Civil Rights Act but for the Voting Rights Act in 1965.[49] Despite his lukewarm comment, he, too, approved the Correctional Rehabilitation Study Act.

Switzer was gratified with her victory. "We want to get the job done—and fast," she told Congress. "I am not awfully enthusiastic about waiting three years to do something."

# THE MANY FACES
# OF PRISON PLASTIC

Experts Say That Crime Can Be Skin Deep—*St. Petersburg Independent*, 1966

Elimination of Scars Aids Criminal Reform—*Boston Globe*, 1966[1]

Inside a small restaurant just off the highway, eighteen-year-old Larry smiled politely at diners as he moved from table to table, handing out menus. He approached a small table at the side of the room where two forty-something white men sat, both dressed in sleek tuxedo jackets.[2] They waved him away; they were fine with their coffee. Larry nodded and turned around when one of the men whispered to the other, "How does he get a job at a place like this with *that* thing on his face?" His voice was low but pitched to carry. Larry spun around, his face darkening. "You want to say that to my face?" The man stood up, laughed, and tapped his cheek. Larry grabbed his shirttails and swung at him, sending him sprawling back into his chair. Then his manager appeared and wrestled him away, ordering him to the back room. "Sir, are you okay?"

"That boy is crazy! He attacked me out of nowhere! Why do you hire a dangerous thug like that?"

Once he calmed the situation and comped the men their meal, the manager dealt with Larry. "That behavior is not acceptable at this establishment," he said. "You're fired."

"You didn't hear what he was saying," Larry protested, his finger grazing the thick scar that bisected his right cheek from ear to chin.

"I don't care what they said. You don't act that way around customers."

Larry left, growling. Why did all his jobs seem to end like this? He stomped to his car, loosened his tie, and pulled onto the highway. His shoulders relaxed; driving always soothed him; his white Austin Healy, a sporty British import, was the only thing that gave him joy these days. Then the auto dealer called—Larry

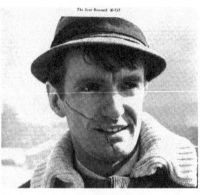

Movie still from *The Scar Beneath*, produced by the Vocational Rehabilitation Administration, 1964. *Courtesy National Archives and Records Administration*

was behind on his car payments. Larry begged for more time but they were firm: pay up or we repossess the car. He looked around hopelessly. He had no savings, no money coming in. . . . But it wasn't his fault! He didn't ask to be treated unkindly! It was time someone paid. He bought a $1.98 toy gun, pulled a stocking over his face, and marched into the nearest bank, waving it in the air. "Fill this up," he told the teller, handing her a paper bag. "Nobody follow me!" A quick-thinking employee wrote down Larry's license plate and sent it to the police. They traced him to his house, where they arrested him, still dressed in the white shirt and black tie he'd worn waiting tables.

Douglas Lipton anxiously surveyed the room as *The Scar Beneath* rolled, trying to gauge the guards' reactions. The assembled officers were bathed in light from the film projector, and it was hard to read their facial expressions. A few seemed engrossed in the movie, but many looked bored, quietly chatting to a neighbor. Did they think he couldn't see them in the low light or did they just not care? That don't-care attitude was precisely why he'd shown them this movie—there'd been multiple viewings—but he didn't know if it would be enough to get through to them.[3]

And he needed to; the guards were proving the biggest holdup to the project. He kept stressing that to the wardens, but it hadn't translated into behavioral changes among the everyday guards. Their dismissive outlook was in keeping with the old-fashioned principle that correctional officers knew more about the inmates than psychologists or social workers, since they spent significantly more time with them.

"When the chips are down and hell is breaking loose, people do not call a psychiatrist, they call the police," noted forensic psychiatrist Melvin Heller in *The Prison Journal.* "It's just one of the things that must be recognized about the altruistic impulses that occur in almost all of us."[4]

The Rikers Island guards didn't understand why mental health staff were allowed to keep their interviews confidential and regarded Lipton's team as impractical idealists that posed a security risk. In return, his team had charged the correctional staff with being unnecessarily punitive and anti-education and rehabilitation.

"You research people come in here like you own the place" was a common refrain. Kurtzberg and Cavior were forced to assume the role of enforcer; not only did they proctor the tests, but they had to physically prevent the guards from rifling through the inmates' completed tests. Another concern was the guards' reluctance to allow the inmates privacy during the psychological tests. Over and over, the pair reminded them to stop reading over inmates' shoulders; if the men felt they were being judged, they might alter their answers.

Onscreen, Larry was getting into trouble again, this time inside the jail. A kindly guard matches him with a vocational counselor who lends a sympathetic ear to Larry's stories of being scorned and dismissed due to his facial scar. Perhaps we can help you with that, he tells Larry, but first, you must help yourself. Larry enrolled in the prison's college classes and participated in group therapy—to "smooth out the scar in his personality," his counselor says. A visiting plastic surgeon removes his scar, and Larry is ecstatic with his new look. At the movie's close, Larry is out of prison, happily ensconced in a professional office job, and friendly with his colleagues.

The picture faded to black, and "Produced by the Vocational Rehabilitation Administration," flashed across the screen; this was another of Commissioner Switzer's side projects. *The Scar Beneath* had been well received so far; the National Institute of Mental Health called it "absorbing," "convincing," and "an excellent job of explaining why some people commit crimes." The *CNA Bulletin* also approved; "Scarred face—scarred mind?" it wrote. "Very fine film," commented the *American Journal of Correction.* The movie aired on the nation's educational television[5] channel and was shown to women's groups and volunteer organizations across the United States, the intent being to convey how behavioral science could help reform offenders.[6]

Lipton gestured to the projectionist to stop the tape and flipped on the lights. Was that interest and compassion he spied in some of their faces? Hopefully, they'd empathized with Larry's plight.

"Does anyone have any questions?"

The officers shrugged.

"No questions?"

The lukewarm reception on Rikers Island wasn't echoed by the rest of America. Thanks to the positive media coverage and Mary Switzer's congressional pronouncements, the Surgical and Social Rehabilitation (SSR) project reputation was rising. Lipton and Lewin's letter trays were flooded with letters from penologists, plastic surgeons, psychologists, politicians, and progressively higher profile institutions. "I will be glad to be better acquainted with this study, which seems to be a quite original one," wrote Paul Cornil, the secretary general from Brussels.[7] A plastic surgeon from McGill University in Montreal inquired on behalf of the Canadian Mental Health Board, which was interested in running a similar project, he said. Letters arrived from the Smithsonian, the U.S. Disciplinary Barracks, and seventeen countries, as far afield as Australia and Israel.[8]

Lewin especially enjoyed the letter from Maryland's director of corrections, which was addressed to "Martin Lewin," almost as amusing as the time the *Detroit Press* referred to him as "Dr. Marvin Herwin."[9]

All the correspondence essentially asked the same questions; did their plastic surgery program successfully solve the recidivism problem? The pair were courted by criminologists and invited to speak at events and attend private dinners with senators and governors. The attention was especially flattering for Lipton, as he'd never been wooed like this before. He accepted as many invitations as he could.

Back in their Union Square office, Norman Cavior and Richard Kurtzberg felt increasingly distant from Lipton. There always had been some divide; he was their boss, after all, and most days Lipton wore a suit—the formality necessary for his administrative meetings—whereas they sported more casual attire. Lipton had always divided his time between the Union Square office and Rikers Island, but recently it felt like he spent less and less time at the project's headquarters. Even with him gone, their office had grown crowded with new additions to the team, mostly staffers hot-desking from external agencies, a rotating roster of social workers, medical case workers, and field service agents.

Cavior clicked with Samir Hakki, a field worker from the social services team. Hakki's job was to check up on inmates, conduct follow-up interviews, and help facilitate their care with the city's agencies. After work, they often dined at one another's houses—their wives got on well, too, which was nice. The Hakkis introduced the Caviors to the food of Samir's birthplace: shredded boiled chicken simmered in a paste of walnuts and stale bread with a side of sour cream. "This is Circassian chicken," Hakki told Cavior, who asked for seconds.

Hakki was a definite upside to the SSR work, but the junior psychologists still felt unmoored. At lunch, they bought hot dogs from a vendor on Union Square's north side and walked around the park, trying to figure out a solution. They wanted to be self-sufficient, but they still needed Lipton's input. Perhaps he'll pay more attention when the media circus dies down, they decided. Regardless, the pressure was on. The latest project report to Washington, D.C., noted that they were still two months behind schedule.

Cavior enjoyed the work, but as it was far more demanding, it was harder to balance his job with his evening college classes, his postgrad work, and quality time with his wife and friends. He was the only Spanish speaker on the project, a skill which required him to be on Rikers Island more than Kurtzberg. The ferry sometimes proved a hassle, what with worker strikes and equipment breakdowns. On a bad day, that journey might take an exhausting one to two hours each way.

So much was stacked against them that sometimes it felt like a losing battle. Take Joe Smith, a small, wiry inmate who'd requested needle track removal. His scars gave people the wrong impression, he'd told Cavior; people judged him before he'd even opened his mouth. Smith cleared the surgical screen, two psychological screens, and appeared an ideal candidate; he was motivated, cognizant of potential complications, exhibited a positive forward-thinking reason for the operation.

Smith didn't show up for the next barrage of psychological tests or the one after that. Cavior could write off a single absence as officer incompetency, but two was suspicious. Had Smith been paroled and he hadn't been informed? Nope, he's still here, the warden told him. He was puzzled as to what had changed. He chased him down, determined to understand why someone with so much enthusiasm—and potential—had dropped out of their study. He located Smith in the officer's dining room, clearing the tables after the lunch rush, a washcloth at his hip.

"What happened? You were so excited about the surgery."

"I got a real good job here," Smith explained; waiter jobs were one of the most coveted work assignments in the jail. The work was easy, the food was *much* better than the general mess hall (inmates weren't supposed to eat there, but everyone did), and working there gave him an extra "in" with the guards. "It's almost like I'm not in jail."

Smith *did* want his tracks removed—he still loved the idea—and had taken time off for his first interview, and the one following. But with more scheduled, he was informed that if he skipped any more shifts, he'd be reassigned. "That's why I quit," he said. "I got six months left here, and I don't want to spend that time sitting in my cell . . . just going crazy."

Cavior pursed his lips and inclined his head. He didn't like it, but he couldn't blame him. Their tests, not including the surgical screens or the interviews loaded on top of that, averaged four to five hours, a significant time commitment. Still, it was a blow he didn't need; Smith was the ninety-seventh inmate to quit because their testing was "too intense."

He returned, deflated, back to the intake center. It was isolating working on Rikers; most guards were either indifferent or unfriendly, and the plastic surgeons from Montefiore Hospital were pleasant but distant—not that he saw very much of them as it was. Even when their paths overlapped, they strode around in their lab coats like they were too busy and important to stop and chat.

His favorite plastic surgery resident was Dr. Marvin Shuster, a thirty-five-year-old with a neat brown beard and irascible sense of humor. Whenever their shifts aligned, they'd hang out and shoot the breeze as they waited to see whether the guards would deign to bring them any inmates that day.

"Have you ever thought about having your ears done?" Shuster asked him one afternoon in the fall.

Cavior tilted his head and blinked in confusion.[10]

"Your ears," Shuster repeated, windmilling one hand near his face.

Cavior opened his mouth then closed it. His eyes widened as understanding dawned. "Oh yes," he said. "I mean, no. I mean yes, yes I understand what you're saying, but no I haven't. No, thank you." He was flustered by the abrupt change in conversation and knew his ears had reddened in response.

Shuster shrugged and gave him an easy smile. "Not a problem. Just let me know if you change your mind. It would be on the house."

"Sure, great," Cavior replied, head bobbing up and down like a puppet.

When Shuster glanced away, he self-consciously raised a hand to his ear. He was 80 percent sure Shuster was just messing with him, though his ears *were* larger than other people's, elongated, almost Dumbo-like flappy things that protruded from his face. But they worked well enough, adequately channeling sounds through his tympanic membrane, which was all he asked of them. Their size had never bothered him. In the right light, he fancied, perhaps they could even be viewed as rakish. He shook his head again, a half grin on his face. I guess that's just part of being a plastic surgeon, he thought. When you spend that much time appraising and perfecting people's appearances, can you ever turn that off?

He didn't need—or want—the surgery; he looked just fine, he thought. He might never walk the catwalk, but he reckoned he was the second-best looker on his team. Doug, with his boyish charm and sharp suits, came in first. Besides, he was number one with the person who mattered most, his darling wife Helene.

Helene had his back in every way that mattered. Some people thought it was odd that he spent so much time with prisoners and were concerned about the danger, but Helene never questioned it. She knew he'd tell her if he felt threatened or uncomfortable and trusted him enough to let him decide that for himself. They were Bronx kids, after all, born and raised, with the run of the city since they were small. Age ten, and they were taking the subway into Manhattan unsupervised; Cavior had admired the bright lights on Broadway and the culture of Greenwich Village, whereas Helene hung out at the museums and ice skated in Central Park. They'd never been threatened or scared—New York City was home. It wasn't that crime didn't exist, but they hadn't seen it during their childhood sojourns. Poverty, they recognized: the noses and arms that healed crooked because no one could afford a doctor, the ragged men lying by the dumpsters, the dull-eyed children picking through scraps, and the dead-eyed women shooting up on stoops.

Being poor wasn't a crime, but sometimes it felt that way in New York. His work, perhaps, might offer one solution to that misery, a starting point, at least. What he was doing mattered, he told himself; he gave men—and now, a few women—a chance at a different life. It was more than just making them beautiful—it was about how that beauty could improve their everyday lives. Was there anything more American than self-improvement? It was a national movement these days! How had the First Lady put it in her *Keep America Beautiful* speech?[11] "The drive for national beauty has many facets," Ladybird Johnson had said. "Ugliness breeds ugliness." To be sure, the *Keep America Beautiful* campaign focused on the beautification of the country's forests and cities, but it wasn't a stretch to apply her premise to the nation's people.

The poverty epidemic had another unhappy consequence: addiction. With nothing else to lose, many turned to drugs, finding solace in a chemical fugue. There were few detox programs, and those that existed were heavily oversubscribed.

In 1961, the Association for Psychiatric Treatment of Offenders estimated some thirty thousand addicts roamed the streets of New York City; "a gloomy picture," they called it.[12] By 1965, this had risen to somewhere between one and two hundred thousand. Aluminum foil, needles, and other debris littered the sidewalks and city parks. Drug deals took place in broad daylight, with dealers regularly using children as couriers. The slums expanded and spilled onto Fifth Avenue. Citizens diverted their eyes for fear of reprisals. The city was floundering.

> Our cities are stalked by people changed by the need for narcotics to animals more dangerous than in any jungle.—letter from concerned resident Louise Goodwin, *New York Herald Tribune*, 1965[13]

Numerous tactics were used to try and stem this flow; school boards increased antidrug education in schools, parishes, and community centers. The city commissioned televised public service announcements in which battered ex-junkies warned kids about going down their tragic path. It ran methadone experiments to ease withdrawal symptoms. It even offered voluntary jail time for people trying to kick the habit: in the1950s, a full ward inside Rikers Island infirmary was reserved for self-committed, otherwise law-abiding men hoping to detox in the big house.[14]

Anna Kross had quickly put a stop to that; correctional stays were for the convicted and should not double as a "dry" ward. But the uncomfortable intersection was hard to ignore, as more than half of her inmates struggled with addiction, and, often enough, that was the reason for their convictions, whether it was possession, dealing, or thieving to finance their supply. "Dope addicts don't belong in jail," she told the press. "They need help. Treat them as a medical, social problem and a health problem, not as a crime."

In her view, social services needed to step up more. "When an addict comes out of a hospital or a prison, the chances are he'll have no job and nobody to greet him but a pusher," she said.[15] For her, this was the biggest roadblock to recovery. Mayor Wagner professed his support, but she took it with a pinch of salt; a few years back he'd described addicts as "depraved and reckless."

But even Wagner admitted that it would help if New Yorkers understood that addiction was a disease in itself—and if they stopped racializing it. Television shows, newscasts, and movies depicted the stereotypical addict as a "Black hoodlum from Harlem," which led to discriminatory policing and enforcement. For the administration, rebranding addiction as a medical problem rather than a criminal one was a big ask. To change the narrative, numerous correctional agencies reached out to the press, seeing journalists as the best way to disseminate this concept, often offering them unprecedented levels of access.

"What is the addict like? Can he be cured? What kind of threat does he represent to society?" intoned journalist Walter Cronkite in the opening sequence of *The Addicted.*[16] He dove into the topic, exploring what drives a person to addiction, and how his or her community responds. His reflections were eye-opening. "Violence, sex, and murder are not consistent with the dope fiend, either with his personality or the chemical effect of the drug itself as it spreads though his body," he told viewers. Despite the belief that addicts were dangerous, the effects of their drugs tended to be soporific. Their "dangerous" behavior was a fallacy.

"You're at ease. The last thing you want to do is get up out of the chair," a white male addict told the camera. "You're certainly not entertaining the violence that's attributed to us." Cronkite cut to a tearful mother who shared that her doctor wouldn't treat her child's addiction, despite both parties begging for help. A gruff factory owner expressed shock that one of his employees had a drug problem. "I never had any experience with drug addicts before," he told Cronkite. "I was under the impression that they were wide-eyed and disheveled individuals. But Fred appeared to me to be an honest, hardworking young kid and worked out very well here."

Cronkite hammered the point home in other reports. Anyone can be an addict, he stressed; it's not related to age, race, or employment status, though the intersection can play a role. "There's no discrimination, they tell you, then a white boy right behind me, with less qualifications will get accepted for the job," a Black addict told him. "Things like that you can't reconcile. What can you do about this color thing? There's nothing you can do. Drugs do seem to soothe these things, to make you better prepared to accept them."

But there was only so much the media could do; it was hard to elicit sympathy and understanding when so much of the correctional world still had such a punitive, almost medieval, approach to offenders. In Delaware in 1962, a nineteen-year-old white man broke his probation, and, as punishment, the judge sentenced him to twenty public lashes with a cat-o'-nine-tails. His appeal went all the way to Delaware's high court, which upheld his sentence.

"Public whipping does not constitute cruel and unusual punishment," the court ruled.[17] The following year, a bill requesting the authority to whip juvenile delinquents was introduced in Michigan. "It's time we quit theorizing about what causes delinquency and do something to curb it," announced the bill's sponsor, Democratic State Representative[18] Arthur Law. New York had outlawed whipping in 1847. But its trouble with addicts was mirrored in every state.

Dear Dr. Brothers,

I am twenty-six and not yet married. I think it is my nose. It is too large and has a slight hook. . . .—Miss M.

Dear Miss M.,

Physicians and psychologist have many different views on plastic surgery. There is one thing I can tell you: I have never heard of a girl not getting married because of her nose. If you are not married at the age of twenty-six it's because you have not found the right man, or there is something else wrong, perhaps with your personality.—Dr. Joyce Brothers[19]

The high number of addicts incarcerated on Rikers Island was causing huge headaches for the SSR team. They'd chosen to admit addicts to the study—they wanted to be representative of the jail population as a whole, they decided—and at last count, almost 60 percent of their subjects fell into that bucket. What they hadn't accounted for was the additional behavioral problems unique to addicts and former addicts.

Most of the addicts on Rikers Island began using when they were young— really young: 16 percent admitted to "using" before they turned ten, and 58 percent shared that they were between eleven and fifteen years old when they had their first hit. Less than a fifth of the addicts had graduated from high school, many dropping out before fifth grade. This limited their job prospects. However, even in the menial work available, Black and Hispanic addicts earned significantly less than the white addicts.

Aside from that casual racism, the dearth of career opportunities for the addicts went a long way toward explaining their situation. Low-paying mediocre jobs were increasingly more competitive, as technology edged out workers and jobs declined. But even securing one of these wasn't enough to prevent a relapse; these jobs weren't steppingstones to a career—they were a stopgap. These marginal jobs encouraged recidivism; most led nowhere in terms of opportunities.

The team analyzed the salary range of the addicts and found their weekly income rarely exceeded $80. But something didn't add up, because at the same time, the inmates reported spending around $105 a week on smack. That explained the high number of property crimes among the incarcerated.

The paroled addicts had been of particular concern to the team; 25 percent of addicts were known to return to drugs on their first day of release. Escorting them to the hospital had reduced the dropout rate, but once on the wards, contentious situations weren't uncommon. Fred Marshall's behavior wasn't an anomaly.

Things got hairy even before their operations; often, after arriving at the hospital, the former offenders would need to fill out preadmission paperwork. Despite the lengthy preapproval process the SSR team had initiated with the hospital, a preexisting ruling by the city government stated that no city-funded patient could receive cosmetic surgery. Accordingly, multiple subjects were turned away at this stage, and Lewin had to petition the department of hospitals for an amendment, after even more subjects were lost.

The next problem was the financial investigation, a standard discovery process when the city was covering a patient's stay. At this juncture, the ex-cons were quizzed about their assets and those of their family. The men were suspicious of these asks; after months on Rikers Island, they held a grudge against those in authority. What was the hospital really trying to find out? Was it going to go after their parents? Their children? Many refused to participate, thereby disqualifying themselves for financial support and with it the SSR study. It took another round of interminable meetings and phone calls to get the administrative staff to skip this part.

Their troubles continued. One night, Lewin received a phone call from a hysterical nurse; some of the SSR patients had smuggled in alcohol and marijuana and were partying on Morrisania's hospital ward, Montefiore Hospital's city-owned affiliate. There were thirty civilian patients on the ward, and a few had joined in the festivities—the rest were irate about the disturbance. This happened a few times. It wasn't always clear if the alcohol and drugs came from addicts or just from ex-cons who were celebrating their freedom, but the addicts were blamed regardless.

Then there were the reports of subjects heckling other patients and being needy and demanding with the nurses. Some claimed excessive pain and greedily built up their drug supply on Montefiore's dime. Only 30 percent of those admitted caused problems, but their behavior smeared all future SSR patients.

It was of growing concern for Lewin. He needed the medical staff to support the ex-cons not to reject them. The nursing team were adapting their care in distressing ways; mainly overusing sedatives on the more unmanageable patients. "We gave large doses of methadone or barbiturates, tranquilizers and anti-histamines. The patient was kept in a sedated state," one report read. They'd improved the subject's behavior, which had the side effect of continuing his psychological reliance on narcotics.

Occasionally, the staff biases toward ex-cons and their separate biases toward addicts coalesced into an outpouring of anger. "They should be refused admission for plastic surgery if they're still addicted," some of the nurses told

Lewin, their faces red. He smiled wearily and explained—again—the reason for their enrollment and their surgeries.

Paroled addicts were even more capricious and prone to lying about their health and their post-release activities than other ex-cons. "They could potentially skew our entire study," Lewin informed Lipton. "We have a real problem here." He doubted they'd follow the instructed aftercare—or even keep their appointments. "We'll factor this into our data," Lipton replied; they'd have to separate the results for addicts versus nonaddicts.

Throughout 1965, many of the bankers, attorneys, and self-proclaimed big shots who frequented New York's gentlemen's clubs—along with the busboys, barkeeps, and braggarts at the working men's clubs—considered themselves to be connoisseurs of the female form. Those who were more refined discussed beauty as a "cultural condition," elevating the idea that certain qualities and features were a westernized aesthetic, whereas others merely opined that they were breasts, butt, or legs guys. Such conversations soared into a cacophony that March when eighteen-year-old Jennifer Jackson from Chicago's South Side was crowned *Playboy*'s Playmate of the Month.

Jackson measured in at 36–23–36 and was five feet eight, the text next to her picture revealed. Jackson smiled suggestively from the centerfold, her eyes dark and mysterious, her thick brown hair styled in a tidy flipped bob, her Black skin gleaming.[20] Jackson was *Playboy*'s first Black centerfold. *Playboy* received hate mail, some of which the magazine published in subsequent issues. "Integration has reached into schools, all forms of business, and now it seems to have taken over *Playboy*," complained a letter signed "Concord College Students, Athens, West Virginia."

> At the risk of being labeled bigots, racists, reactionaries and sundry other things currently in vogue we entreat you to return to your time-tested format of Playmates selection which is more in line with the thinking of the vast majority of your readers.—Interested readers, University of Maryland

"Stay in your own lane," decried her detractors. "You didn't see black women in the Miss America pageant, did you? Let them have their own magazines." Hugh Hefner, *Playboy*'s founder and editor, ignored such remarks; he celebrated all shades of women, and admitted all races to his clubs (though only those who could afford it). "We are outspoken foes of segregation," Hefner wrote in 1961.[21] "We are actively involved in the fight to see the end of all racial inequalities in our time."

Black bodies were also under scrutiny in the *Negro Digest*. "It is not news to anyone that lighter color Negroes consider themselves a shade superior to the dark ones," wrote author Thomas O. Echewa.[22] "They perform plastic surgery on their features. I don't have much patience with the people who are trying to be white but can't quite make it!"

Food for thought indeed, Lewin thought, as he tried to place his plastic surgery work within the cultural context. There was also news on the criminal cosmetic surgery front. Dr. Edward Lewison—a Canadian plastic surgeon with a name eerily similar to his own—had a new paper out in the *Canadian Medical Association Journal*.[23] Lewison's report comprised a ten-year analysis of his plastic surgery work on 450 prisoners in the Oakalla prison farm.

Lewison calculated a 42 percent recidivism rate for inmates who received plastic surgery compared to 75 percent of the general prison population. He focused primarily on nasal surgeries, with a few chin implants, scar removals, and the like; in his view, the more visible the deformity, the more likely it was to cause social harm. "Man has always had an innate desire to look like his fellows, and not to appear peculiar," he remarked. His data wasn't as scrupulous as Lewin's, but since Lewison had worked at the prison for more than a decade, it was relatively easy for him to identify which, if any, of his patients returned. "A physical defect, although usually only a contributory factor, can be a dominant cause of criminal behavior," Lewison summarized in his paper. "Removal of such defects makes these individuals more confident on their re-entry."

There was positive news out of Illinois, too. Dr. John Pick announced a twenty-four-year follow-up of his original surgical study showing a 20 percent reduction in inmate recidivism over time. One small problem arose, Pick noted; some inmates since had developed criminal specialties—bettering themselves through illegal rather than legal channels. The overall thrust remained positive, which was a relief for Lewin and Lipton. In some cases, they heard stories that were almost too positive. In Michigan, an inmate reportedly refused parole so as to have a facelift.[24] Another Michigan inmate's surgery was cited by his parole board as a reason for his release.[25] The most peculiar of these stories originated in North Carolina, where a judge *intentionally* jailed a man to give him access to facial plastic surgery.[26] Still, things looked good, and there was national public support for these types of procedures.

Then, during the summer of 1965, a kid from Cleveland, Ohio, became national news.

Sixteen-year-old Frank Burdel Jr. had a long history of running afoul of authority. It was hard to trust any adult, after all, when your da' was beating on your
ma every night. His teachers complained that he was rude in class, and his
friends whined that his teasing went too far; no one wanted to play against him
in football. The cops got involved when he was twelve years old, small things at
first, petty thefts, vandalism, loitering. Then, when Burdel was newly thirteen,
he took a sharp spill off his bike. The fall bruised his knee and hip and carved
a jagged scar across the right side of his face. His attitude grew worse and his
crimes escalated: he broke into garages in his neighborhood, he hot-wired cars,
and his punches grew harder. He adopted a swaggering walk, gelled his hair,
and dressed in dark black leather, a cut between Elvis and a greaser. He terrorized the neighborhood kids who looked up to him in awe.

He had a special knack for hot-wiring cars and could have one purring in
under two minutes. Burdel floored them around town, dumping them in empty
lots when he grew bored. After multiple run-ins with the police, he was sent to
juvenile hall in Columbus, Ohio. Burdel saw this as a challenge; during Christmas break one year, he hot-wired the reverend's automobile and escaped.[27] He
wasn't found for a week.[28] Back inside, he talked circles around the psychiatrists
and continued disrupting the jail's education classes. Then he threw the staff a
bone. "All this is because of my scar," he told them. "It's why I act out so much.
. . . I can't get a girlfriend and kids make fun of me."

The sympathetic—and desperate—staff arranged for Burdel's scar to be
treated by a plastic surgeon in Cleveland. The papers were full of stories about
how plastic surgery could reform a personality, and they hoped it would adjust
the boy's attitude. He was granted temporary parole to stay with his parents,
who lived close to Parma Community Hospital.

When he checked in, he was assigned to surgical nurse Barbara Ann Ambrose to help him with his paperwork and medical scripts. He was smitten
with Ambrose and tried to charm her—"Want to go out for a date after this?"
he asked. Ambrose didn't reciprocate—"You're sixteen and I'm twenty-three,"
she reminded him.

His surgery went well, his scar excised and his cheek smoothed out, and he
was booked for a post-op visit a few weeks later. Home alone, Burdel brooded
about Ambrose's rejection, about having to return to juvenile hall, about his
deadbeat dad and his mother's new loser husband. He raided his stepdad's
liquor cabinet, stashing the bottles in his car, and drove to the local strip mall.
Drunk and angry, he used a bottle to break into a random car in the lot, hot-

wired it, and drove away. When it stalled, a few streets later, he cursed, kicked it, then jimmied his way into another car. He parked it by the hospital and sat in the lot for a few hours, the engine idling.

Around 10:30 p.m., Ambrose exited; she'd finished her shift for the day. Burdel waved her over, and she walked to the car, a quizzical expression on her face. "I'm in trouble," he told her. "I don't know what to do." She sighed and got into the car. "Let's talk about this," she said. "I'm sure we can figure this out." He started the engine—"Here is fine," she said quickly—but he ignored her and drove up Main Street. "I want to talk somewhere quieter," he said, pulling into the deserted lot of a local high school. "Want some wine?"

"No," she told him. "Look, we really should get back to the hospital. It won't be so bad if you return to juvenile hall. Look how great your face is now!" Burdel glowered then leaned in for a kiss. Ambrose pushed him away. "Frank, no!" she said. He tried again. "Stop it!"

He glared at her—wasn't he good enough now that his face was smooth and perfect?—and punched her straight in the jaw. He raped her on the backseat. When he was done, he looked at her bruised, tear-stricken face and panicked. "This isn't going to look good," he thought. His hands closed around her neck, choking her till she went limp.[29] He dumped her body in the gravel lot of Kiddie Park, a local amusement park.

When Ambrose didn't return home, her mother called the hospital and then the police. Burdel was arrested. The murder was so brutal that the juvenile court passed him over to the adult court for trial.[30] At first, he protested his innocence.[31] "She died from epilepsy and I panicked," he claimed.[32]

He shortly rescinded his statement[33] and received two concurrent life sentences.

"Plastic Surgery Failed Its Task, Youth Convicted," reported the Associated Press.[34] The public was furious. Who thought it was a good idea to let a violent youth roam free for two weeks? Why was Burdel getting plastic surgery—*free* plastic surgery—to begin with? If these do-gooders had just left well enough alone, Barbara Ann Ambrose would still be alive! Other stories of surgically enhanced criminals gone wrong surfaced. In an English detention center, nineteen-year-old Michael Stratford had his large nose chiseled down by reform-minded surgeons. Once paroled, over the subsequent six months, he sexually assaulted thirteen women, aged four to seventy-five years old before he was caught.[35] During his trial, Stratford admitted he'd committed twelve additional offenses; "I have a grudge against all women," he told the judge. If anything, his nasal surgery had made it easier for him to lure his victims. In the United States, many on the FBI's Ten Most Wanted list had reportedly had plastic surgery.[36]

The public furor over Burdel, Stratford, and other miscreants was the last thing that the SSR team needed. As each scandal went public, their concerns increased. As the hospital procedures became more standardized, their work had shifted to the social welfare side. They'd expected that connecting group one, which received plastic surgery and social welfare services, and group three, which was assigned social welfare services alone, would be the most straightforward part of the project. Kurtzberg and Cavior were quickly relieved of that notion.

The social and vocational services offered included help with welfare benefits, housing accommodations, job placement, legal aid, medical help, parole liaison, work training, and drug rehabilitation, and numerous city agencies were involved in this process.

However, the already beleaguered community and social service agencies of New York balked at the addition of two hundred–some clients. The sudden influx was too much, they argued. They couldn't be expected to stop helping their lawful clients to make space for these ex-cons. The caseworkers were suspicious of the former inmates' motivations. "We don't think they're serious about this," they told Kurtzberg; in their opinion, the ex-cons planned to use their welfare checks for drugs. They dismissed them without aid. Some welfare officers cited the ex-cons' attitudes as the reason for their refusal; their application was too "passive," they explained. "They need to convince us they want this," a welfare officer told Kurtzberg. For some, the rejection provoked angry responses: loudly insisting their cases be assessed and knocking things over for attention.

Men showed up at the Union Square office to complain. "I went there, like you told me," one said. "They turned me away—they said they weren't seeing anyone from Rikers anymore." "They accepted me . . . but then they took away my benefits," claimed another. His benefits had been rescinded as he'd refused to stay at the "junk houses" recommended by the welfare worker, and he'd forgotten to inform them of his new address. "They aren't giving me enough cash to live," groused a third man; the food allowance was budgeted on being able to cook and prepare food, but most cheap rooms had no cooking facilities.

Frustrated by the clear disconnect between the men's needs and the help provided, Kurtzberg and Cavior went to meet the social welfare staff in person. They had to do something about the project's 30 percent dropout rate. The senior social staffers were dismissive. "We don't have to cooperate," they informed the duo. "We will help these men—when we have availability. They're difficult, and they just want money for drugs. You can't trust an addict."

"Everyone deserves food and housing," argued Kurtzberg, who was met with a shrug. Housing was one of the most immediate problems for ex-cons, especially for their enrolled addicts, many whose families refused to take them in. "Can you at least share the case files of the last three subjects, so we can try and figure something else out for them?" The welfare agent consulted his notes and shook his head. "I'm afraid that's not possible. Says here that your access has been revoked. You should look into that." Kurtzberg turned away in disgust. The pair had more luck with the junior welfare staff. "We'll do our best to help," they informed them; "Just send them our way, and we'll clear some space in our schedules." Sadly, these helpful aides were in the minority.

On the vocational side, Kurtzberg and Cavior were intent on placing the men in suitable jobs or equivalent educational and work-training programs. Cavior tried placing Louis Taylor, a Black inmate, into the Better Essential Skills Training Program (BEST), a pathway to work program sponsored by the city's department of labor. However, Taylor read at a fifth-grade level, which precluded him from entry to all but the heavy vehicle driving course, which was a no-go, as his criminal record made him ineligible to receive the chauffeur's license the course was geared to. Another training program limited eligibility to sixteen- to twenty-one-year-olds, whereas another was open only to people with hand or arm deformities.

Frustrated, the pair met with the Correctional Vocational Rehabilitation Service (CVRS), a state employment agency designed specifically for placing ex-cons after release. Here, too, there were holdups, mainly around participants' addiction status. Some CVRS staff refused outright to work with addicts. "It was difficult to decide whether to counsel the offender or to do an immediate job placement," employment consultant Arthur Mann wrote in the *Employment Service Review* newsletter.[37] "It was found most require immediate job referral because they have no financial resources." In return, many of the ex-cons were wary of accepting a position through CVRS, concerned about the potential of discriminatory behavior from their new employers, who'd be aware of their criminal history. It's happened before, they told the SSR team. Even when both sides were willing, the ex-cons' lack of education and work experience meant that few received placements.

It was a wake-up call for Cavior and Kurtzberg. They knew there were difficulties in reassimilating once released, but the nitty-gritty of it—the tiny granular indignities suffered day in and out, the struggles of simply existing in an unwelcome world—had eluded them till now.

They reported their struggles to Lipton, who ran it up the chain; with Washington, D.C., on his back, he wanted all the boxes checked. He made calls.

More calls. Follow-up calls. Their problems rose up the chain, all the way to Mary Switzer in Washington, D.C., and Anna Kross in New York City. "This isn't sustainable," Lipton told them; the way things were, inmates were set up to fail. Switzer was furious about the lack of cooperation Lipton had received.

She demanded a meeting of the interagency heads, ordering them to hammer out a solution. Douglas Lipton presented, emphasizing the issues the project was having and appealing to their sense of decency—and oversight: "The president is watching what we're doing! We need to live up to his expectations." After much back and forth, the interagency heads negotiated an agreement; they would tell their junior staff to be more accommodating, and this bottleneck would end. It wasn't perfect cooperation, but it was a step in the right direction.

This worked out well for Fred Marshall, who was placed in a detoxification program once he'd healed from his surgery. So far, only nine ex-cons, including Marshall, had begun treatment, despite twenty-eight requests. The holdup had been a combination of clerical errors, overbooking, and program shortages. Marshall's program combined one-on-one counseling with group meetings and periodic check-ins.

At Marshall's six-month follow-up interview, he was upbeat. "I'm less self-conscious," he told Cavior. "I really want to beat this thing for good. I still think about drugs, but I don't do them—I just think of all the good things in my life instead." His new focus was on finding himself a job.

Marshall's interview and testing took a little more than four hours. When he left, Cavior walked over to where Lipton and Kurtzberg were conversing to tell them about Marshall's progress. His smile faltered at their expressions. "We just got word from the social services team," Lipton informed him. Three of their subjects were dead. One by suicide, one by drug overdose, and one had been stabbed to death.

There were shakeups happening at a departmental level as well.[38] Mayor Robert Wagner was succeeded as mayor by John Lindsay, a forty-three-year-old, six-foot-four stout Republican from the Upper East Side.[39]

Mayor Lindsay ran on a platform of social reform and police oversight, courting citizens of color, but his ascendance to mayor was not easy. His first day in office coincided with the beginning of a city-wide transit strike, which brought New York to a standstill for twelve days. The economic losses were so staggering that Lindsay quickly acceded to most of the strikers' demands, allocating approximately $43 million to increase salaries, sanitation, policing, and more.[40] Once elected, he quickly cleaned shop, replacing Wagner's commissioners with his own.

By April 1966, Commissioner Anna Kross was the only original Wagner appointee remaining.[41] She summoned Douglas Lipton, along with the rest of her correctional chiefs for an all-hands meeting. "I'm leaving," she told them. "I'm seventy-five years old, and it's time to step down." She'd renewed her position twice already. "I'm not going to disappear," she assured the distraught faces around her—she would be available as a correctional consultant for the department. "You haven't seen the end of me," she joked. Lipton cheered and applauded along with the rest, but his mind was racing furiously. Losing Commissioner Kross was a blow for the department—and for his project. Without her championing the SSR, would it lose its departmental backing and status?

Her replacement was George F. McGrath, a forty-nine-year-old lawyer from Boston. Till last year, he'd worked as the corrections commissioner for Massachusetts before being fired ignominiously after a wave of scandals that included escape attempts[42] and inmate overdoses.[43] Rumors suggested that he was a penal reformist, but no one knew for certain. One thing they knew for sure: McGrath was not a New Yorker commented the dailies. This is what happens when you put a Republican in charge, another asserted. Would an outsider like McGrath care about the city the way Kross did? She'd grown up in the city's slums and lived and breathed New York. Why hadn't the new mayor chosen a local candidate? the papers demanded.

McGrath had been personally solicited by Mayor Lindsay, persuaded to leave his home city for $25,000 a year—a starting salary that was 25 percent higher than Kross's after twelve years on the job.[44] New Yorkers mourned her departure; her plain-speaking manner, brusque kindness, and willingness to call out her own department had won her fans at every level of society. "Thank you for your long, constructive, and rewarding service," Mayor Lindsay told her at McGrath's swearing-in ceremony.

Initially, it looked like the SSR team had been worrying unnecessarily. Commissioner McGrath was fascinated with the plastic surgery project and impressed that seventy-three ex-cons had received surgical treatment so far. He threw his support behind the project. "We have had interest from seventeen states and six foreign countries," he informed the press.

But the new commissioner's attention was quickly diverted elsewhere. Two months into his term, questions arose as to the legality of his hiring—McGrath had lived outside of New York when he was hired, and it appeared as though Mayor Lindsay had appointed him unlawfully.[45]

Lindsay disagreed, and to demonstrate his continued support for McGrath, he boosted his salary to $30,000, now 50 percent higher than his predecessor. Lindsay defended the raise. "We have to have this kind of talent," he said; according to him, the old salaries were "not competitive" with the paychecks that private businesses offered. McGrath was tight-lipped. His lack of comment spoke volumes to the SSR team; he'd support them during the good times but when things went south, he wouldn't have their back. By now, the team knew the question was *when*, rather than if, the next issue would arise.

Seven months after exiting Rikers Island, and six months and twenty-five days since his needle tracks were surgically removed, Bill Cooper hopped out of a yellow cab outside 64 University Place. Richard Kurtzberg was waiting on the sidewalk for him; he walked over to the cab, paid the driver, and then beckoned Cooper inside.

They traipsed up the stairs to the SSR's office, and Kurtzberg directed Cooper to a seat in the corner. There was a new desk in the office; after much cajoling, Lipton had used the remaining portion of the grant to hire some part-time

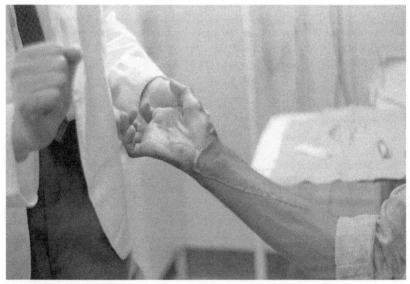

Photograph of inmate's needle track removal plastic surgery at Sing Sing Prison, 1961. *Courtesy of McGovern Historical Center, Texas Medical Center Library*

field aides, along with Carole Ferguson, their first female employee, a twenty-one-year-old school psychology student from New York University. Ferguson was a few years behind Kurtzberg in school but on the same track, and he'd recruited her to fill a part-time research assistant position.

Kurtzberg escorted Cooper to a seat by his desk and asked how he was feeling. Cooper shrugged. "My arm stings. It doesn't seem to be healing," he said, removing his jacket to reveal a crusted yellow bandage on his forearm. He peeled a small square back with a dirty finger, and a sour smell seeped out. Across the room, Carole Ferguson made a strangled sound and sneezed twice.

"Have you been following the aftercare provided?" Kurtzberg asked Cooper.

"Yes," Cooper said. He'd wrapped and rewrapped the wound, just like they'd said.

"So to be clear, you did *change* the bandages?"

"I rewrapped it!"

"I see." Kurtzberg sighed internally and fished in his desk drawer for the surgical supplies that Montefiore had sent them. "Why don't we rewrap it again, with some antiseptic, and this time, we'll use fresh bandages? It's best to change the bandages every time you rewrap the wound. You can take some of these home with you," he said patiently.

"Fine."

He gingerly peeled off the bandage, revealing the weeping wound beneath. There was no hint of the obscene tattoo and telltale needle tracks that had once covered Cooper's forearm, instead there was a glaring red, raised scar where a large strip of skin had been excised. The wound had been closed with stainless steel wire, and silk sutures held the skin in place as it healed. Dr. Lewin had warned Cooper—and Kurtzberg—of this outcome. Sometimes there were too many tracks to excise—in those cases, removal essentially required stripping the skin from the entire limb.

Kurtzberg painstakingly washed and dressed the wound, instructing Cooper to watch what he was doing so he could repeat it at home. Then he began the interview, moving through his checklist question by question.

"Age?"

"Thirty-one years old."

"Ethnic group?"

"Black."

"Occupation?"

"Artist."

"Marital status?"

"Married but separated six years ago. Would like to patch things up."

"You have been 'on the street' now a while. How many places other than [address given] have you lived since you got out?"

Cooper shrugged. "Maybe two," he said. "It depends. I don't always want to stay at my folks'."

"Now I'm going to ask you about your friends, y'know, guys you hang around with, go around with."

"Go ahead," Cooper said.

"How many of them did you first meet at Rikers Island? How many of them are working? How many of them are drug addicts?"

"A few have drug problems," Cooper admitted. But he'd known them a long time. He didn't hang out with anyone from Rikers.

Kurtzberg moved onto the final interview section reserved for ex-offenders from groups one and two only.[46]

"During your hospital stay, what do you feel was most pleasant?"

Cooper smiled. "It was wonderful," he said, his eyes lighting up. "The food was really good, the nurses were sweet, and there was space for me to paint. They even helped me get canvas and brushes."

Kurtzberg looked at his notes. Cooper had been housed in a four-person room in Montefiore Hospital, where there were plentiful amenities and activities, with radios and TVs in every lounge. No wonder it had felt like a vacation! Cooper had no formal art training but had enrolled in a training therapy program connected to an urban poverty agency, which included art.

"How do you feel it looks now? Are you pleased?"

"I've lost the self-consciousness I had before because of the tracks," Cooper told him. He covered the bandage with his jacket sleeve. "It's still healing," he said, "but people don't treat me like I'm a junkie; they ask how I'm feeling! I haven't touched the stuff all year."

When the interview was done, Kurtzberg shook his hand and escorted him to the door. "Come visit me if you like, doc," Cooper told him. "I'll do you a good rate on a painting."

Carole Ferguson was quiet as Cooper left, but as soon as the door closed behind him, she spoke up. "That terrible patch of skin on his arm . . . it looks so wrong," she told the team. "Just seeing it felt . . . I don't . . . I don't know if the surgeons cut corners because he's an ex-con, but . . . if they were really interested in the cosmetic aspect, you wouldn't do it that way."[47]

Kurtzberg acknowledged her comment but said nothing. Cavior looked up and then back down. Ferguson sighed, picked up her purse, and went outside for some fresh air. It felt good to get out of that dirty, dusty space. Not that the men cared, she thought. They seemed perfectly content to work in that filth—to change weeping bandages in that filth—to see that poor man's arm in that . . .

Ferguson walked around the small square, thinking furiously. When Kurtzberg had first told her about the job, she'd imagined that the office would be in a nice brownstone or perhaps a Soho-style glass paneled loft, something light filled and airy. It was within walking distance from her Fifth Avenue dorm, a high rise she shared with three other girls, and his offer felt like a great—and convenient—opportunity. Instead, she'd found herself outside a dilapidated building with cracks in the brickwork and scuffs where the paint had flaked off. She walked up the dark, narrow stairs and sat at the small desk assigned to her in the corner of the room. She looked around, taking in the overflowing ashtrays, wilted apple cores, and discarded coffee cups. A light layer of grime seemed to cover everything, and the windows were cloudy with dust.

Still, she'd been captivated by the concept of their research. She knew from experience how much one's looks impacted one's behavior toward others; she was a woman in a male-dominated field, after all! She'd experienced so many sexist microaggressions and inappropriate come-ons from strangers, students, and peers that she'd lost count. It was so easy for people to assume certain things about you because of how you looked. She'd been excited to study the effect of surgery on behavior . . . but now—now that she'd seen Cooper's arm and the other men and women's photographs—she wasn't so sure.

The overarching goals of the SSR project didn't mesh with the everyday workings of the study. She'd never considered just *how* a tattoo or needle track would be removed, but she hadn't expected huge, rectangular swaths of skin to be stripped from their forearms or back in the process.[48] Sure, there was no drug or gang stigma attached to those raw pieces of skin, but the quality of those procedures . . . seeing that open gaping skin on Cooper's arm had almost brought her breakfast up.

Inside the office, Cavior looked guiltily at his desk. Ferguson had a point about the aesthetic outcome. There *were* better, more visually pleasing ways to clear tattoos and scars; some lasers and acids were very effective at removal and created more acceptable levels of scarring. However, Dr. Lewin had made the call not to use these methods in treating the inmates—such techniques involved multiple sessions at periodic intervals that were dependent on the continued motivation and cooperation of the subject. "Therefore, they are not considered appropriate for this project," he'd informed them, despite calling the scars resulting from the excisions "conspicuous and unattractive." Nonetheless, Lewin still considered the ugly scar a net win, and it was hard to argue with his reasoning. "The concrete esthetic outcome of a procedure will be variously interpreted by the patients and surgeon," Lewin wrote in a memo. "The question of improvement is thus broadened to become one of whether surgical procedure will produce a significant change in societal reactions to the individual, as well as changes in the individual's perception of himself."

Lewin was looking at the big picture, but the members of the SSR team were focused on gathering the data. Dropouts were still an ongoing issue. Some ex-cons suddenly would go silent and unreachable for no obvious reasons. Others were so unhappy with their surgery that they refused to attend any more interviews. Even those with positive outcomes would stop checking in, busy with work or family or friends. Those cases, technically surgical success stories, had to be stripped from their data; without completing the follow-ups required, those individuals had invalidated themselves from the study. Their follow-ups were integral to the project's success—the data, not the anecdotal stories, would demonstrate the success or failure of the experiment. And despite Kross's wishes and the push they'd made in the women's jails, it was becoming clear that this would be a study of male prisoners. Almost forty women had received surgery, but sign-ups remained low; their data could not be included in their final tally.

Other times, despite the SSR team's best efforts, the data was not as "clean" as they'd like it, thanks to men like Jose Rodriguez, a small-time burglar who'd requested tattoo removal. He'd been assigned to the surgery-only group but as part of his admission had been visited by one of the team's social workers. He'd shared his cigarettes, and when Rodriguez recovered, he tracked the man down and badgered him to find Rodriguez a job.

"I'm sorry, but you have not been assigned to receive extra vocational services," the worker informed him, but Rodriguez was persistent. "You got my friend a factory job," he said, referencing another SSR subject in the surgery-and-services group. "I want a job like that. Help me, too, friend." The worker initially resisted, but Rodriguez was tenacious, and he eventually called the factory and placed him. "He wore me down," the worker told Kurtzberg. "I'm a human being, how could I say no?"

Sadly, they cut Rodriguez's data from their study.

⌒⌒

Most summers, Lewin packed in volunteering expeditions to Eastern Europe, South Vietnam, and Israel, where he worked with war-wounded men and women and children with facial deformities. The days were grueling but necessary; when he saw the glazed looks and blackened, flaking skin of small children, he couldn't *not* be there.[49] He spent two months in Vietnam, working with Medico, a nonprofit medical foundation, training local surgeons and performing necessary plastic surgery operations. He was shaken by the wounds he saw; 20 percent of civilian casualties were children! Their injuries were worse than those on the battlefields of World War I. "The images of badly burned children with shattered faces and limbs stayed with me a long time," he wrote to a friend in New York. "My duties gave me so much satisfaction that I did not get tired."

There was drama brewing when he returned to Montefiore. During his daily rounds, the head nurse pulled him aside.[50]

"There's . . . an issue with one of the convict patients," she confided.

"Ex-con," Lewin reminded her.

"Yes, uh, ex-con patients."

"Well?"

"It's about Dennis, Dennis Jordan."

"Oh, Dennis." Lewin was pleased with how the young man's operation had gone; he'd slimmed his nose, built up his chin with a bone graft, and smoothed his skin. He'd healed very nicely, and the change was quite remarkable. "Yes, he's quite the success story."

The nurse twisted her hands. "That's . . . yes . . . well, that's sort of the problem."

Lewin looked at her.

"Well, Dennis is . . . his . . . his appearance is much improved," she told him. "We all think so. All the nursing staff do." She looked meaningfully at him.

He tilted his head to one side, puzzled.

The nurse sighed. "Well, maybe one of us—she's not on shift right now—thinks that a little bit too much."

"Oh." Lewin's eyes widened. The news threw him, but the more he thought about it, the better he felt. Jordan had asked to be "Kirk Douglas" attractive, and if the nurses agreed, well, that was proof his work had been successful.

"Well, uh, keep me informed," he said. "Very good."

The SSR team had planned for a six-month and a twelve-month follow-up with their subjects; however, the various delays made it clear that that was only achievable with a project extension. Lipton filed for a grant extension: "The need for this extra time . . . [is] to permit testing for statistically significant differences between our four groups."[51]

In July, the Department of Health, Education, and Welfare in Washington, D.C., awarded the project an additional $124,118. The new round of funding gave them some flexibility with their outreach. They switched from cajoling and pleading the ex-cons to attend follow-ups to offering them a $10 fee for participation, paid on arrival. This was not a bribe, the staff explained—it was because they understood that the men might have to miss work or lose income due to the interview. Attendance rose accordingly, but even this incentive only cut the attrition rate from 30 percent to 20 percent. Lipton fretted about the numbers; hundreds of men and forty women had now had surgery, but less than a quarter of them could be counted in their final tally. He hoped the Vocational Rehabilitation Administration (VRA) did not regret funding this project.

However, in Washington, D.C., the VRA had bigger issues to worry about than Lipton's small plastic surgery project. For the last couple of years, the organization poured money into various rehabilitative research projects, and so far, it had little return on its investment. Even when there was a good result, the programs were rarely ever replicated, which frustrated Commissioner Mary Switzer to no end. What was the point of funding these findings if the groundbreaking discoveries they uncovered remained siloed—making them basically useless?[52]

What was the point of developing programs and collecting their data if she wasn't able to scale it? she wondered. Some early-stage projects based around housing and delinquency troubles had shown remarkable results, but no one was utilizing this potential. No outside organizations used that data to shape their own offerings.

To shake this up, Switzer formed the Research Utilization Task Force, charging the team with identifying and analyzing the most significant studies published in corrections.[53] They were to develop a large-scale plan of action about how to best integrate those findings into corrections as a whole.[54]

Generally within the administration, it's common for the commissioner to take a backseat when task forces are formed. Switzer disagreed, worried that if she wasn't hands-on, she'd re-create the issue she was trying to avoid: another arm of the government cut off from its brain. Instead, she took a different tack.

Not only was her task force instructed to assemble and analyze the various studies, but they were required to file a monthly progress report as well. With one caveat: their reports needed to be written in a very particular manner, she decreed. She wanted to see research summaries of each study assessed as well as actionable recommendations—and these briefs were to be kept to a maximum of two pages. *Two pages*, she repeated. Their reports would be circulated to all staff, in and out of the department. The task force was befuddled by her directives, but she was firm.

Switzer kindly explained her reasoning: it was straightforward, she told them. Researchers—no offense!—were a wordy bunch, and she knew that correctional staff, social workers, and all other arms of the bureau disliked wading through reams of reports.[55] Keeping them trim and tight would, she hoped, mean that the team's findings would, at the very least, be skimmed by the people she was trying to reach. "Practitioners can keep abreast of research despite little time for reading," her research director noted.

Despite the popularity of the shortened reports and the task force's diligence, six months on, few of their recommendations had been implemented.

# 9

# CHANGING PLACES
# AND FACES

Beautified Ex-Convicts Repeat Less—*New York Times*, 1966[1]

Does the Face Make the Criminal?—*Observer Sun*, 1967[2]

L ife was very different when you were thin, mused Fred Marshall, as he strolled down 125th Street in Harlem. He wasn't thin-thin, but compared to his previous 280-pound bulk, he felt lighter than he had in years. His torso was still crisscrossed with bright red scars, but he'd been promised they'd fade over time. They looked less obvious on Black skin than white, he told himself; one time that being Black was a bonus! In all other ways, his Blackness worked against him.

No one in New York City was hiring; at least, they weren't hiring *him*. Fat *or* thin. Small wonder 40 percent of Blacks in New York lived below the poverty line compared to 12 percent of whites. Storekeepers eyed Marshall suspiciously and security guards trailed him in stores. Everyone was on edge. Cities across the country were imploding. Marshall was turned down for one job after another. They were mostly factory jobs, the kind of gigs he wasn't really that interested in, but it was frustrating to get rejection after rejection. Bored and broke, he stared at the four walls of the room he'd been allocated, struggling to sleep. It was a hot summer, and his room reeked of body odor and stale smoke. The honks and hums of the streets seeped through the thin walls. He woke up feeling tired and unsettled.

With nothing to do, he aimlessly walked the neighborhood until he reached a certain street corner and shambled to a stop. Surely one small hit wouldn't hurt? Just a small one to help pass the time, till one of those jobs called back with an offer? He'd been so good for so long—one wouldn't hurt, would it? Marshall shot up in a small alleyway just off the main drag and leaned against the door frame as the drugs flooded his system. He shut his eyes, waiting for that familiar blur to overtake him. *This is the last time*, he vowed, but two days later he was back there again. And again.

Marshall reenrolled in another detoxification program but quit after a few days. Around 80 percent of people in the program were under eighteen! It was pointless, he told his caseworker. What was the benefit to staying clean? He'd tried that, and look where it had got him. He felt bad about disappointing the Surgical and Social Rehabilitation (SSR) project staff; they'd been so kind and were the first who'd seen him as a person, not a number, in a long time—but they were just two nice white men who didn't get it. They couldn't help with the systemic racism and injustice that ruled America. Two weeks later, he was arrested for possession and sent back to Rikers Island.[3]

The SSR team were notified of Marshall's drug relapse and readmission to Rikers Island. They were all disappointed. He'd shown so much promise. They felt like they'd managed to reach him, to help him. Douglas Lipton took the news particularly hard. He'd been wondering if it was foolish to attempt surgical work on addicts in general. The experiment was about improving one's self-image and, with that, social acceptance. Though personal appearance mattered to addicts, *nothing* mattered to them as much as their drugs. With addicts making up such a large proportion of Rikers Island inmates—and inmates in jails and prisons across America and abroad—he was unsure if their plastic surgery project could effect any change for this population.

The precise causes for addiction were also unclear to him. He understood what drew people to drugs: lack of opportunity, poverty, and so on, but why were some men able to take one hit and put it down and others with similar economic backgrounds were catapulted into a downward spiral? Lipton dusted off his graduate school textbooks and skimmed the pages on addiction and delinquency. One data point stood out to him: how someone was raised seemed to have the largest corresponding impact as to whether he or she would develop an addictive personality. Trauma, especially during childhood, had a significant influence on later-life behavior.

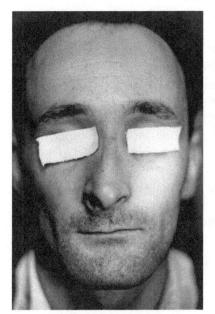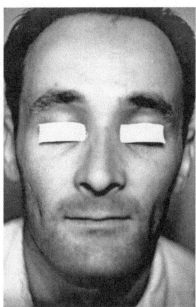

Before and after Rikers Island rhinoplasty. *Courtesy of the Archives at Montefiore Medical Center*

"There's a connection there," he told his friends over dinner one night. Intrigued, they asked him to expound on his theory at their local Toastmasters club—they're always looking for articulate speakers, they said. Lipton happily accepted; he found community feedback and discussions a helpful way to identify the crux of a problem. In front of a hundred or so people in the Teaneck Toastmaster's club, he explored the genesis of juvenile delinquents and drug addicts. "Broken homes are not always responsible . . . but more often than not, a child from an unhappy home gets into trouble," he said.[4] "Parents should give their children a set of values of what is right from wrong."

More invitations followed, and Lipton found himself a regular on the community circuit, lecturing about addiction in an American Legion Hall one night[5] and police brutality toward addicts at the Democratic Club on another.[6] It was a refreshing change to be involved in this type of education, to spend a few hours without worrying if his subjects were following their surgical aftercare program or causing trouble at the hospital. A few weeks before, an inmate at the Women's House of Detention had asked for breast enlargement surgery, and he'd turned her down; she already had a pair of breasts and that type of cosmetic work wasn't covered by their experiment. She'd looked so deflated when he'd said no.[7] Lectures and conferences were a great way to keep his mind occupied.

Psychologists weren't supposed to let their work life bleed into their home life, but everyone did, a little.

Then Governor Nelson Rockefeller's office reached out. Lipton had met some of his staff at a recent criminological conference, but he wasn't sure what the fifty-nine-year-old governor of New York wanted. Still, you didn't say no when he called. They met downtown. The governor was shorter than he expected—he looked taller on television—but he cut an imposing figure, a well-tailored double-breasted suit draping his broad shoulders. He gave Lipton a wide smile when he saw him. "Hi, fella," he said. "I've heard good things about you."

The governor cut straight to the point. "I want to stamp out New York's drug problem," he told him, "and I'm assembling a team of the best criminal and addiction experts to do that." Last year he'd established the Governors Special Committee on Crime Offenders to explore innovative approaches to recidivism, community participation, and to draft new legislation.[8] "It will be a lot of work," he warned, "but you'll be making a difference on a much bigger scale." He offered Lipton the position of assistant director of crime control planning. "Think it over," his aides said. "Let us know soon." "Of course," Lipton replied, stunned.

Lipton considered the offer on his drive home. Rockefeller was a Republican, whereas he voted Democrat, but the governor was a *moderate* Republican, so that could be okay. He turned the idea over and over in his head. He didn't want to let the SSR team down, but they were getting closer to endgame every day. He had to think about what his career would look like once the project was completed. He was paid more than Chaneles, but he could already see that his pay was unlikely to increase, the new commissioner suffering the same funding cuts that Commissioner Kross had to deal with.

Meanwhile, the governor had become a force to be reckoned with in New York City's corrections circuit. He'd passed one bill that extended parole to all county jails and another that allowed first offenders the vote.

Lipton was still mulling the job offer over later that week when the phone rang in his office; it was Sydney Schanberg from the *New York Times*.[9] Somehow, Schanberg had gotten ahold of the SSR's monthly reports and was publishing a story about their plastic surgery project. Would Lipton like to comment?

"It's too early—we're still gathering our data," Lipton told him, but Schanberg was insistent. "Tell me about some of the cases," he asked. "Was anyone excluded based on their offense?"

"No one was excluded," Lipton told him. "The only people we cut were those who didn't pass the physical or psychological screens."

"I'd like to know more about your data," Schanberg said, scanning the report. "It says here that preliminary results indicate that disfigured inmates who do not receive surgery recidivate at a 10 percent higher rate than those with surgery?"

"That's correct," Lipton replied, "however, we believe the difference may be larger if we exclude the addicts in the study. We don't do as well with addicts, because they have a compulsion we can't do anything for," he added.

"Are you seeing a correlation between appearance and criminality?"

"A guy may have started in crime before he got his scar," Lipton said. "But if there is any rehabilitative chance for him, it certainly is handicapped by his disfigurement."

The story ran on the front page of the *New York Times* on Monday, August 22, 1966.[10]

It sealed the deal for Lipton. He rang Rockefeller's office; he'd be honored to accept the position, he said.

~~

Dear Father,

I was sentenced for two years for theft. I am very bitter because I feel I was sentenced wrong. Without a lawyer, aid, or anything I just left from doing four months and I was out four weeks. Why did I go back to drugs and prost[itution]? Because when I left here I had no money nor anything and these people put me in the streets like an animal. With nowhere to go and no one to turn to I had to go back to my old friends, and what have you, please help me.—Ethel Cooley, 11th floor dorm, Women's House of Detention, 1965[11]

~~

With Lipton gone, Richard Kurtzberg assumed control of the SSR project—and the backlash that went with the role. The project now had three directors in less than three years—not a good look. The *New York Times* article was just the start; it prompted a deluge of news stories about the still-unfinished study, which led to a number of crank calls and letters. Some were vicious. "How can you take this valuable surgery and give it away to rotten scumbags?" a man with a rumbling Midwest accent complained. "You should be ashamed of yourselves. I don't know how you can sleep at night."[12]

Kurtzberg learned to ignore the negative feedback. He didn't let it bother him; the overall response had been positive. There was always grumbling about how inmates received benefits that "honest" folk didn't, but generally this talk was from the people who didn't differentiate between sending someone to prison as a punishment versus sending them to prison to *be* punished. Across America, the latter group was getting louder.

"Federal judges and the U.S. Supreme Court insist on coddling the criminal," complained fifty-six-year-old Kenneth Donecker in the reader's letters section of the *Fort-Worth Star Telegram*.[13] "Let us put an end to this farce." The media stirred the pot as well. "The philosophy that the criminal must be protected from the consequences of his own acts, even at the expense of society, is making great advances in the current state legislature," slammed an editorial in the *Post-Standard*.[14]

Kurtzberg's full attention focused on assembling, cleaning, and crunching the project data. Montefiore Hospital was still admitting new patients from Rikers Island, but the cutoff point for the study had passed—anyone treated after October 1966 would not be included in their data. Their study design was based on a six-month and twelve-month follow-up, and there was not enough time to include late additions. A shame, he thought, seeing as how they'd just about got it running smoothly now, but it couldn't be helped.

He tasked research assistant Carole Ferguson to chase down leads, and most of her time was spent making call after call to locate their absentee subjects. She worked her way down the list, ringing social workers, welfare officers, and the hospital administrator to confirm appointments, attendance, behavior, and any changes in address. From there, she cross-referenced the Department of Correction to see if any new offenses had occurred, documenting each call with meticulous notes. It was a monotonous process; necessary, she knew, but the daily grind wore her down. She comforted herself with the bigger picture: after all, it was *always* the funny-looking kids that were picked on at the playground. No wonder they lashed out as adults! She'd acclimatized to the graphic photographs that accompanied most files, the pages of weeping skin and raw, red flesh, but occasionally a new picture appeared that made her stomach clench.

But it's necessary, she reassured herself—weren't the papers constantly going on about the increase in crime and all the horrible things happening in the city since Mayor John Lindsay took the reins? Crime in New York City was up 6.5 percent from last year[15]—or maybe even higher. It was hard to know what to believe. The police commissioner told the press that New York City crime rose a "statistical 72.1 percent" in 1966. Sure, he'd attributed the spike to the rollout of their new data-reporting tool, but even so. Meanwhile, the FBI attributed the increase in violence to the ease of access to firearms.[16] Ferguson just wanted to feel safe in her city!

For all the commotion about New York's spiking crime rate, Norman Cavior hadn't really noticed much change in the neighborhoods he frequented. The same bums lay around in Union Square, panhandling or shooting up, the same decaying tenements teetered on the brink of collapse in Lower East Side, the same trash and graffiti covered the city's sidewalks where he lived in Queens. There was still economic poverty, addiction, discrimination—despite the civil rights movement, it felt like much of New York remained segregated down color lines, with whites firmly at the top. It was always one step forward and two steps back. New York State *finally* struck down vagrancy—"being without visible means of support"—as a crime, declaring it unconstitutional, and the next week it was all "compulsory rehabilitation," with talk of addicts being forcefully committed to maximum security units for detoxing.[17] In both cases, Black men were affected disproportionately.

Most Wednesdays at around 8:00 p.m., Cavior headed to the Palladium Ballroom, between East Fourteenth Street and Third Avenue, to blow off steam on the dance floor. Wednesday nights were generally salsa, with some Latin and Dominican fusion thrown in. It was a mostly Hispanic crowd, but they were friendly—anyone who was happy losing themselves to the beat was fine in their book. They kept the lights low and the music loud. Whenever Cavior danced, he forgot about his problems; for a brief, beautiful time, it was just him, the music, and his dance partner. One week, the Palladium announced a special guest, a Cuban vocalist with the most fantastic range. Cavior lost himself in her voice as he whirled around the room, hot, sweaty, and happy.[18]

Then the room pitched into darkness, all the lights blinking out as one. The music stopped midbeat. He froze, awkwardly scanning the room to understand what was happening. He could hear thuds and shouts, and a man near him dropped something heavy on the floor. Then the house lights turned on, and he blinked; everywhere he looked, there was a uniformed cop. They stood against the walls, walked across the emptying dance floor, climbed onto the bandstand, all dressed in their crisp New York Police Department blues. Some knelt to collect the dropped items—he caught a glimpse of a knife and a gun in their evidence bags—while even more cops were patting men down against a wall.

On stage, the Cuban singer was protesting something they'd told her, her delicate arms waving in the air, but the officers didn't react. Sullenly, she held out her hands to be cuffed, and they walked her haltingly out the venue. "Immigración," someone whispered. Cavior swallowed, smoothed down the front of his shirt, and walked toward the exit. A few officers looked him up and down as he passed, but they waved him on—*he* wasn't their target. Later, as he revved his motorbike across the Williamsburg Bridge, he realized the police had stopped only the Hispanic and Black revelers.

Racist discrimination and color bias had become a serious issue in the SSR experiment. Three days after one of their subjects, Kenneth Smith, a twenty-five-year-old Black man, was discharged from Montefiore Hospital, a white bandage taped across his healing nasal bones, he was arrested for consorting and taken to jail. Smith was outraged by the cop's accusation. He'd been sitting on a park bench and catching up with his brother—not doing anything nefarious, he told the SSR staff. They held him overnight before releasing him and dismissing the charge, but Smith was shaken. His face was still bruised from his operation, his eyes ringed in yellow and purple, and his cheeks swollen. He wasn't in any condition to push back, he told them. The fellow in the cell next to his had complained, and he'd seen two officers drag him out and beat him with their nightsticks. "You can call us when something like this happens," the SSR staffers told him, horrified by his treatment. "You should never have been arrested."

A few weeks after that incident, Smith, now free of his bandages, was lined up inside a welfare center, hoping to persuade them to increase his benefits when two women in line began screaming at one another. One woman grabbed the other's hair and tried to swing her around by it, and the other retaliated by raking her nails down the woman's arm. A small crowd gathered around the brawling pair. Administrators called the police to break up the tussle. The cops separated the women, cuffed them—and then arrested Smith, as well, on the charge of "disorderly conduct." Two days later, Smith went to court for his hearing. "I arrested him because he looked guilty," explained the officer. The judge, a white man in his mid-fifties, laughed and dismissed the charge.[19]

"The general white community has told us in a million different ways that God and nature made a mistake when it came to the fashioning of us and ours," wrote Abbey Lincoln in the *Negro Digest*.[20] "At best, we are made to feel we are poor imitations and excuses for white women."

Other SSR participants shared similar stories. A number in the services-only group complained about police harassment, both verbal and physical. They weren't doing anything, they said—just minding their own business. A few times, the team were able to track down the harassing officers and interview them. The cops tended to be defensive, saying the subject had seemed suspicious and they were just doing their job, but a few commented that the men's facial scars or caved-in noses had initially raised their concerns.

This behavior was reflective of the overall state of affairs in America. After centuries of abuse, people were pushing back against police brutality and entrenched racism. In July 1967, a Black cab driver in Newark—about a twenty-five-minute drive from Michael Lewin's home—was pulled over for a traffic violation and arrested by white cops. They beat him so badly that they had to drag him by his legs into the station. This sparked a five-day protest that escalated into urban warfare, with fire bombing, snipers roaming the streets, and looting, as residents cowered in their homes. The police were issued shotguns and ordered to "fire when necessary." It left twenty-six people dead and 1,100 injured and caused $10 million in damages.[21] Similar riots took place in Spanish Harlem, Chicago, and Los Angeles.

Dr. Michael Lewin was horrified by the violence on both sides. He supported the protesters but condemned the violence. When he received the SSR's debrief about Kenneth Smith and other subjects he felt guilty. This is how he was treated, someone who'd *had* plastic surgery? What about all the inmates who'd requested it but had been directed into the nonsurgery groups? It wasn't fair that the men who, through no fault of their own, had randomly not been allocated plastic surgery were suffering the consequences of their own faces, when he could have helped them.

Twelve hundred miles from New York, in a small surgical office in Kansas City, plastic surgeon Dr. Frank W. Masters was mulling his next move. So far, he had spent his career jumping from one random interest to the next; he'd done a deep dive into the physiology of people struck by lightning,[22] analyzed the benefits of bioreagents in surgery, and examined in vitro immunity to tetanus.[23] It was time to turn his attention to something new.

During the last few years, Masters had noticed an uptick of cosmetic surgery clients requesting tiny defect corrections: a nasal bridge that was 0.01 percent higher than preferred or a jaw that wasn't perfectly symmetrical. It was puzzling—his services were not cheap, and it seemed like a lot of expense for such a subtle change. "The aphorism, a man's face is his fortune, reflects society's constant attention to the overall affect created by personal appearance," he wrote in the *Journal of the Kansas Medical Society*.[24] "Social reflection may also be predicated on appearance. The weak chin is widely accepted as evidence of weakness of character."

For Masters, the requests for these minor, insignificant changes signified something larger, the greater attention that people were paying to their physical appearance. Masters believed that these feelings of inferiority had been carefully crafted and fanned by corporations in order to benefit from people's insecurities.

"The multibillion dollar cosmetic industry has molded public opinion by a constant flood of advertising, until the entire nation has become so cognizant of the effect of appearance, that all facets of society spend a considerable portion of their earnings in this constant search for beauty of face and figure," he commented.

He ended his journal article with an observation on the state of the world. "Since society tends to deny its prejudices, those affected with aesthetic deformity soon become well aware of hostile social attitudes but are unable to combat these prejudices."

It was the ultimate catch-22, he thought; the less attractive were treated poorly because of their looks, but people refused to admit that their bias had made them act so, attributing their behavior to an imagined "fault" about that person. He'd seen this play out, time and time again, when angry, sullen patients metamorphosed into smiling, charming adults once their ears or nose or breasts had been altered. There was a clear psychosocial element to his work—but that was often pooh-poohed by those who attributed it to vanity alone.

This is what he would explore next, he decided: whether he could find a way to conclusively demonstrate appearance bias. He reached out to the psychiatry department at the University of Kansas to gauge interest in collaborating. He clicked with psychiatrist Donald Greaves, whose research also veered toward the more esoteric end of the spectrum. Greaves had investigated phantom pregnancy, narcissists, and music therapy. It was a perfect match. Together, they plotted how to best measure appearance-based social rejection. They settled on criminals as a substratum of society that were broadly demonized.

They sourced male and female mug shots from five police departments across Miami, Baltimore, Los Angeles, Kansas City, and St. Louis, collecting some 11,285 photographs in total. Next, they catalogued any and all facial deformities displayed in the pictures, which included facial scars, crooked or broken noses, protruding ears, acne, receding chins, and more. They cross-referenced their data against seven thousand photographs of the general public; 60 percent of mug shots featured a facial defect compared to 20 percent of the public photos.

The mug shots were then categorized into different criminal "buckets" to assess if certain features related to specific criminal activity. The results were surprising: 43.7 percent of murderers had facial defects, the most common features being protruding ears, nasal deformities, and recessive chins.

Rapists also rated high on the scale, with 61.5 percent having facial defects, with large ears, acne, facial scars, and weak chins being the most common. Masters also looked at suicides, which he considered a "complex act of self-aggression." The data was startling. He found that 70 percent of suicides (attempted and otherwise) had facial defects. Many within this group had referenced their unhappiness with their face or body in their suicide notes. *Would cosmetic surgery have given them the will to live?* he wondered. They coined their investigation the Quasimodo complex, in reference to the hunchback of Notre Dame, and published their results in the *British Journal of Plastic Surgery*, complete with illustrative bar charts.[25] "It's by no means conclusive, but the increased incidence of disfigurement among the criminals evaluated gives some objective credence to the Quasimodo complex as a clinical entity," they wrote. "Modern society has placed such a premium on appearance that those afflicted with aesthetic deformity become well aware of hostile social attitudes."

Even with these caveats, Masters worried about how his work might be interpreted. He didn't want people to assume he was promoting the existence of Lombroso-like "criminal types." "By no means can this be interpreted as evidence that an individual's facial defect led him into a specific crime," he wrote. "The 40 percent overall differential in incidence is significant evidence only that a difference between the general public and the criminal exists."

Satisfied with his analysis, Masters moved on to his next project, designing a new treatment for burn victims, unaware of the penological tornado he'd created.

~~~~

[A]mong the criminals evaluated, [it] gives some objective credence to the thesis that the Quasimodo complex exists as a clinical entity.—*Abstracts on Criminology and Penology*[26]

American plastic surgeons have been trying to put the matter on to a more scientific footing.—*The New Scientist*[27]

[F]rom America comes a piece of criminological research which suggests there is a correlation between facial deformities and criminality.—*Justice of the Peace and Local Government Review*[28]

Does the Face Make the Criminal?—*The Observer*[29]

The furor surrounding the "Quasimodo complex" was the *last* thing that Richard Kurtzberg needed. The whole point of the SSR study was that it was based on science and logic, but the Masters and Greaves paper—although appearing statistically accurate (they hadn't included their methodology or how they'd correlated their data)—was a return to the nineteenth-century premise of eugenics and the notion of the "born criminal." Even with their caveat and acknowledgment that most deformities were *not* congenital, their work still hit close enough to home to be uncomfortable.

But there wasn't time to entertain the impact the paper might have on the penological and political arena. It was crunch time for the project, and Kurtzberg was swamped. Carole Ferguson had quit due to a heavy college course load and with Lipton gone, he was severely short-staffed. With pages of data to drill through, Kurtzberg, Cavior, and Lewin entreated their wives to help, and as a group they compiled, calculated, and rechecked their data.

"We are particularly grateful for the professional and technical assistance offered by family members," Kurtzberg wrote on the project's acknowledgments page. "Helene Cavior aided in data analysis, Berta Lewin reviewed manuscripts, and Evelyn Kurtzberg provided psychological consultation." By July 27, 1967, they'd crafted a 192-page preliminary report that covered their three-year Surgical and Social Rehabilitation of Adult Offenders study.

Their report was detailed enough that Wallace Mandell, now lead investigator on the project, felt comfortable presenting it during a two-day correctional research seminar in Washington, D.C., hosted by the Vocational Rehabilitation Administration.[30] Commissioner Switzer had invited the top penal researchers in America to attend, hoping that their collectively shared wisdom would broaden the field.

The silver-haired Switzer opened the seminar with some well-chosen remarks. "We need desperately to make our correctional system truly correctional," she told the attendees. "Ineffective programs must be discarded. New programs must be developed and tested. We must find out what works and what does not work to rehabilitate offenders. It is time to capture this elusive paradise. The primary objective of this meeting is to identify broad areas for research and to discuss how this research can be stimulated and conducted."

Mandell listened intently as his peers shared their progress. A statewide survey on public crime was underway, as requested by President Johnson under the auspices of Switzer's organization. In Portland, there was an alcoholic offender project, and in Tulsa, delinquency was being tackled with a supervised study program in schools. Here, the researchers admitted there had been difficulties beyond the students' behavioral problems; generally, their holdup was administrative "middlemen" who didn't communicate properly with outside agencies.

Mandell grimaced sympathetically; he knew what that was like! Then it was his turn at the podium. In the audience, George F. McGrath, New York City's latest corrections commissioner leaned forward in his chair, eager to hear the latest on the project.

Mandell cleared his throat and launched into a brief overview of their study. "We set out to answer the question: can a program of rehabilitation services be developed around cosmetic surgery for offenders?" he said.[31] "We started off with the hypothesis that surgical and social rehabilitation would cut down on recidivism." They'd intentionally chosen Rikers Island subjects, he explained; much of the recent correctional research ignored the jail population, believing that the average six- to nine-month terms weren't long enough to rehabilitate someone.

"However, it wasn't the jail setting that proved most challenging," he continued; it was finding the right personnel and interagency cooperation. It's not just inmates who are stigmatized, he explained—so too are the people who work in corrections.[32] "Agencies fear that by dealing with prison institutions or its inmate population, they too will be stigmatized." Wry smiles appeared on the faces in the audience, and Mandell nodded in acknowledgment. "We need to address this problem," he continued. "It is wasteful for single agencies to attempt evaluative research alone."[33]

Then he smiled broadly. "But that's not what you want to hear about right now, is it? You want to know the results, albeit the preliminary ones, of the plastic surgery project." Heads nodded in agreement. "Through monumental effort, we now have complete and corroborated follow-up appointments on 168 subjects," he announced. "Lo and behold, recidivism in the surgery group is 49 percent during the one-year follow-up. In the nonsurgery group, it is 66 percent." Mandell smiled self-consciously as the room broke into applause. "The aftermath of this study is yet to be seen," he continued—the full results and a detailed statistical analysis would be presented in December.

Commissioner Switzer was pleased to hear Mandell's update. She hoped for positive outcomes for all of her projects but knew that wasn't always the possible. His good news was the clincher she'd needed to push her rehabilitative agenda during Congress's appropriations hearings. She'd requested an additional $3.2 million to fund 130 new projects.[34]

"Miss Switzer, would you be good enough to justify for us the fascinating provision of plastic surgery for facial disfigurement?" asked Senator Jacob Javits, during the Department of Labor, Health, Education, and Welfare hearings.

"It was surprising to discover the number of people in prisons and reformatories, particularly young people, whose delinquency appears to be very directly related to some physical disability. Our project is not only physically successful, but also psychologically," she replied. "It has been tremendously successful."

"I approve enormously," Javitz said, motioning for her to elaborate.

Montefiore was not the only plastic surgery recidivism project, Switzer explained. "Georgia, for example, has for a number of years taken cases out of the federal penitentiary in Atlanta that need plastic surgery and provided it. Other states have been doing it, too, but the Montefiore project can be looked at as an example of what can be accomplished through this method."

By December 1967, the SSR dataset in its entirety had been compiled. One of Montefiore Hospital's largest conference rooms was reserved, and invitations to correctional rehabilitation researchers, sociologists, psychologists, wardens, officers, and analysts were mailed across the United States and Canada. It was showtime.

Early Wednesday morning, on the December 6, 1967, more than seventy plastic surgeons, sociologists, and corrections workers descended on New York City, their ties ironed, trousers pressed, and shoes shined, ready to attend the inaugural three-day event: the Montefiore Conference on Correctional Plastic Surgery. Dr. Frank Masters flew in from Kansas City, and Dr. Edward Lewison flew in from Vancouver, in addition to representatives from prison plastic surgery programs in Texas, North Carolina, Minnesota, Oregon, Ohio, California, and Michigan. It was a veritable who's who of the plastic surgery prison space.

Douglas Lipton and Richard Kurtzberg stood near the front of the room and exchanged excited grins. There was something uniquely wonderful about seeing a research project to fruition. And what better way to do so than with the world's first correctional cosmetic surgery conference? Lipton was attending in a dual role; both as a representative from the governor's criminal committee and as SSR's former director. Once all the guests had arrived, the weak coffee refilled, and basic pleasantries exchanged, people began shuffling to their seats.

William Usdane, the assistant commissioner from the U.S. Department of Health, Education, and Welfare, walked onto the stage to present the keynote address. "Miss Mary E. Switzer sends warm greetings to the conference," he said; unfortunately, she'd been swept into Senate meetings and would be unable to join them. He gave the assembled a rundown of their three-day itinerary: the proceedings would be a mixture of speakers, paper presentations, and small breakout groups.

"We hope that this conference will give us a model for the future," he concluded. There was polite applause, which rose in volume when the next speaker stood: Dr. Michael Lewin, who smiled genially at the crowd.

"In this day and age, plastic surgeons must learn to cooperate with behavioral scientists in tackling social ills," he declared. "Physical defects can be a strong contributive factor in antisocial behavior . . . [but] the causes of antisocial behavior are multiple and interrelated. The physical factor is obviously but one aspect of this many-faceted problem. What is important is an objective evaluation of the effectiveness of these programs. Is this approach significant enough to warrant the investment of public funds?"[35]

He walked the audience through his work at Sing Sing then launched into the reasoning behind the Rikers study. "The claims of success in the literature are most divergent," he explained. "Most of the authors report a reduction in recidivism rate, although there are wide discrepancies," hence the reason for the SSR and its strict control groups and demographic data collection.[36]

He smiled, retrieved his reading glasses from his pocket, and broke down the data. The team had used chi-square, z-tests, and Fisher's exact tests to measure the statistical differences among the groups. Due to the number of addicts enrolled, they had separated the data in their final analysis.

"The nonaddict group showed clear gains following surgery," he announced; those who'd received plastic surgery alone had a recidivism rate of 30 percent compared to 56 percent of the control group. The plastic surgery and vocational services group had a 33 percent recidivism rate. There had been some surprises, he admitted: for one, the services-only cohort had an 89 percent recidivism rate. Combined, the recidivism rate for plastic surgery treatment was 32 percent compared to 65 percent for the nonsurgical groups.

A murmur of confusion ran through the room. Lewin directed their attention to external research findings assembled by Kurtzberg and Lipton, which reported that similar kinds of counseling and placement techniques could have a null or even negative effect when applied to problem populations. They'd estimated that would be the cause of the increase in offenses for the services-only cohort.

There were no statistically significant reductions for addicts who received plastic surgery, he continued, but they had found, generally speaking, that the addicts who had their facial defects removed tended to recidivate less than those who had their needle tracks excised. The majority of former offenders was, at minimum, partially satisfied with the work, he concluded.

Douglas Lipton replaced Lewin onstage to provide the economic breakdown of their project. "The cost of plastic surgery is estimated at $575 per case, or $57,500 for one hundred cases, based on a six-day hospital stay with no fee to the surgeon," he said. The data showed that an estimated two hundred of New York City's inmates would both desire and be accepted for plastic surgery on any given day. "These findings have practical, as well as scientific significance," he added; New York City paid $4,577 a year to house one inmate, or $457,700 a year to house one hundred inmates. "If plastic surgery were administered to one hundred nonaddict disfigured inmates, the best estimate is that only thirty-two of them would return as compared with sixty-eight of one hundred without surgery." The cost of maintaining the additional thirty-six prisoners would be $164,416.60 for one year. "The resultant savings to society, in only one year, would already be far more than the cost of plastic surgery."[37]

There were no major findings in the other areas, he added; plastic surgery had not played a major role in the ex-cons' subsequent employment status, though 32 percent of subjects who had gained work reported an increase in salary compared to 19 percent of the control group. "It's not statistically significant, but it is encouraging." There had been some small differences in recidivism behavior based on the race of the participants: Black men who received plastic surgery, from both the addict and nonaddict groups, had a 22 percent lower recidivism rate than the control group, whereas white subjects dropped only 13 percent.[38]

Over lunch, Lipton found himself besieged with more questions. He answered as many as he could. Yes, they had started with a much bigger sample size: 663 inmates had passed the physical screens, but due to significant dropouts (explained in the report!) they'd lost 123 men after they'd completed their surgeries, and 213 additional surgically approved subjects had quit during the psychological screens. Yes, he did think there was a real benefit. No, he didn't think there would be former cons on the catwalk! Yes, undoubtedly changes would need to be made when looking at prisons versus jails.

After lunch, a new presenter took the stage, seventy-year-old Richard Mc-Gee, who'd spent the best part of the last four decades in corrections. He'd been a warden at Rikers Island in the 1930s, acting commissioner of correction for New York in the 1940s, and director of corrections in California until 1961. Today, he wore his Institute for the Study of Crime and Delinquency hat. He expressed concern about the establishment of prison surgery programs.

"From the standpoint of a correctional administrator, I would feel we were embarking on a costly program not unaccompanied by risks," he said, including surgical failure, administrative issues, legal authority, patient consent, mental health of patient, selection criteria, and public disapproval. "That elusive thing we call public opinion should not be ignored," McGee continued. "Who is likely to be critical in the event of failure of miscarriage of the procedures? Looked at superficially, this comes under the head of a 'soft' approach to crime and criminals."[39]

Regardless, McGee concluded, much of this conference discussion was theoretical. "The use of these techniques will not, in the immediate future, be widely employed anyway, if for no other reason than the scarcity of competent surgeons. A second reason why this is not and will not be widely used is because of the general reluctance of legislative bodies to make adequate funds available."

Lipton and Lewin exchanged looks. McGee's words had cast a pall on the room, dimming enthusiasm. It wasn't that he was wrong, Lipton thought—it was a fact that corrections had been historically tight with its funds. It was true in McGee's day, and in Anna Kross's day, and even now, it varied wildly from state to state. But history didn't have to repeat itself. Lipton was in the administration now, working on the legislature. He knew Governor Rockefeller was putting serious money toward this problem, as was President Johnson. McGee seemed mired in the past, whereas they were thinking of the future.

By the end of the conference, the mood had lightened. Three days of lunching, drinking, and discussing the vagaries of different state programs had pushed the majority back in the positive box.

Post-conference, a special ten-page report was issued by the U.S. Bureau of Prisons, *Guidelines for Plastic Surgery Program in Corrections*, outlining the process of setting up such a program and providing a step-by-step worksheet for interested jails and prisons.[40] Its recommendations included reaching out to plastic surgery training schools: "Surgeons are usually interested in cooperating in such programs," it explained.

The Bureau of Prisons emphasized that in an ideal situation, this program would be run from a prison hospital; it was cheaper than a civilian hospital, and the surgical outcomes tended to be better—with one caveat. "New techniques for tattoo removal must be developed," it stated. "The removal and appearance of scar is often much worse than the tattoo itself. Subjects with this are the most dissatisfied and have the highest rate of recidivism." Unlike jails, the more restrictive state and federal prisons allowed surgeons the assurance that full aftercare could be provided to all patients. The *Guidelines for Plastic Surgery Program in Corrections* pamphlet was widely distributed across the United States.

With this governmental stamp of approval, more of these programs were green-lighted. Correctional officers and rehabilitative staff finally had the data needed to push these programs through. The SSR pilot was viewed as the model for future surgical work. The study's findings were adapted and built on, many programs excluded addicts and alcoholics based on the SSR data.

In general, the media's coverage of the conference supported the growth of prison plastic surgery programs, if with a side of snark. "The theory that thieves are all hulking brutes with monkey brows and stick out ears died a half century ago," commented reporter Tom Tiede in the *Herald Journal*. "But evidence again, is that in some cases unsightly physical characteristics may at least contribute to a criminal's delinquency."[41]

The project's psychologists were the toast of the criminological world, their attendance requested at conferences worldwide. Dr. Michael Lewin was pleased with the outcome; his hunch had been scientifically validated. He published a report about his process in *AORN Journal*.[42] "Plastic surgery services offer the promise of becoming an important adjunct in the social rehabilitation of the public offender," he wrote. There was more to be explored here, he thought. This was just the beginning. For one, it raised the question of whether plastic surgery as a life improvement program should be limited to inmates.

"It could also be effective in the prevention of potential criminality. Plastic surgery services should be made available to various underprivileged groups, especially underprivileged adolescents," he mused.

# 10

# TEENAGE DIRTBAGS OR PROM QUEENS IN THE MAKING?

World Bids Adieu to a Violent Year; City Gets Snowfall—
*New York Times*, 1968[1]

State Convicts Receiving Plastic Surgery New Look—*Daily Sentinel*, 1968[2]

In early January 1968, Micheline Douglas winked at herself in the mirror, flipped her platinum blond hair, and admired the taut lines of her face and the smooth expanse of her forehead.[3] She looked—and felt!—like herself again. She'd missed that feeling. Micheline was used to being adored, even exalted; in the 1940s and 1950s she high-kicked her way through off-Broadway shows, her stage name outlined in lights. Depending on her mood, she'd gone by Gypsy Marie, Cachita Valdez, and Micheline Bonet. Sometimes she'd drape herself around the microphone, sling a guitar over her shoulder, and belt out a torch number; the applause and the attention had made her feel giddy. She thought it would never end. But work dried up as she got older, as her skin grew lax and stomach sagged. At fifty years old, she felt like her life was over; she was just a dried-up nobody.

Everything she owned was crammed into a poky Manhattan hotel room—one of those miserable single rooms that welfare referred you to—which she shared with her ex-husband; neither could afford to leave. Her eighteen-year-old son made up the shortfall in rent from her welfare checks. But then, like a miracle, she'd heard that Medicaid covered cosmetic surgery. She visited a plastic surgeon and requested a face-lift—she'd wanted one for years but never dreamed she could afford it. The surgeon checked; Micheline was right, cosmetic surgery *was* covered by Medicaid, and there were no rules governing its use. Postsurgery, he billed Medicaid $1,300. "I feel fifteen years younger and twenty-five pounds thinner," she told a *Herald Statesman* reporter. "My friends are amazed. Strangers have written to me and asked where to have it done. I want to get back into theatrics and get off welfare."

In her small hotel room, she struck a pose for the reporter's photographer, pursing her lips and raising one eyebrow, reveling in the attention. News of her face-lift had gone viral, covered by newspapers across America, with everyone offering their opinion.

Two years prior, plastic surgeons had begged to delay Medicaid's implementation until a co-pay could be agreed upon, citing fears of "excessive utilization."[4] For many, Micheline's fresh face was a slap in the face to taxpayers courtesy of an administration that had foisted its liberal policies to the forefront, prioritizing those who contributed little to society and heavily taxing working-class folk.

It was a slippery slope, warned pundits; Micheline claimed she needed her rejuvenation for psychological and employment reasons, but where would it end? "Most logical thinkers might agree that the new-faced actress has no more a guarantee for success in the theater than the remodeled wife would have in keeping her husband," argued a *Herald Statesman* editor. "All paid for by the taxpayer who often can't afford such luxuries himself."[5] The editor of the *Chicago Tribune* was equally verbose.[6] "Medicaid is an example of what can be foisted on the country by an insistent and overbearing administration," he complained. "The bill rolled through the houses like a Sherman tank in a field of goldenrod."

Still, no one could deny that there were significant benefits related to cosmetic surgery. A study from Johns Hopkins University reported that 55 percent of its postoperative cosmetic patients experienced some type of positive life event shortly after their operations, from new jobs to salary increases, marriage proposals, promotions, and new romantic relationships.[7] But public opinion was too strong to counter, and in January 1968, Medicare updated its policies to exclude "plastic surgery for cosmetic reasons." "Surgery for cosmetic reasons is out,"[8] reported the Newspaper Enterprise Association.[9] Dental care was also removed from the bill, making surgical self-improvement out of reach for many.[10]

Two days after the Montefiore Conference on Correctional Plastic Surgery wrapped up, Leo Munick, a thirty-six-year-old plastic surgeon from Cincinnati, flew back home. Munick had enjoyed the event immensely—it was always pleasant to be surrounded by like-minded individuals, and the breadth of skill and knowledge of the those in attendance was humbling. Their discussions had clarified some of his own thoughts, and it felt reassuring to have his own theories verified by men with a lot more experience.

Munick had entered the correctional cosmetic space in a roundabout manner. Two years earlier, as a newly minted surgeon, he'd begun the process of getting himself established in the city. It was slow going; he had to build a clientele, get referrals . . . everything took time. He filled his free hours with biking; he loved the feel of gravel below him and seeing the open road expand in front of him. People gave him the side-eye—a surgeon on a bike!—but he didn't care.

Then, unexpectedly, he received a call from Robert Jones, a psychologist at the Hamilton County juvenile court. "I'm working on a dissertation about the effect of using cosmetic surgery to correct deformities among juvenile delinquents," he told him. "Would you be interested in being a part of this?"[11]

Munick was speechless; this was something he'd never considered before. "It would just be part time," Jones said. "I want to see if cosmetic improvement can change delinquents' behavior, perhaps even make them productive members of the community. This would be under Judge Benjamin Schwartz's oversight."

Munick considered the proposal. He'd never met Judge Schwartz, but he'd read enough about him to know he was an unorthodox progressive—you couldn't live in Cincinnati without the eccentric man popping up in a column or as a talking head in a news spot. The judge had a range of opinions on *everything*; one day it was dire warnings about the *Beatles* threatening children's morality;[12] on another he'd be telling defendants that "appropriate hair length was a requisite of proper decorum for his courtroom," insisting they have a haircut before coming before him again. He sentenced delinquents to job training rather than jail and personally founded Bob Hope House, a group home and sanctuary for delinquent and abandoned boys.[13]

The judge's résumé was impressive, thought Munick. His interest in surgery was surprising, but not completely out of left field. For the last year, Munick had serviced inmates at the local prison with minor surgical work, the adult inmates, that is. He'd never considered there might be a need with the juvenile cohort. *Perhaps I should have*, he thought; in his opinion, by the time a child was seventeen, his or her personality was pretty much set in stone. His fledgling private practice included a number of children.

Jones offered little renumeration—he'd cover costs, but that was it—but Munick had chosen his profession to help people, not to make money. "Okay, I'm in," he told Jones. Judge Schwartz was pleased to have Munick on board.

During his years on the bench, he'd noticed that many of the problem children who came before him had visible facial defects. Recently, he'd been questioning whether they were somehow related to the youths' behavior. With Munick's assistance, they could start to test that theory and de facto become the first "problem child" plastic surgery program in America. Schwartz switched up his sentencing; from now on, if youths appeared who would benefit from Munick's scalpel, they'd be sentenced to plastic surgery, subject to physician and parental approval. Their other charges would be reduced accordingly. He chose not to discriminate by their criminal acts, focusing on what was facially fixable instead.

Slowly, the sentenced kids trickled into Munick's office. They ranged from twelve years old to eighteen, the younger children accompanied by their parents or guardians. Most showed up alone. There was a white fourteen-year-old "wise guy" with one oddly protruding ear. A Black fifteen-year-old boy who politely asked Munick to remove the vivid knife scar that ran from his lip to his chin; it would help him get into college, he explained. A Black girl who was bothered by the deep acne scars on her face. A white boy who wanted liposuction on his breasts. A teenage white girl with an overly large nose. He listened to each request and, after checking their vitals and examining the affected areas, informed them whether their requests were feasible, and assessed whether they had realistic expectations of what could be achieved with treatment.[14] He operated on his one day off each week.

The court psychologists did most of the follow-ups on his patient, and the court sent him updates. Munick was pleased to hear how his patients were faring. Prior to surgery, "Betty the bird" (due to her beaky nose and small, pointed chin) had been so miserable about her appearance that she regularly skipped school. She was friendless, with grades so poor she was on the verge of expulsion. A dramatic change occurred, Jones informed him. "Betty's grades have improved, she has a circle of friends, and she now works in a pizzeria," activities that were unthinkable prior to her operation.[15]

The *Cincinnati Enquirer* reached out for comment: why is this program so important? "Children, especially teenagers, look in the mirror twenty times a day," Munick explained.[16] "They are both extremely sensitive about their appearance and extremely ruthless toward each other." That's why help at this juncture was so important for shaping their long-term personality. "I think I can say right here that the project has been a huge success. After correction, the rate of relapse, I am told, is only one in fifty." It's not a panacea for solving the juvenile delinquency problem, but it is encouraging, he added.

Munick's experiments with juvenile delinquents were unique, but starting in the 1960s, there was an upswing in the number of cosmetic surgery operations performed on law-abiding, consenting children.[17] In these cases, it was less about prevention of current or future criminal behavior and more about improving the child's acceptance by society and themselves.

"Those who are the against so-called cosmetic surgery, may be against giving a child a happy adult life," claimed one columnist.[18] A growing body of psychiatrists posited that childhood was the optimum time for such operations. "Body image is an essential source of personal identity for the adolescent," reported Dr. Norman Knorr, a plastic surgeon from Johns Hopkins Hospital in Baltimore, Maryland.[19] He recommended treating children before they reached adulthood, because the postoperative management—emotional and physical— was more effective for those "in the formative stages of adolescence."

With cosmetic surgery still a luxury service, numerous individuals and organizations tried to plug the Medicare gap, both pre- and post-amendment. In New York, the eccentric philanthropist Stanley Slotkin offered free cosmetic surgery to people he considered "in need." This included breast implants for single mothers who moonlighted as exotic dancers, face-lifts for aging women who struggled in the competitive workforce, and "Dumbo" surgery for big-eared teens on the cusp of reform school.[20]

In South Dakota, birthplace of Hollywood blond darlings Mamie Van Doren and Cheryl Ladd, providing children in need with cosmetic surgery was a high priority. The Jaycettes, a statewide leadership and community service group, held frequent fundraisers to pay for their operations. All children who were unhappy with their appearance qualified, but those who were most likely to be socially or psychologically handicapped by their defect were prioritized.[21]

Six-year-old Sheri was a perfect example; most days, she could be found sobbing about the dark brown birthmark on her nose, her mother informed the Jaycettes. Kids teased her and called her names. The Jaycettes funded her operation; Sherri's brown splotch was excised and replaced with a skin graft from her abdomen.[22] The state was proud of this program; so proud, in fact, that in 1967, the state governor declared the second week in October as "National Cosmetic Surgery Week," to support the Jaycettes.[23]

"Parents may tell Johnny Big Nose or Gloria Big Ears that 'it's what's inside that counts,' but it is now recognized that what's outside may be adversely affected by the nonconformist outside packaging," reported the Associated

Press.[24] Children, it seemed, just like the adults who raised them, were equally conscious about being viewed as attractive. There was some dissent; in Florida, juvenile court director Don Sellas felt surgery was too simplistic. "Plastic surgery for juveniles is not a salvation," he objected. "Other needs must be met first."[25]

In New York City, bolstered by the success of the Surgical and Social Rehabilitation (SSR) project pilot and the reception to its December conference, Michael Lewin petitioned the state to expand the program. In early 1968, New York State granted the surgeon (and his associates) full permission to extend their beautification services to sixteen- to eighteen-year-old inmates. Lewin was pleased that the powers that be had seen sense—or enough data—to recognize something that felt glaringly obvious; by far, the biggest impact appearance had on behavior was among children and teenagers more than any other age group. These developmental years impacted the social relationships, behavior, and communication skills that they'd carry with them for the rest of their lives.

Across America, the effects of the Rikers Island SSR project were far reaching. Twenty-three state prisons and seven federal facilities ran comprehensive plastic surgery programs. Many of the new programs included juvenile surgery in their rehabilitation remit. However, even as the majority of American penologists adopted, or were considering, the surgical approach to recidivism, the catalyst for this interest, Rikers Island, was in jeopardy.

By all accounts, the Rikers Island pilot had been an unprecedented success, both in curbing recidivism and by building connections among different support agencies. To make the SSR program sustainable in the long term, the researchers, corrections officers, and plastic surgeons needed to scale their findings and treat a larger portion of the inmate population.

This was the result that Michael Lewin had worked toward—and something he still believed in—but as his responsibilities at Montefiore Hospital increased, his time grew increasingly short. During the decade he'd been at Montefiore, he'd grown its nonexistent plastic surgery residency into one of the premier training programs in the nation, and his resident rotations and array of junior doctors had swelled accordingly. He was also a regular on the conference circuit, flying to three or four countries a year for a week or more of networking with his peers. He liked to make a vacation of it, bringing his wife along; conference itineraries generally involved days of fine dining and tours of local hotspots and surgery facilities, plus the occasional lecture. It was fascinating to see how plastic surgeons went about their business in non-Western settings; in Russia, he'd been amused to see a hairdryer used to dry the splint for a rhinoplasty! The Russian army encouraged soldiers with protruding ears or overly large noses to undergo plastic surgery, the surgeons told him. Appearance was everything in their post-Stalin world.

Back in Manhattan, he had less and less time to give to his various projects, his days split among his plastic surgery and training duties at Montefiore, his work at its newly established cleft palate clinic, and his membership obligations to the fifteen or so medical societies to which he belonged, in addition to his volunteering duties. By now, he estimated that he'd operated on more than one thousand men, women, and children, and he wanted to share what he learned with his students. He'd found that the biggest problem in regard to surgical outcome related to the emotional state of the patients and their expectations. The psychological rather than the physical is a bigger issue than inadequate care, he lectured. "Beware of the aging patient who comes in with clippings to emphasize her stage triumphs at eighteen," he wrote in his lesson plan. "The surgeon should be enthusiastic but modest in describing the anticipated results."

As Lewin's interest in the psychological state of his patients grew, he deprioritized his visits to Rikers Island. He still sent his residents to the jail and to prisons upstate, but he was increasingly less involved with the running of the program. As Lewin's calendar filled, his dinners with Anna Kross dropped from every month or so to less than once a year.

On the corrections front, New York's new corrections commissioner, George F. McGrath, though amenable to continuing plastic surgery on released ex-cons, was no Anna Kross. McGrath's name just didn't inspire people or elicit action the way that Kross's had. People railed against crime in the city and laughed at his response. He shared a helicopter to Rikers Island with Mayor Lindsay and strolled the isle contemplatively.[26] Rikers was more expensive to run than initially thought, and the revolving door was in constant motion. Reports were piling up on his desk, everyone suggesting a new, different way to "solve" recidivism.

One report suggested that improving the quality of care might change inmates' behaviors: "Institutions could be improved at little cost by the use of brighter interior painting," it read. "Food preparation techniques could also be vastly improved." McGrath's aides scanned and ignored most suggestions. The city's crime rate continued its upward climb—and the jails filled accordingly—around ten thousand residents were behind bars each day. McGrath blamed this spike on the shortage of economic opportunities; one report noted that one in eight of the city's teen workforce was unemployed—a large number of them Black—and their frustration was showing.[27]

On Rikers Island, the Adolescent Remand Shelter was bulging at the seams. Its eight three-tiered concrete-and-steel blocks were designed to hold 1,920 youths but regularly housed more. The windowless cells opened onto a long gray corridor, the gloom alleviated by a bare bulb. The walls were scrawled with various statements, including "Make love not war," and "Give acid a chance."[28]

The behavior of juvenile delinquents overshadowed every one of the approximately one million youths who lived in the five boroughs.[29] Teenage street violence had surged along with theft, and both rich and poor neighborhoods were targeted, their homes ransacked, and their belongings carried off by thieves who never even tripped their alarms.[30] Some homes were hit multiple times a week.[31]

Men and boys were disappearing across the city, off to jail or the military, whether drafted or willingly enrolled, where they were shipped overseas to Vietnam.[32] Metal bars appeared on windows and doorframes. Fathers wept as the names of the dead filled the dailies; mothers wailed as they swept broken glass and syringes off their stoops. Unease with their leadership soared, as did the reluctance to follow rules.

"Excessively high intake and prisoner population levels are a continuing problem, resulting in daily over capacity," McGrath noted in his annual report.[33] Troubled, he rang Anna Kross for advice, but found her engrossed in her own projects.

Aged seventy-seven, she'd accidentally become a New York style icon thanks to a surprising shift in fashion. For decades, Kross had clomped about the city encased in chunky, comfortable Oxfords from Murray Space Shoes.[34] Their arch support was the best in the business, she believed, but their clunky utilitarian style had been mocked and viewed as orthopedic. Overnight, New York's fashionistas had decreed her molded toe space shoes the height of style. Kross was name-checked alongside Steve McQueen and Greta Garbo in the papers' glowing write-ups of the "space shoe style icons." It was an unexpected and unwanted honor.

Her retirement was every bit as jam-packed as her work life had been. Kross hosted monthly lectures about the changing role of women in the city's various high schools[35] and was an active member of ten-odd social and welfare boards. She thought about the cosmetic surgery project sometimes, but that was controlled by the Department of Correction and out of her hands. Anyway, there were far more pressing matters in New York to keep her busy.

She was pleased to hear from McGrath; after years in corrections, it had been an adjustment to take a step back. She listened to his litany of complaints. It seems that your most pressing issue, right now, is the overcrowding, she told him. She thought hard. How about repurposing some cargo ships into floating prisons as a temporary solution? Just while more accommodation was being built.[36] Perhaps, said McGrath, immediately discounting her idea. "The disease in this business is cynicism," he told the *New York Times*; after guards see the same faces return over and over, they "succumb to it."[37] He didn't want a stop-gap; he wanted a solution! But there were never any easy answers in corrections.

In February 1968, New Yorkers received further confirmation of how rotten their administration could be. Overnight, the sanitation workers union had approved a strike, its members frustrated by the low pay and meager benefits they received. Residents woke to find refuse piled high on the streets, piles that got larger by the day. Uptown streets turned into slums, and slums became shanty-towns.[38] The stench of eggs and feces wafted across the city, from the jaws of the Hudson on the West Side to the gray East River and up and down the wealthy tree-lined enclave of Fifth Avenue.

Michael Lewin was stunned by the sight as he exited Grand Central terminal on the second day of the strike. He waded through chest-high garbage and crunched through the beer cans, eggshells, and milk cartons that littered the sidewalks, slowly making his way uptown. The street outside the entrance to Montefiore Hospital was mercifully clear—the one "public good" concession the strikers had made—but public transit was untenable. Everyone arrived late. He drove to work for the rest of the month.

Three days in, thirty thousand tons of trash littered the street. Five days later it had grown to one hundred thousand putrid tons, attracting flies and oozing onto people's shoes and skin.[39] No one was unaffected. The Big Apple's grid-locked design always had highlighted the inequities of the promised American Dream, with its poorest denizens shoulder to shoulder with the Rockefeller and Carnegie dynasties, an aspirational jab to immigrants that, with enough work, they too could walk those marble floors, but for most, it was just another lie. America *was* the land of opportunity—for those who were rich, white, and well-connected. Now, those same dynasties—accustomed to keeping the slums and smells away with their retinue of guards, groundskeepers, and staff—couldn't buy their way out of the stench and shit.

It took ten days before Mayor Lindsay acceded to the union's demands, after begging Governor Nelson Rockefeller for help with the mess. Things didn't improve once the stench subsided; in fact, the city's troubles were only beginning. In March, a rapist and murderer who'd been spared the electric chair by the governor escaped from prison and attacked a married couple, raping the woman as her bound husband struggled in the adjoining room.[40] A teenage sniper in Central Park killed one woman and injured three more.[41] An eighteen-year-old arsonist whose Bronx fireball injured nineteen people, including fifteen children,[42] was sentenced to a maximum of five years. The increasingly foreboding headlines and dire news reports triggered new levels of hysteria to New York City.

Juveniles, a broadly defined term encapsulating anyone under nineteen years of age, were the new bugaboo.[43] They're the new "problem for society," bemoaned the dailies.[44] The data surrounding the dangers of delinquents flip-flopped depending the newspaper or radio show—on Monday, the papers reported that 13 percent of all crimes were committed by youths aged eleven to seventeen years; by Friday they'd ominously state that 30 percent of all arrests were for minors according to FBI data.[45] The attorney general announced that 84 percent of all cars stolen were by youths under eighteen. The furor eclipsed all common sense; in San Jose, California, a three-year-old and a five-year-old boy were arrested for arson.[46]

Money poured into fixing the "juvenile" problem. The annual cost for New York's public and private services for juvenile delinquents aged sixteen to nineteen amounted to $35 million per year. At a national level, President Lyndon Johnson proposed the Juvenile Delinquency Prevention and Control Act, which focused on diverting youths from jails through deeper community involvement and social programs that focused on keeping children with their families.[47] "One in every six young men under eighteen will be taken to juvenile court for at least one offense this year. Our nation can help to cure these social ills if we pledge our continuing stewardship of our greatest wealth—our young people," he told Congress. "Crimes increase as the channels of opportunity are limited and social mobility is foreclosed."[48]

The president advocated for an intersectional approach to crime. "The reason we passed three hundred conservation bills and added forty-six national parks was so that little boy wouldn't go off and smoke pot or become a juvenile delinquent or a murderer at twelve or fourteen. . . . [I]nstead he will have someplace to go and play and enjoy the beauty of nature."[49] Beauty can fix things, continued the president. "This is a more beautiful country than it was four years ago."

FBI Director Edgar Hoover was less enthused about his proposition, criticizing Johnson's "tendency to ignore punishment as a deterrent,"—this was "coddling of criminals," he complained to the president's Crime Commission.[50] Nonetheless, Congress authorized a bill providing $150 million to states to implement a targeted juvenile delinquency prevention plan. A number of youth-focused experimental projects were initiated. In New Jersey, police recruited a local "mom squad" to patrol near the schools, instructing them to walk or drive around their local streets, calling out any malingerers.[51]

Another experiment, run under the auspices of the National Institute of Mental Health, investigated whether juvenile delinquents could be identified prior to offending and, if so, at what age.[52] Eleanor T. Glueck, a child psychologist and delinquency researcher from Harvard University, observed the social behavior of two- and three-year-old boys in New York. Some were more rambunctious than others, but Glueck announced that this age group was too young to identify any criminal traits; there were just too many variables, she said. However, five- and six-year-old boys were another ballgame. She scored a group of 301 boys via her "delinquent traits" design. Based on these results, she said she was comfortable sorting 72 percent of the children involved into a potential delinquent or nondelinquent bucket. If we can find them earlier, perhaps we can treat them earlier, she surmised.

Those advertisements for . . . flesh-colored bandages are merely a profitable manifestation of a common assumption amongst white folks: White skin is what human flesh is supposed to look like.—*New York Times*, 1968[53]

Sexual assaults and rapes had also increased in New York City. Its women were scared—and angry. They were sick of being told how to dress, how to talk, how to live—and then being attacked anyway. Even the civil rights movement sweeping the nation treated Black women as an underclass. It was time for a change. Enter New York Radical Women, a feminist group founded in January 1968. "Liberation of women," its manifesto stated: they wanted equal rights, equal pay, and to stop being valued only as ornamental sex objects.

When the Miss America pageant came to Atlantic City that fall, the organization saw red. New York Radical Women issued a statement to the press that invited women everywhere to join them in protest on the day of the contest.[54] "The pageant contestants epitomize the roles we are all forced to play as women. The parade down the runway blares the metaphor of the 4-H Club county fair, where nervous animals are judged for teeth, fleece, etc. . . . So are women in our society forced daily to compete for male approval, enslaved by ludicrous 'beauty' standards we are conditioned to take seriously," they wrote.

The statement also highlighted the racial inequities the pageant perpetrated. "We protest racism with roses. Since its inception in 1921, the pageant has not had one Black finalist. There has never been a Puerto Rican, Alaskan, Hawaiian, or Mexican-American winner. Nor has there ever been a *true* Miss America—an American Indian."

On the day of the pageant, some five hundred women marched up and down the boardwalk outside Boardwalk Hall. They held signs—"All women are beautiful," and "Miss America makes money for *Revlon*. Revlon makes bullet casings for *war*!" and "Let's judge ourselves as people!"

"They're a bunch of nuts," pageant director Albert Marks told WNYC radio. "I wonder how many of them, if they had a man, would have the time to do what they're doing."[55]

A few blocks from the boardwalk inside Atlantic City's Ritz-Carlton in front of roughly two hundred people, nineteen-year-old Saundra Williams was announced as the inaugural Miss Black America.[56] She trembled as the host draped her in a cream-colored cape, passed her a red velvet scepter, and then carefully placed a large rhinestone crown atop her natural curls. "The curvy, hazel-eyed co-ed edged out seven other black beauties," the *New York Times* reported. She didn't care about the protest at the main pageant, she told reporters; she was just happy she got to take part in *this* pageant.

Miss Black America was the brainchild of J. Morris Anderson, a wealthy businessman from Philadelphia. The genesis was a conversation with his two daughters about what they'd like to be when they grew up. "Miss America!" they replied. He was saddened by their answer; that pageant eliminated them by default, its rules stating that "contestants must be of good health, and the white race." Even when those rules shifted in the 1950s, entering was a zero-sum game for Black women.

Miss Black America was his way of changing that; racism would not ruin his daughters' dreams.[57] No television cameras captured Williams's winning performance—she performed the Fiji, a traditional African dance, for her talent and spoke about the need for greater inclusivity in the interview portion—as all the mainstream broadcast media attention was laser focused on the show up the road.

Inside the official Miss America hall, Judith Anne Ford, a blond-haired, blue-eyed, 36–24½–36, eighteen-year-old lifeguard from rural Illinois was crowned Miss America. Ford gasped as she received the requisite sash, staff, and crown in front of eighteen thousand attendees. Millions more watched the proceedings on their televisions at home. Her diamond-studded crown sparkled under the spotlights. During the press conference that followed, she was asked how she felt about the Miss America crown theoretically being awarded to a Black woman in the future. Ford paused to consider her answer. "That's fine," she answered, "if she's the prettiest and the talented and best qualified . . . not just because she's a Negro." Ford giggled self-consciously. "I hate to make my opinion on these things as it's so controversial."[58]

⌒

In Washington, D.C., Mary Switzer's team were wrapping up a national survey of American attitudes regarding criminals and related reform services, interviewing one thousand adults and two hundred youths for this project. The survey had been initiated by a personal request from President Johnson; "It's imperative that we have a better understanding of what our nation thinks," he'd told her. Nationally, the crime rate was up 16 percent since the previous year, with a 27 percent increase in robberies and a 12 percent growth in murders, and Johnson needed to gauge public sentiment.[59]

Switzer understood; in order to help, you first had to understand what the pain points were. Her department published its findings in a slim book titled *The Public Looks at Crime and Correction*.[60] The thirty-five-page volume assessed the public's understanding of the correctional system as a whole. The researchers had tried to ensure that every group was represented: 51 percent of those surveyed were white, 40 percent were Black, and 9 percent were from other minority groups.

What they discovered was sobering; so much so that Switzer instructed the book be prefaced with a warning: "Many readers of this report will find some of the facts it presents disillusioning, even saddening," it read. "Society as a whole is not tolerant of the presence of the returned offender. If we are laboring under illusions, it is time we were nudged into awareness of reality."

Researchers disclosed that 89 percent of Americans believed that the country's crime rate had either risen or plateaued during the previous year. White Americans attributed criminal behavior to poverty, a poor environment, and shoddy parenting, whereas Black participants cited unemployment, lack of education, welfare, and poverty as the biggest driver of crime.

Twenty-seven percent of all respondents claimed that their media consumption had informed them of the spike in crime. "Just read your paper. Every night it's this shooting or that robbery," a sixty-one-year-old laborer from Pennsylvania told Switzer's staff. "Also, the crime rate has risen because of all the bad programs on TV. A child sees all this killing and soon grows up to think it's okay."

Black citizens also placed significantly less trust than whites in the police, with 32 percent believing that jailed folks were treated fairly compared to 71 percent of white people. "We have a dual justice system," explained a forty-two-year-old Black teacher from Baltimore. "If financially adequate then you can get off easy. If not, you are one of the masses that feel the sting of justice." Such responses, the researchers knew, were based on Black people's lived experience; not only was there wealth inequity, but there was color inequity too. Black kids were disproportionately arrested more than white kids, and, if sentenced, received second-class treatment and longer sentences.[61] Leaked reports from the juvenile halls in the South found that Black kids were regularly beaten and barred from rehabilitative programs.[62]

However, both Black and white respondents opposed raising taxes to fund rehabilitative projects for criminals. Of bigger concern was defense funding and schools, they explained. If money *had* to go into the corrections sphere, it should prioritize forcing criminals to behave, they opined. However, the treatment of juvenile delinquents was exempt from this; most approved funneling funding into school intervention treatments.

At SSR's headquarters, a slim letter arrived from Washington, D.C. Richard Kurtzberg ran his finger over the edge and slit it open. He scanned the page; his request for funding to extend the SSR project another year had been denied. Funds had been diverted elsewhere, the letter explained. His efforts were deeply appreciated, and plastic surgeons were still welcome at Rikers Island—and at the state's prisons—but, save a few special cases, their directives were to work on the medical rather than cosmetic side of surgery.

Kurtzberg put the letter down. So this was it, he thought. He'd hoped to document the ex-con's recidivism rate over two years, three years, even five years, and increase the subject pool as well. But now, well. . . . He sighed. There was no point in appealing the decision, the Department of Health, Education, and Welfare wasn't known for compromise once it made a decision. It probably funneled its funds into some sort of delinquency program. That was all anyone talked of these days.

It wasn't a shock that Commissioner McGrath hadn't fought harder for the program; he seemed to back rehabilitation as long as it was useful for him. "Behavioral people are so permissively oriented that they resent any controls," McGrath told the press.[63]

In addition, Rikers Island, always a problematic jail, was a hot mess right now. In July 1968, eighty white inmates inside cell block five had armed themselves with chair legs, mop handles, and knives made from filed-down spoons and attacked six Black prisoners, whose "offense" was daring to eat lunch at a picnic table in "white-only" territory.[64] One man was in a coma—"He will always be a vegetable," his doctor reported—and the rest of the victims were hospitalized.[65] "A racial attack," the papers called it, and justifiably so. The jail complex likely didn't want any more attention.

Dejected by the project's end, the SSR staff sought other opportunities. Kurtzberg washed his hands of the corrections world and was hired as a school psychologist by a high school in Westchester County, New York. Wallace Mandell remained head of the Staten Island Mental Health Society research division and doubled down on his research on disadvantaged youth, hoping that these studies required less hand-holding. Norman Cavior was accepted into the clinical psychology doctoral program at the University of Houston.

Cavior was sad to leave New York, his mother, his dancing, and the overall vibrancy of the city, but Houston was the only program he got in. The city felt low key compared to Manhattan. His classes kept him busy, but he couldn't get the Rikers Island experiment out of his mind. There were so many parallels within the college system! The prettiest girls and the most rugged men were so obviously more advantaged than their peers. Professors paid them more attention, and they got better treatment in the library and the cafeterias. The appearance hierarchy was also present among the department heads; the more attractive staff tended to be given greater responsibilities and were paid better than their average-looking colleagues.

In developmental psychology, Cavior's professor tasked each student with completing a research project on a topic of their choosing. In a small seminar room, his professor quizzed each student, one by one, about his or her past experiences in the field. When it was Cavior's turn, he brought up the plastic surgery project and its investigation into the role of appearance bias in society: "When you perform plastic surgery to alter someone's appearance, does that make a psychological difference? What role does physical attractiveness play in everyday life?"

His professor looked intrigued, but many of his classmates were upset. You can't reduce someone to their physical features, they complained. Our work is about treating the *mind*, not the body. Some glanced down at their own bodies, wondering how their own features had influenced the course of their lives, triggered by his words. "You should go deeper into this line of inquiry," his professor advised; that his students were perturbed enough to quarrel over this suggested that there was a lot more to unpack in this area. "It's an interesting research space," he told Cavior; compared to other biases on the spectrum, little research existed on beauty bias.

Cavior nodded thoughtfully. He spent the next couple of months figuring out what part of the attractiveness equation to dive into. It would be helpful to understand whether there was a universal agreement about what counted as attractive, he thought. Did race make a difference? What about personality; did someone's attractiveness score change if you became friends? At faculty parties, Cavior was peppered with questions from his colleague's wives, clamoring to hear his discoveries. Appearance is such a taboo subject, they told him guiltily; they had to pretend their looks didn't matter to avoid appearing vain or shallow—but their looks factored in to where they were today. Cavior smiled and told them his research was progressing nicely, thanks to his wife. Helene taught at a local school and had facilitated access to the students for Cavior. He'd been granted permission from parents and the school board to run a small study.

Early one morning, he drove to the elementary school with Helene, who escorted him to his assigned classroom. One at a time, the entire class of fifth grade boys shuffled through the room. He directed each child to stand on the same marked spot on the ground and instructed them to look straight ahead, unsmiling. "Stay as still as possible," he asked, snapping a Polaroid of each.[66] He wanted the images as standardized as possible.

A few weeks later, Cavior returned to the school and met with a different fifth grade class. He made copies of the photographs taken on his first visit, and he distributed them to the class. "I'd like you to look at these pictures and sort them into five categories," he urged them. "The categories I'd like you to sort them into are as follows: very attractive, attractive, average, unattractive, and very unattractive." The results were startling. Time and time again, fifth graders assigned the exact same photos to the same piles. There was little variation. "The phrase 'beauty is in the eye of the beholder' turns out to be a lot of baloney," he marveled to his professor.

"I'd be interested to see if these findings cross cultural lines," his professor remarked. Cavior pursed his lips in agreement; that was an interesting proposition. He visited a similarly sized elementary school, located just over the Rio Grande in Mexico, and repeated the experiment. The results were almost identical. Skin color, it seemed, was irrelevant to children's grading of beauty; their highest scores unequivocally correlated to facial symmetry.[67]

Meanwhile, inside the cavernous capitol building in Albany in upstate New York, Douglas Lipton was putting in the hours in his new job as the deputy assistant director of state, office of crime control planning. It was an exciting time to be in government, he found—a lot more was happening here than it seemed from the outside. The legislature had passed a revision to the Penal Law and the Code of Criminal Procedure, and everyone was adjusting. For the first time, men who visited prostitutes were equally culpable as those they solicited and could be charged with a crime. And that was just the beginning.[68]

However, Lipton's job was more complicated than expected, primarily because the goalposts kept changing and the overlap between departments was unclear. On any given week, the state head of the narcotic control commission might march into the office and sound off compassionately: "Being an addict is not a violation of law in New York!" then a week later earnestly tell staffers that they had to "mount an all-out war" on addicts.

It was clear from the beginning, however, that addressing the state's drug problem would be a large part of his role. He was tasked with creating an in-depth accounting of the state's narcotic predicament and designing legislature that addressed it. Lipton pushed back; addiction is not that straightforward, he explained; it deeply intersected with economic inequality, racism, mental health issues, and poor self-esteem. Heroin, in particular, had become the fall guy for a raft of racist and classist policies and attitudes. You could not plan a one-size-fits-all solution. Put that in the report, his superiors told him.

As Lipton dug into the statewide data, he was struck by its similarities to New York City. Somehow, he'd thought that the drug problem might be a localized issue, a big city problem. But the issues at Rikers Island scaled to the whole state. Overall, treatment programs were sparse. Here, too, the majority of offenses committed by addicts were for low-level thefts, crimes that enabled them to score again.

Some addicts even reported that *unsuccessful* crimes were their goals; it was easier to score drugs in the state's prisons and jails, they said. Some drugs arrived by way of an inmate's digestive system. Other times, drugs were smuggled in by guards or visitors, concealed in orifices, or creatively melted into Hershey bars or woven into braids. It was a sad, sad state of affairs. In the end, it was all so *pointless*, he thought. These men and women and children turned to drugs because there was nothing better in their lives. They needed medical help, social help, psychological help, but instead they were locked up with rapists and murderers.

Altering the drug laws might help, he thought; as it stood, they were far too broad, encompassing heroin, cocaine, morphine, and cannabis under one umbrella. Legalization of all drugs might go a long way toward solving this problem, he told his coworkers. If narcotics were legal, the state could control the supply. His colleagues looked skeptical, but he shrugged it off. Perhaps if he could show the administrators how this would help, they might take it more seriously.

At his desk, he mapped out what legalization would look like in a detailed memo. He wrote the first draft of a piece of legislature that advocated for the legalization of cannabis, figuring that would be the best drug to start with. He outlined the benefits of legalization: taxes, public health and safety, more restrictive for minors. He'd made a good case, he thought, but his work was dismissed.

There's no way the public—or the governor—will go for this, the director told him. "But I have another job for you—I want you to be the point man for a new project: collating and reporting an overview of the most promising recidivism programs in existence. Governor Rockefeller has made this a top priority." Of course, Lipton acquiesced, frantically trying to figure out how much more of his time this would entail. Somehow, he had to source, vet, and assess an exhaustive number of recidivism studies, in addition to his narcotic investigations, plus a never-ending multitude of administrative chores. It was too much for one person.

He hired two junior researchers to assist him: Judith Wilks, a New York University criminology professor, and Robert Martinson, an adjunct sociology professor from City College. Wilks had a traditional academic background, but Martinson's history was more eccentric. In his twenties, he'd cut ties with his family when they objected to his Black wife. He'd been a Freedom Rider and spent thirty-nine days in a Mississippi prison, some of it in solitary confinement, for protesting racism. "We were stripped by the guards . . . and walked barefoot, two by two, into our cages and stood there embarrassed, naked, outraged," Martinson wrote in *The Nation* magazine.[69] "It is impossible to prepare anyone for the humiliating, brutal atmosphere of even the best prison." Martinson was an unconventional hire, but Lipton hoped he'd bring a fresh perspective to their work. The blend of multiple backgrounds and personalities was what had made the SSR project work so well. Plus, Martinson was charming, a natural storyteller, a breath of fresh air from the government grind.

By June, the recidivism work was still in progress, but his narcotics analysis was ready to present to the corrections community. Lipton's findings were included in a 328-page dark blue volume titled *Preliminary Report of the Governor's Special Committee on Criminal Offenders*.[70] A sketch of a blindfolded Lady Liberty was printed on the cover. The book began by flattering the administration's rehabilitative programs: "It has weak spots, but on the whole, New York is widely recognized as outstanding."

The rest of the text took a stronger stance on the issues at hand, in particular the concept of recidivism. "The term recidivism means nothing more than an *omnibus concept*, that whenever used must be accompanied by definition," it stated. Context was everything, the book elaborated; recidivism had become an umbrella term that encompassed probation and parole failures, new crimes, arrests for new crimes, convictions for new crimes, major crimes, minor crimes, repetition of the *same* crime, a revocation. Essentially, whenever recidivism was discussed, no one had any clear understanding of what *kind* of recidivism was on the table.

Due to this, recidivism studies weren't an apple-to-apple comparison. Another important discovery was that a "do no harm" approach should always be on criminologists' minds. In some cases, physically intensive rehabilitation treatments such as chemotherapy for withdrawal and cosmetic surgery for the scarred could increase reoffending rates. In 1969, *Plastic Surgery for Public Offenders Guidelines* had been amended to clarify that treatment must be "purely voluntary" and have a sound legal basis.[71]

For youths, the book recommended that the "status of juvenile delinquent be merged with the general category of child in need of supervision," placing this group under social welfare agencies instead of the Department of Correction. The volume ended with a promise that the next edition would provide a comprehensive analysis of effective recidivism programs.

The balance had shifted in Washington, D.C. In August 1967, the Vocational Rehabilitation Administration was disbanded, its services subsumed into a new, larger department called Social and Rehabilitation Services (SRS), which covered welfare, aging, and rehabilitative services—the idea being to stamp out fragmentation of care. Mary Switzer's title changed from commissioner to administrator of the new bureau, a role that came with a lot more power. "I went to bed one night with a budget of more than $300 million and when I awoke it was $6 billion dollars," she told a friend.[72] Even so, it was a daunting task. The attitudes of her own staff needed adjusting. "There is still a strong desire to cling to traditional ways, and to continue to select clients with whom our predominantly white middle-class counselors feel most comfortable," she wrote in a memo.

As the Nixon administration loomed, Switzer began lobbying to keep her position. It wasn't unheard of for certain chiefs to remain in charge, regardless of political affiliation, and the SRS was surely a bipartisan issue, she thought. Everyone knew how dedicated she was to rehabilitation. Her job was her life! She'd never married, her cat, Snowshoes, her only companion.[73] Nixon's administration was unmoved, and on December 17, 1969, she was forced to resign; she'd exit the bureau in February. She published her good-bye statement in the bureau's February 28 newsletter. "We must continue to break the barriers of fears, of differences," she wrote. "The most tragic development of the 70s for the disabled, the aged, the poor, and our children, would be if their government failed them."[74]

The next eighteen months were busy ones for Lipton, Martinson, and Wilks. Their desks creaked with books and stacked folders teetered in piles, with more sheafs of paper arriving each week. They sorted through hundreds of studies, all dated between January 1, 1945, and December 31, 1967. Each had to be evaluated on whether its research could translate to incarcerated New Yorkers. Hundreds more papers were scanned and discarded by the trio due to faulty research, poor science, or vague data that didn't meet their selection criteria. On the job, they were tireless, focused, and motivated, but Lipton and Wilkes were able to shake it off by the time they got to their cars. They soon realized that Robert Martinson didn't have an off switch.

Martinson was passionate about their project, but his behavior was erratic—he'd often pull all-nighters and was found napping in his chair when they clattered in the next morning. Other times, he shouted and railed about the inequity of it all, throwing books and papers he considered "biased" on the floor. "They're full of lies," he told Lipton. "So many of these reports, the authors just care about being right, not if their work actually makes a difference," he said. When riled, he strode about the building, lecturing staff from other departments, who then complained to Lipton. A few times, Martinson had clambered on top of his chair, furious he wasn't getting the respect he deserved. Lipton talked him down. "Whoa, there," Lipton said, concerned the man would injure himself. Eccentricity was one thing, but Martinson was extreme. Lipton thought about firing him, but the completion date for their first draft was winter 1969; there wasn't enough time to train and brief someone else and still make their deadline.

The trio's final tally included 231 methodologically sound social science reports spanning 1945 to 1967. The team spent months crunching the data and checking and rechecking the statistics, resulting in 285 findings, due to the fact that more than one variable was assessed. They measured the variable outcomes (recidivism, community adjustment, personality and attitude change, etc.) against eleven treatment methods, including probation, imprisonment, counseling, group methods, and medical methods. Lipton was adamant that they cross every $t$ and check every box.

The SSR project was part of their analysis and he reexamined the data. With a fresh perspective, it was less cut-and-dried than he'd thought. There were several problems in their initial comparisons; for one assessment, the group receiving surgery and the group with surgery and services had been combined, their data compared with the surgery-free groups. "These comparisons underestimate the effects of surgery for addicts and overestimate these effects for nonaddicts," he wrote. "The cutting points in these comparisons are determined by the idea the surgery is the treatment, and casework given alone is not." He summarized by saying that further research was needed in this area and qualified that "addicts and nonaddicts do appear to stay out of prison significantly longer if they have undergone surgery."[75] Nonaddicts who received surgery were the sweet spot here, with a 30 percent recidivism rate compared to an 88.9 percent rate for services alone. In particular, nonaddicts who had facial disfigurements treated remained crime-free longer.

In early 1970, Lipton delivered the first draft of their findings to Governor Rockefeller, who'd been waiting impatiently for their results.[76] Rockefeller eyeballed the 1,400-page, two-and-a-half-pound report sitting on his desk, sighed, and waded in. His brow furrowed as he skimmed the pages. Overall, the team's findings were inconclusive. They'd provided an overview of every study, along with detailed notes about the research methods that were used. The report was structured as a presentation rather than summation, allowing readers to make up their own minds for each evaluation.

Governor Rockefeller was disappointed. Their data didn't look good—it wasn't the sort of metrics he wanted associated with him. "It's really more about interpretation," Lipton cautioned, but Rockefeller had stopped listening.

Their study was killed, and Lipton and his team were told that their work was not to be published nor publicly discussed. It was disheartening; they delivered what had been asked of them: the point of data analysis was to represent all sides of the story. Lipton had thought better of the governor. His boss told him to drop it. Martinson and Wilks were let go. Wilks was resigned by the news, but Martinson was incensed. "It is what it is," Lipton told him.

His own prospects in the administration looked shaky. He'd given two years of his life to the governor but had never been promoted—and, with the governor's current disapproval of his work, maybe he never would. "Assistant director is as high as you'll go here," a friend told him. Lipton was stung. He grew increasingly unhappy about the direction Rockefeller's legislation was taking and, on a wider scale, the larger problem of power in America.

When President Richard Nixon replaced President Johnson on January 20, 1969, he'd instigated a wave of strong, Republican-minded anticrime sanctions. Nixon's campaign had been a fire and brimstone attack against the "liberals'" relaxed attitude toward law and order, and he'd explicitly promised a tougher approach to America's drug and crime problem. He declared that drugs were "public enemy number one" and pledged to be "tough on crime."

Rockefeller, once a staunch proponent of criminal reform, leaned in to President Nixon's edicts, angling for a spot in his cabinet. New York established mandatory minimum life sentences for drug users and dealers and stripped judges of the autonomy to direct first-time offenders to community or probation services instead. This change, in addition to Rockefeller's stop-and-frisk and "no-knock" laws—both of which disproportionately targeted poor Blacks—created a statewide return to the punitive approach toward corrections.

Pushed to the end of his tether and seeing no other options, Lipton quit the state office of crime control planning. He was hired by the Drug Abuse Research unit, a fledgling team of five under the auspices of New York State. He ramped up hiring, employing 115 people during the course of six months. Lipton made it a point to hire former addicts or inmates whenever an appropriate position came up; he'd seen how hard it was for employers to take a chance on them, and he wanted to make that process easier. Plus, it was good for the more "straight-laced" members of his staff to see that once an addict, not *always* an addict.

The frenzied discussion surrounding juvenile delinquents of the 1960s bled into the 1970s with juvenile delinquency reaching an all-time high. In 1970, 1,052,000 juvenile cases were processed by U.S. courts, with three million more youths arrested and released without charge.[77] The authorities threw

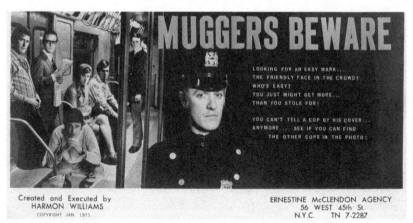

"Muggers Beware" subway poster showing an undercover officer on the subway, 1971. *Collection JVL: Mayor John V. Lindsay, Courtesy Municipal Archives, City of New York*

everything they had at this problem, including the Scared Straight program, in which high schoolers toured their local prisons and talked with grizzled convicts who shared lurid tales of prison life—a warning of what might happen if they weren't careful. Death was another option, both on the street or inside the city's jails and prisons. Three hundred men had died inside New York City's jails during the last six years, with guard brutalization attributed to their demise.

For many, however, crime was often the end result of poverty. It was a tough time to be a teen; jobs were scarce and employers were unenthusiastic about hiring young and inexperienced employees, especially those from the slums. A survey by the Congress Subcommittee on Employment, Manpower, and Poverty found that a full third of employers avoided hiring those twenty-one and younger.[78] "A man changes jobs three times in a lifetime," an employer told a researcher. "I don't want to get him on the first one." Those living in poverty lacked information about job openings and how to approach interview situations. This handicap, in addition to race and gender, caused Black girls to experience the highest rate of joblessness.

Teenage runaways and addicts grouped together in the East Village and downtown Manhattan; there was safety in numbers. "I sleep on rooftops, crash pads," a young white runaway told a documentary reporter, her acne reflecting off the camera lens. She'd been in New York three months now, she explained, moving from alley to alley, anywhere she could get a hit. "I'll sell baking products for skag if I have to, it's that desperate," she confided.

"You gotta watch out for weird people in the park here," her friend, another runaway, added.

"I'd like to leave New York City if I can," the girl said, a little mournfully. "Nowhere to go though. . . . In five years I'll probably be in a state penitentiary."[79]

On the medical side, Dr. Munick and Dr. Lewin's theory about plastic surgery benefiting a younger population was embraced. Criminologists believed that surgically treating juveniles would be more effective than treating adults, as criminal tendencies were established in youth. Congress funneled $2 billion dollars to the Department of Justice, with the remit that it be used to remake the juvenile justice system. Plastic surgery was included on the agenda.[80]

Mid-1970, Norman Cavior completed his doctorate and was hired by West Virginia University (WVU) as an assistant professor in the psychology department. The college was located in Morgantown, deep in coal-mining country, where the social calendar revolved around Friday-night football and Sunday services.

But what the city lacked in theaters and arts, it made up for in hippy culture. Cavior was enchanted by the collegiate atmosphere he found. WVU's students wore their hair long, strummed their guitars on the grass, and marched up University Avenue to protest racism. Cavior shucked his smart shoes for sandals and dressed in loose pants. He attended faculty parties at which his colleagues passed joints around, the room heady with the smell of marijuana and hashish, and pies—cherry, raspberry, and boysenberry—brought out when the inevitable munchies occurred. This never would have happened in New York—at least, not on this scale, he thought. WVU was its own liberal bubble in a red-leaning state. His students adored him; he was the most playful of their professors, and they were endlessly fascinated by his research on physical attractiveness.[81]

"In almost every outcome of importance, it's better if you're attractive," he lectured, smiling at his seminar group. "I'm only about a six out of ten on this scale!" He winked at the class as he pinched an inch at his stomach. Those pies added up. Every day brought new ideas for research. "Is beauty really in the eye of the beholder?" he asked the class. "Does attractiveness correlate to popularity among kids? What role does it play in dating and marriage? How about the courtroom? Is there a relationship between appearance and adolescent criminality? Is anyone interested in working with me on these projects?" Hands shot up around the room.

He paired up with Ramona Howard, a twenty-four-year-old Black student on the psychology PhD track, to tackle the juvenile delinquency question: could criminality be inferred from a youth's appearance? Howard rang the local schools till she found one that agreed to send over its senior yearbook photos to be used as a baseline comparison. She received seventy-eight photographs of its male seniors—the entire graduating class that year. Every boy was white and wore his hair short.

Robert F. Kennedy Youth Center, a federal prison for delinquent boys situated three miles from campus, supplied the duo with 103 photographs of white juvenile delinquents aged sixteen to twenty-one years old. The boys had similar hairstyles to the high school seniors. Their photographs had been taken using a photo vending machine at the center and printed on white 2- × 1.5-inch cardstock. Only the cardstock differed.[82]

Cavior and Howard's hypothesis was that the jailed boys would be regarded as less attractive than the high school seniors. They distributed copies of the delinquents' photos to a class of sixty (all white) freshman and sophomores—thirty men and thirty women—who were taking Introduction to Psychology. They assigned the high school senior photos to another sixty students with the same gender breakdown. Neither group received any information about the origins of the photos, and each group was asked to rate the pictures for attractiveness on a scale of one to five, with five representing extreme attractiveness.

They gathered the data and analyzed it in Cavior's office: 9 percent of the jailed kids were rated three or above compared to 37 percent of the high schoolers. It was clear that children with different levels of attractiveness were treated differently. Howard was shocked. "That's such a large difference," she told Cavior. "How can it . . . why does . . . what do *you* think about it?" Cavior was unsurprised by the results. "It's complicated," he told her, "you have to look beyond the concept that 'all delinquents are unappealing.'" For one, a person's appearance intersects with economic wealth, social situations, access to health care, and more, he explained. Their appearance might also have contributed to their sentence; research found that judges regularly doled out harsher sentences to the less attractive. Then there was the prison itself; incarceration, which disproportionately targeted poor and minority groups, could cause decreased attractiveness due to the quality of food, lack of exercise and sunshine, and other restrictions.

"Low physical attractiveness in children contributes to careers of deviancy," he wrote in the *Journal of Abnormal Psychology*.[83] "Lack of attractiveness may play a role in antisocial behavior."

Howard was intrigued by their findings but wanted to go deeper. She was troubled by the exclusion of Black kids from their study, she told Cavior. Nationwide, Black inmates were beginning to outstrip white prisoners. It was true that white inmates far outnumbered Black ones in West Virginia at almost six to one, but with only 4 percent of the state's population Black, that was still far larger than expected.[84] "I completely agree," Cavior told her—he'd wanted to include Black delinquents in their assessment, but with most of the student body white, it hadn't seemed fair. Howard drummed her heels on the floor. Not good enough. "I'll reach out to my contacts in Georgia," she said; she'd source a selection of Black evaluators to rate their next batch of pictures.

Cavior called the prison to request photographs of their Black delinquents; he received fifty-six pictures. Howard added fifty-six photographs of Black high-school seniors from Atlanta to the pile. They shuffled them together and showed them to three fresh groups of evaluators: sixty Black male and female undergrads at WVU with 50/50 gender split; thirty white WVU graduate students with a 50/50 gender split; and a group of thirty Black men and women comprised of teachers from Georgia, WVU faculty, and students. Each group was asked to rate the photographs from one to five.

Of the high school seniors, 77 percent received a two or higher compared to 45 percent of the Black delinquents. Both the Black and white evaluators graded the lighter-skinned Black children as more attractive. Their data showed that collectively the Black delinquents had darker skin tones than the Black high school kids. Surprisingly, they found that white evaluators gave higher physical attractiveness scores to Black subjects than Black evaluators. Cavior hypothesized that this might be due to "whites rating the black pictures from a position of defensiveness," an area that needed further study. Howard was saddened; her family had brought her up to embrace "black is beautiful," and it was hard to see that not everyone thought that way.

"Black has been devalued in the black community. . . . They've been socialized to accept the white world and white standards of beauty," their report stated.

Year after year, the emphasis "surgical" correction for juveniles grew stronger. In Chicago, a white plastic surgeon, Harvey Zarem, set up free plastic surgery clinics for youths, which were intentionally located in Black neighborhoods on the premise that Black delinquents might reform if their features were smoothed out. "Plastic surgery will not solve all youth's problems in the ghetto, but it may solve some," he told *Jet* magazine.[85]

This belief made its way into policy. In 1972, the youth development team of the U.S. Department of Health, Education, and Welfare added plastic surgery for unattractive adolescents to its social care tool kit.[86] It was a new addition to its nationwide youth services program, which broadly covered psychological services, GED tutoring, job placement, and early prevention programs like Kiddie Kamps.[87] It was hoped that surgery, or a combination of services, would effect a long-term change on troubled youths.

"By 1977, almost $1.5 billion could be saved in official court costs," reported Robert J. Gemignani, the commissioner of the Youth Development and Delinquency training program at the National Symposium on Law Enforcement Science and Technology.[88]

This was far from the first time that doctors had targeted children's bodies for treatment, but it was the first time it was fully adopted as national policy. The notion appealed for many reasons: for one, the Cinderella redemption story was symbolic of the American Dream, and it was a (mostly) one-stop shop, after all, it was far more effective—and quicker—to give someone a new nose or chin than to spend years providing counseling, welfare, and the necessary social follow-ups.

Not everyone agreed with the "surgery for social problems" philosophy. At Johns Hopkins University in Baltimore, plastic surgeon Dr. Jon Meyer tested this hypothesis on twenty-one youths aged twelve- to twenty-one years old, theorizing that, "the improvement would be reinforced by less scapegoating from his family and peers, with a decrease in social isolation," he wrote in a paper published by the *Plastic and Reconstructive Surgery Journal*.[89] However, Meyer was surprised to observe no discernible differences in the youths' behavior. "Plastic surgery appears to be no more effective in achieving positive change than nonsurgical intervention," he reported. In Missouri, Dr. Eugene Kissling, psychology director of St. Louis Juvenile Court, refuted the notion. There is little relationship between a juvenile's appearance and juvenile delinquency, he told the *St. Louis Post-Dispatch*.[90] Psychologists should prioritize juveniles' interpersonal relationships, *not* their looks.

But Kissling and Meyer's voices, among other critics, were quashed, their sample sizes too small, their concerns invalid, the opposition said. The popular viewpoint was that plastic surgery worked wonders for juveniles—the context being that if they didn't receive it while they were young, "you'll be paying psychiatrists to straighten out their psyche later," according to Dr. Peter Steinchron in his nationally syndicated advice column. Some psychologists even posited that *not* providing children with cosmetic surgery was akin to child abuse; and, as popular theory went, unhappy children grow up to be criminally minded adults.

From their respective institutions, Norman Cavior and Douglas Lipton were wary of this narrative, but their work had become more and more removed from affecting this type of correctional policy.

# 11

# HARD PASS

## The "Nothing Works" Problem

Plastic Surgery Made Us Better Teachers—*Instructor*, 1969[1]

Plastic Surgery Now as Acceptable as Wigs—*Press Democrat*, 1970[2]

Welcome to Fear City—New York City Council for Public Safety pamphlet for tourists, 1975[3]

You want to look halfway well-dressed. . . . God knows you've lost your identity, you don't want to go around looking like a complete freak. You feel enough like a freak being in there—Peggy Russell, inmate at women's prison, Tipton, Missouri, 1975[4]

On June 16, 1970, four months after Mary Switzer had been forced out of the Department of Health, Education, and Welfare, fifty-two-year-old Jessica Mitford found herself hurtling through Washington, D.C., in the back of a police van. Mitford flinched as the van took a corner too fast, jostling her against the other eight female prisoners stuffed next to her. She grimaced as the cool metal cuffs grazed her wrists. They would leave marks, she thought.

The other women were also restrained, though a few had their feet shackled and the lone murderess of their group was draped in chains. Two of the prisoners were Black and the rest, like Mitford, were white. Some giggled uneasily as the van picked up speed. She glanced around; she was probably the oldest here, she thought, bracing her back against her seat for the next turn, though, judging by the careworn faces of her companions, many had significantly more experience of incarceration. The van shuddered to a stop, and the doors were jerked open by a uniformed officer.[5]

Mitford blinked as her eyes readjusted, taking in the gloomy brick building on North Capitol Street, the only female detention center in Washington, D.C. Female guards hurried the group out of the van, keys clanking, and rushed the women into a large gray reception room. One guard grasped Mitford by the arm and directed her to a counter at the side of the room. Her handbag was removed, its contents upended on the desk. Her lipstick tube and compact were roughly examined. She was shuffled to another guard, who rolled her fingers in ink and pressed them on a sheet of paper. Then she stood in front of a screen and stared, unsmiling, as a bulb flashed. She turned to the side and the process repeated. Then she was searched; rough hands smoothed down the outline of her clothes and rifled through her thin gray hair for lice and contraband. "Now, strip."

Mitford's fingers trembled as she undid her shirt and slowly slipped off her skirt. She'd known this was part of the booking process, but it was so demeaning, so unseemly. No one but her husband had seen her naked body in decades!

"Bend over, spread cheeks."

Once the new arrivals were processed, the group was marched through a narrow corridor into the main detention center. An eerie, muffled wail reverberated through the room. "A broken air conditioner?" Mitford wondered aloud. Her guards shook their heads. "Nope, that's just Viola in Adjustment. She's mental, always bothering the other inmates."

Mitford was taken to her cell, and the door slammed shut behind her. She looked mournfully at the small cubicle and its two wilted-looking beds. It smelled stale and earthy. "Hello," her roommate, a slim Black woman, said with a shy smile. "I'm Della." She was thirty years old and serving a six-month sentence for soliciting. "You got off lightly," she informed Mitford; normally they'd perform a vaginal examination and douse you with Lysol.

"What do we do with our free time? Is there vocational training?" Mitford asked. Della laughed. There are "eight old broken-down typewriters somewhere," she said, and that was it. Mitford's face dropped. An hour later, she was yanked out of her cell by another guard. "You've been called before the disciplinary committee," the guard told her. "I haven't done anything! I just got here!" The guard shrugged. The stern-faced committee members told Mitford that she'd been accused of kissing another inmate. "That's a lie!" Her denial was ignored, and they pronounced judgment: "Ten days in Adjustment!"

Adjustment was a dark, narrow corridor tucked away at the back of the detention center, which held eight solitary confinement cells, each with a bed and a lidless toilet that flushed from the outside. Mitford was forced to strip again. This time, the officer didn't return her bra, wedding ring, and cigarettes. She wasn't allowed books, either, the guards told her. Then, a wrinkle. The adjustment cells were full. But a sentence was a sentence. . . . Her guard sighed, unlocked one of the doors, and squeezed Mitford into an occupied cell. Her new bunkie was Tina, who'd been sequestered for fighting the other inmates. It was hard to make out what Tina was saying over the plaintive screams emanating from another cell a few doors down. "That's our juvenile," Tina explained. "She's seventeen." Mitford looked skeptical. Seventeen years old and in solitary confinement? That made no sense. Ninety minutes later, another guard unlocked the cell and pulled Mitford out. She was free to go.

"What did you think?" one of the officers asked as they escorted her to the reception room to reclaim her belongings.

Mitford gave the guard a small, thin smile. After all, she wasn't a real inmate. Mitford and the eight "prisoners" she'd arrived with had been sent here to observe the inner working of the jail as part of a Crime and Correction workshop. Her group included five reporters, a lawyer, a social worker, a policewoman, and a drug counselor. A similar van filled with state judges and prosecutors had been sent to the men's prison.

It had not been a pleasant experience. Still, she was pleased that she'd had the chance to experience it, unpleasantness and all. This was the first time she'd been allowed to spend unsupervised time with real prisoners. Every other jail and prison she'd contacted had refused access, even after she sued—and won!—the right to enter. The more the prisons pushed back, the more convinced she became that there was something bad brewing in corrections. How were the inmates treated? What conditions did they live in? What was their care really like? Why were there so many unexplained deaths each year?

Now, she had glimpsed what life behind bars was like—albeit an extrasanitized experience in which the inmates had been warned to be on their best behavior—and she saw just how problematic the correctional system was. The wailing girl in adjustment really was seventeen years old, confirmed an administrator. Ideally, she would have been placed in the medical ward, but all beds were taken. Minors weren't allowed to be housed with adults, so she'd been locked up in solitary. She could mingle with the rest of the women when she turned eighteen in three months. "Aren't you afraid she'll go completely insane by then?" Mitford asked. The administrator shrugged. "There is a danger." Mitford recorded her comment in her reporter's notebook.

⌒⌒

Mitford's forays into the incarceration space were part of a wider examination of prisoner care. Despite good intentions, the American prison system as a whole had become a fetid, dank locus of corruption and unsanitary conditions. President Nixon's preventative detention policies had filled jails and prisons to bursting, and in New York City, things had rapidly escalated. Rikers Island was more crowded than ever, at 75 percent over capacity.

The tension between white and Black inmates grew unmanageable, as did the violent outbursts in the yard. Stories leaked out about sexual abuse and rape, savage, racist beatings by the guards, and an unexplainable suicide epidemic. "It's a dumping ground," a social work student from New York University (NYU) told the media, slamming the poor food, medical care, and general inadequacy of all facilities on the island.[6] "Some of us have clients who have not been outdoors in six months."

The problems put the city's corrections commissioner, George F. McGrath, on the defensive. The NYU students were "immature young people," he told reporters. They'd been "manipulated by prisoners" due to their inexperience. In the city, citizens complained of police brutality and corruption and demanded sweeping reforms.

McGrath's pressure came from within the administration as well. The New York State Senate Committee on Penal Institutions issued a report that described the Tombs, a jail for men in downtown Manhattan, "less humane than our public zoos." This escalated into a four-day riot in 1970, in which guards were held hostage by inmates seeking better "care." Things deteriorated further when the leaders of the riot were confined to indefinite solitary, and the Legal Aid Society filed a lawsuit alleging conditions at the Tombs in Manhattan constituted "cruel and unusual punishment" and deprived inmates of due process. The city's prisons were now 183 percent over capacity.[7]

In upstate New York, the prisons were equally bad. At Auburn prison, the warden's food budget allocated seventy cents per inmate per day, which comprised three meals a day—a sum that made up less than 7 percent of all Auburn's expenditures.[8] Seventy cents was especially low—federal prisons averaged $1.25 to $1.35 a head, per day, for inmates' food.

Still, seventy cents was a wealth of riches for some inmates. Attica prison, which lay 120 miles east of Auburn, spent sixty-three cents per head,[9] and the state of Texas spent fifteen cents a day per prisoner for non-prison-produced food—about what New York's Clinton prison paid per head in 1914! New York City jails averaged fifty cents a head.[10] "At the zoo chimpanzees are fed for $1.28 a day. Tigers $3 a day," Jessica Mitford wrote in the *Bulletin*. Prisoners everywhere were rioting, the most devastating of those being the 1971 Attica uprising, which left forty-three people dead. An overhaul was long overdue, but it wasn't coming from the government.

Her responsibilities diminished after being forced from office, Mary Switzer, once the highest-ranking woman in government, finally had time to tackle her personal to-do list. Task number one was getting a barrage of medical tests. Her mind was as sharp as ever, but she'd lost weight and her knees troubled her. Sometimes her energy was so low that she used a wheelchair. Tests confirmed she had an incurable cancer. "Keep yourself comfortable," her doctor advised. She deteriorated quickly and passed away at 4:00 a.m. on October 16, 1971. Seven hundred people attended her memorial service.

Life was tumultuous for the rest of America during the early 1970s. As troops returned from Vietnam, the press covered horror stories about the bitter political war being fought for no real purpose. Many of the returning veterans had suffered injuries and indignities and had severe post-traumatic stress disorder. Americans saw the pain in the eyes of the returning soldiers and railed against the administration.

The American economy was growing, but with this came dire warnings from analysts about "overheating"—and inflation grew accordingly. Jobs, which had been on a slow upward trajectory since the mid-1960s, began to decline. Many blamed the lack of employment opportunities on minorities and women; their campaigns for equal rights and pay had left "good, honest, white men" out of work. Every good piece of news—like NASA's introduction of the space shuttle program, for example—was tempered by a political scandal or an oil crisis or a crime wave, news that tended to be extremely racialized.

Despite this upheaval, or perhaps partly because of it, the cosmetic surgery space flourished. In 1971, around one million cosmetic operations were performed, a 6,566 percent increase since 1949.[11] A new era had dawned; investing in cosmetic surgery was now viewed as an investment in one's self. "I had a Jewish nose and I felt it branded me," Sophie, a sixth-grade science teacher, told *Instructor* magazine.[12] After she had it "fixed," she received a promotion from her superintendent. "He'd passed over me before, saying I was too aggressive," she said.

Surgery for men was also increasing, making up around 15 to 20 percent of all operations. They told reporters that they'd opted for face-lifts, nose jobs, and the like to allow them "to stay competitive" in the business world. "The youth cult sweeping corporate suites has pushed many executives into hospital for cosmetic surgery," noted the *New York Times*.[13] The plastic surgery sphere had become less taboo in general, its face-lift helped along by the publicized nose jobs and jaw implants of Hollywood starlets and prominent politicians.

In February 1972, Senator William Proxmire from Wisconsin issued a statement regarding his recent appearance in the Senate. The fifty-six-year-old had turned up for a hearing sporting two black eyes, and, a few weeks later, he walked the halls wearing a large white turban. The reason? He was recovering from a face-lift and a $2,578 hair transplant. "I will still be a semi-baldy, but a little more semi and a little less baldy," his press release stated.[14] The reception to his announcement was mostly positive, if somewhat jeering. "We should not regard Senator Proxmire as vain or foolish," reported the *Lowell Sun*.[15] "He is, rather, a realist."

Few Black Americans opted for plastic surgery—both for economic and cultural reasons, Dr. James Benjamin, one of the few Black plastic surgeons in America, told *Ebony* magazine.[16] Benjamin, the assistant chief of plastic surgery for Walter Reed Army Medical Center, had been surprised by their reluctance. "They seem to have the notion of what God gave me I should leave alone," he said. White people had no such qualms.

The use of cosmetic surgery had grown inside the justice system as well, though the approach and quality of the treatments varied. Tennessee state prison recorded 7.4 procedures per one hundred inmates. White inmates received double the number of plastic surgeries as Black inmates.[17] In Texas prisons, the cosmetic work was folded into the plastic surgery residencies of the University of Texas Medical Branch at Galveston and the Southwestern Medical School. Some 350 operations took place each year. In televised media interviews, Texas inmates professed wild enthusiasm about their cosmetic changes. "I know I can make it, but not because I got a new look," an inmate, his nose, forehead, and ears obscured by white bandages, told CBS. He tapped his head. "It's because I changed what's up here."

Other prisons folded their plastic surgery programs under the broad umbrella of their ongoing medical research. These programs soon developed cracks, due in part to the generally poor conditions of the prisons at large, and horror stories about maltreatment and abuses were leaked to the press.

In Pennsylvania, the Federal Office of Economic Opportunity responded to the leaks by launching an investigation. It commissioned a research report presided over by staff and students of Pennsylvania Law School. The findings, released in August 1972, filled 282 pages. Pennsylvania's eight state prisons all had widespread rat and cockroach infestations, in addition to inadequate medical treatment, a culture of sexual assault, violence, and "an unusually high amount of plastic surgery."[18]

"The prisoners are getting everything from nose jobs to eyebrow lifts," elaborated Carl McConnell, the lead attorney on the report.[19] "They seem to prize very highly the hair transplants." The prisons had no official screening process for these surgeries, McConnell noted. "It is supposedly voluntary," he wrote, with the caveat that although inmates were not paid to undergo surgery, enrolling offered perks such as transfers to more desirable prisons (to use the hospital facilities) or even to "enjoy escape through a few shots of Demerol."

Plastic surgery and otolaryngology[20] residents from Western Pennsylvania Hospital performed the surgeries. The consensus was that the inmates were "practice" for the residents, but both parties were agreeable to this arrangement. There was a pecking order among the surgeons, who often battled over access to inmates; they were eager to practice surgeries that would be useful in their own practices. One surgeon recruited inmates to work with him by offering them "higher shots of painkillers" than other surgeons.

Aside from that clear ethical breach, the investigation uncovered a large number of consent forms. Even the signed ones were cause for concern, as the language was so jargon-heavy and vague it was hard to know whether the inmates understood the potential consequences of what they were signing up for. The quality of the work is generally good, McConnell admitted, but the lack of oversight was a concern.[21]

Beautification aside, the living conditions inside the prisons raised a number of health and human rights concerns. In the kitchen, paint chips that had flaked off the ceiling and walls were regularly found in food storage containers—along with a few instances of urine—along with dirty dishes stacked up in the "clean" section. Many of the cells lacked hot water, heat, and flushing toilets. There was little privacy surrounding sensitive medical records; guards accessed them at whim.[22] In Huntingdon prison, Pennsylvania's oldest correctional facility, inmates with mental health problems were kept in solitary confinement, often locked inside soundproof glass cages for observation.[23]

All of this paled in comparison to the numerous medical experiments happening inside the institutions, which ranged from dermatological trials to experimental drug testing. Again, enrollment in these trials was voluntary, but many paid $10 a day compared to the $1 a day wage earned by working in the prison laundry or woodshop.

Inside Holmesburg prison located in northeast Philadelphia, some of the most egregious experiments had been taking place since the early 1950s. These were led by Dr. Albert Kligman, a professor of dermatology at the University of Pennsylvania.

Funded with hundreds of thousands of dollars from thirty-three of the world's largest drug companies, Kligman had free reign over his subjects. He plied them with huge doses of hormones to test baldness cures and exposed them to herpes, athlete's foot, and staphylococcus bacteria. He covered their faces and backs with high concentrations of Retin-A to test acne treatments,[24] which scorched and scoured their skin, leaving them with forearm-sized burns.

For one study to analyze the absorbency of Johnson & Johnson wound dressings, he paid $5 per wound. Inmates were handed knives and told where to slice their skin. "We had an ethical problem," Kligman told the *Philadelphia Bulletin* in 1966. "How much right do you have to cause risk to a prisoner in medical tests from which he has no direct benefit?" The U.S. Army was another of his corporate clients, requesting that Kligman conduct chemical weapons research. Inmates, the majority of them Black, were injected with dioxin, the active ingredient in Agent Orange. Kligman carefully recorded the severity and onset of side effects, reporting back to the Dow Chemical Company. At one point the FDA blacklisted him for record-keeping discrepancies; he appealed and was reinstated[25] three weeks later. Efforts at oversight were continually blocked—when Philadelphia appointed a prison ombudsman to assess conditions at Holmesburg, the prison denied access, citing undivulged "disqualifying factors."[26]

Overall, there are "grave deficiencies," the law school's report concluded.[27] "Prisoners do not forfeit human rights simply by donning prison garb." Its observations lit a fire under Pennsylvania's governor, who immediately formed a task force, demanding it address these allegations. Nationwide, states were inspired to take a closer look at the treatment of inmates in their care.

Prisoners were lawyering up as well. Riots weren't that effective, but lawyers, well, they couldn't be ignored. More and more prisoners chose the litigation route, thanks to legal help provided by the American Civil Liberties Union (ACLU) and a string of court decisions that had established inmates' legal rights to counsel and appropriate medical care, the most important being the 1964 ruling of Cooper v. Pate, which permitted inmates to sue correctional facilities and staff in federal courts. This fell under the Civil Rights Act, the ruling designed to protect Black inmates from state officials or judges who were members of or affiliated with the Ku Klux Klan, a common occurrence in many southern states. Federal courts assumed the authority to judge misuse of power, which applied to all civil rights of the inmates.[28]

An onslaught of cases hit the courts. In Clinton prison in upstate New York, an inmate sued for $100,000, alleging that the medical staff had discarded his severed ear (which resulted from a prison altercation) with no attempt to reattach it, saying "he didn't need it." In Iowa, two inmates filed for a restraining order to prevent the state-sanctioned use of unqualified inmates providing medical and surgical care. During inmate Phillip McBride's routine nasal surgery, the prison surgeon had instructed his assistant—an inmate—to tap his mallet against McBride's nose. "You hit too hard,"[29] he berated the man as McBride reeled in pain. The special assistant attorney general pushed back against the restraining order, contending that granting their request would "unduly restrict medical services at the penitentiary." And, in Chino prison in California, a male inmate sued the Federal Bureau of Prisons for $200,000 for discontinuing a hair transplant program in the middle of his treatment, leaving him with unsightly patches of hair on his pate.[30]

Flustered by the onslaught of suits, some prisons dropped or downsized their plastic surgery offerings, alongside a reduction on prisoner experiments.

There was also the bigger question as to whether an inmate in an inherently coercive situation can really volunteer for anything, including plastic surgery. Prison reformists didn't think so. Was it true "consent" if inmates believed that opting for surgery or medical studies would improve their chances of early parole? Reformists pushed to shut down exploitative programs, and the Attica prison riot of 1971, along with numerous complaints in prisons across the country, spurred a deeper investigation into prisoner health care. "There are no stringent safeguards," wrote Alvin Bronstein, founder of ACLU National Prison Project.

Bronstein was the reason that journalist Jessica Mitford had endured an unseemly strip search at Washington, D.C.'s house of detention. At his behest, the ACLU had funded her research, hoping that the best-selling author would reveal the prison issues to a mainstream audience.[31]

The more time Mitford spent in this world, the angrier she got. There were so many obvious abuses of power, of human rights violations. She wrote a scathing riposte about the conditions inside California's so-called modern prisons for the *Atlantic*. "The supposed beneficiaries of the new enlightened penology denounce it as bureaucratic window dressing design to impress the public," she wrote. "In some places physical degradation was replaced with psychological degradation."

It became clear to her that there was little oversight around medical research in prisons—to a worrying degree. Companies were capitalizing on inmates' poverty. During the 1970 to 1971 fiscal year, the governor of Florida informed her that 4,122 of its inmates had been involved in sixty medical research projects. They received $108,891.71 for their labor, averaging $26.27 a head.[32] The fruits of their labor made the companies *millions*.

Mitford published an exposé for the *Atlantic* titled "Experiments behind Bars."[33] "Criminals in our penitentiaries are fine experimental material and much cheaper than chimpanzees," she wrote, documenting how much money the companies made off their backs: inmates constituted almost 99 percent of all phase-one drug tests. The inmates viewed their small payments as a largesse, she explained; they suffered through burns, scurvy, and hemorrhages in order to afford phone calls home and cigarettes. She compared the treatment of the physicians to those at Nuremberg, emphasizing that voluntary consent of the subjects was essential in these kinds of experiments. Procedures that happen in prison would never be allowed if the subjects were graduate students, Mitford explained.

Doctors and drug companies disagreed and loudly protested her reporting in the letters page of the following issue.

> Prison based research has advantages which may make it worth the extra effort required to regulate it.—Dr. John Parrish, assistant professor of dermatology, Harvard Medical School[34]

> The element of risk in this kind research is obviously negligible.—Edward Littlejohn, vice president of Pfizer Inc., New York City

> If the element of risk is so negligible, why are convicts required to sign an illegal waiver of their rights to sue for damages if they are disabled by the experiments?—Jessica Mitford

Mitford's follow-up was a 373-page book, *Kind and Usual Punishment: The Prison Business*. Its publication was explosive in the literary world as well as among the general public and the government. Its timing was crucial. The Attica prison riot of 1971, during which forty-three inmates and guards died in a four-day siege, was still fresh in people's minds, and the Tuskegee syphilis study, in which 399 low-income Black men had been subjected to forty years of untreated syphilis by the Centers for Disease Control and the U.S. Public Health Service, remained headline news. The agencies had been interested in the long-term effects of the bacterial disease; by this point, 128 of the subjects had died, either from syphilis or related complications. When the men sought treatment, they were given placebos, yet another abuse of power and disregard for the health of Black bodies.

In the wake of these scandals, the public expressed a new willingness to hear out stories about the shoddy behavior of those in authority. President Nixon's upcoming impeachment had sowed doubt among Americans, making them receptive to stories that revealed what was going on behind the scenes. Change was in the air. *Kind and Usual Punishment* rocketed up the best-seller lists and was short-listed for a National Book Award. Mitford found herself the de facto spokesperson for prison problems.

In light of her book and related stories, the Department of Health, Education, and Welfare created a senate subcommittee to investigate further and to provide guidelines for the broader biomedical research space.[35]

The committee was chaired by Senator Edward Kennedy, a Democrat from Massachusetts. "The burden of developing these products is not equally shared," he announced in one of the early hearings. "When a new drug is tried or a new surgery performed there is considerable risk. That risk is taken most often by the poor, the minority groups, and the institutionalized."

Mitford was the first witness to address the committee. "My findings are, of necessity, only a tiny beginning, a lifting of one corner of the rug," she told them, reiterating her reporting. "If a volunteer becomes seriously ill or dies as a result of the procedures he is subjected to, it is unlikely that this will ever come to anybody's attention."[36]

The Senate was shocked. Multiple agencies sprang into action after the hearings. The American Medical Association created a task force to address the health needs of jail inmates, the Commission on Accreditation of Corrections was formed as an independent adjunct to the American Correctional Association, its focus on maintaining standards and integrity, and on Valentine's Day 1974, Congress announced an immediate funding ban on behavior modification or medical research treatments on inmates[37] (this did not include plastic surgery, which was not considered "experimental").

The magnitude of the stories and abuses that emerged were breathtaking. In Iowa, troublesome inmates were injected with apomorphine, which induced two hours of vomiting. Wisconsin and Connecticut utilized electric shock treatments to rewire pedophiles' sexual preferences. The new ruling wouldn't automatically end *all* behavioral modification programs, but since most were funded by the federal government, it was highly likely they'd shutter.[38]

Subsequently, the National Research Act was signed into law, establishing the National Commission for the Protection of Human Subjects of Biomedical and Behavioral Research. Mitford's book and the Senate hearings had done their job. Frustrated by the bad press and legal problems surrounding medical research, numerous state prison programs closed.

In Pennsylvania, the prison board abolished the clinical research unit. Albert Kligman was given his marching orders, his work inside Holmesburg prison permanently shuttered. Infuriated and a little nervous, Kligman destroyed the data he'd gathered from his experiments. A flurry of inmate lawsuits ensued, all claiming that Kligman had violated their civil rights. One by one, the judge ruled in his favor.

The very fact that they call us inmates, that's like calling a black a n****r or a Jew a k**e. It says that this is a hospital and I'm going to make you well. This isn't a hospital and I'm not flawed, I'm not sick, and there's nothing here being done to make me any better.[39]—inmate serving a forty-year sentence for bank robbery at Marion Federal Penitentiary in southern Illinois, 1975

After being unceremoniously fired from Lipton's recidivism project, Robert Martinson resumed his position in City College's sociology department with a renewed focus on the intersection of crime and policy. He dug into the psychological profiles of inmates and railed against the notion that inmates could be assessed collectively. "We are burdened with timeless abstractions about the 'inmate subculture,' the 'inmate code,' and so forth," he wrote.[40] He grew gloomier the deeper he delved. Solitary confinement, a soul-deadening experience, was being vastly overused, and he felt that the discussion surrounding psychological care increasingly veered toward the ludicrous: wishful thinking rather than reality. If only the public and the politicians could see the *real* recidivism data!

Every month or so, he rang Douglas Lipton, now director of the state's Drug Abuse Control Commission Research (formerly the Narcotic Addiction Control Commission, the National Development and Research Institutes, and

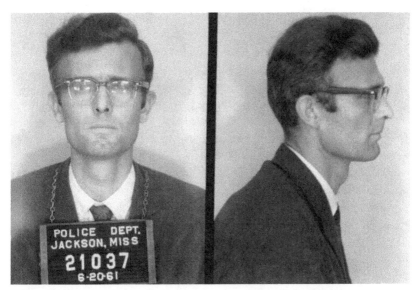

Freedom Rider mug shot of Robert Martinson, 1961. *Courtesy of Mississippi State Sovereignty Commission*

Substance Abuse Services). Lipton's unit had relocated to the sixty-seventh floor of tower two of the World Trade Center, and when he swung around in his chair, he could see all of Manhattan—even the Bronx—laid out before him like a jigsaw puzzle. Martinson badgered him for an update on their report Governor Rockefeller had killed—when were they going to release it?

"Nothing has changed," Lipton told him—as far as he knew, their work had been shelved, and there was nothing that either of them could do about it. You can use what we discovered to influence your own work, he suggested; their studies had influenced the projects he took on. He encouraged Martinson to do the same and avoided his calls.

Martinson tried moving on, but their research haunted him, bleeding into every aspect of his work. He read recidivism roundups from other sociologists and rolled his eyes. He laughed angrily every time he saw a paper that purported to have a new recidivism solution. There had been reports published along the same lines as their killed report, but they lacked the comprehensive scale of the trio's work. The more he read rehabilitation rhetoric, the more bitter and frustrated he became about the energy that was funneled into wasteful projects.[41] He channeled this into fiery conversations with reporters. "There is very little evidence that any prevailing mode of correctional treatment has a decisive effect in reducing recidivism," he told the *Washington Post*,[42] subtly citing their unpublished report. "Rehabilitation is a social myth," he complained to the

*Christian Science Monitor.*[43] He penned a four-part series for the *New Republic* on the paradox of prison reform.[44] "Treatment is a dangerous myth," he wrote, "because it is not true that prison can rehabilitate men, dangerous because their pretense can loose dangerous men upon society."

By 1973, his fury had reached a boiling point. "Pseudo-research fills many correctional journals, helping to justify the fads and fashions that sweep through the field one after the other," he told attendees at the National Conference of Criminal Justice, alluding to their unpublished work. "It would be folly to ignore a body of studies of this kind."[45] He reached out to the *Public Interest*, a neoconservative journal that covered politics and social sciences. Its reports were openly critical of liberals' "over-socialized" policies, and it had published an impressive array of thought leaders. It leaned more pop culture than academic, but the benefit was that it accessed a much larger—and broader—audience. "Would you be interested in publishing the *real* truth about prisoner rehabilitation?" he asked. Intrigued, the journal gave him the go-ahead, and in spring 1974, his thirty-two-page jargon-free treatise, which included a full five pages of footnotes, was published as the *Public Interest*'s cover story. Martinson titled his musings as "What Works? Questions and Answers about Prison Reform."

He opened by airing his grievance that Governor Rockefeller—who was hotly touted as the next vice president of the United States—had refused to allow the publication of his research. "By the spring of 1972, the state had not only failed to publish it, but had also refused to give me permission to publish it on my own," he sniped.

Then he went for the kill. "With few and isolated exceptions, the rehabilitative efforts that have been reported so far have had no appreciable effect on recidivism," he wrote. He qualified his statement by detailing many of the research studies they'd analyzed, from providing educational support for delinquents to a controlled reentry program. "None of this made any difference in recidivism rates," Martinson concluded, softening his words with the caveat that "it is impossible to tell whether this failure lay in the program itself or in the conditions under which it was administered."

He whizzed through multiple rehabilitative processes, ticking them off one by one: Individual counseling? Doesn't work. Group counseling? Doesn't work. Supervision? Doesn't work. Sometimes the rehabilitative programs caused the opposite effect, he added, noting that a study of incarcerated juveniles in California found that they committed *more* crimes after they'd received a combination of therapy, field trips, and work placements. He also found fault with the Surgical and Social Rehabilitation of Adult Offenders experiment. "When one reanalyzes the data, it appears that surgery alone did not make a significant difference." The few studies that reportedly showed a positive effect on recidivism, he labelled "ambiguous" and flawed. "It is just possible that some of our treatment programs are working to some extent, but our research is so bad that it is incapable of telling."

Martinson's report sent shockwaves among policy makers, practitioners, professors, and the popular media globally. His theories were debated on television news shows, challenged on the radio, and chattered about in the commentary pages. Fan mail arrived from across the world. His report wasn't the first to raise such questions; already, there were rumblings that rehabilitation wasn't the lifeboat its proponents had hoped for—but it was the first to break into the mainstream.

"The Martinson Report," as it came to be known, struck a chord with both the left and the right. Liberals were discontented with the lack of oversight in rehabilitation, concerned it was wide open for abuse. They saw Martinson's monograph as validation that rehab needed an overhaul, whereas conservatives viewed his opus as scientific vindication for ending the "soft on crime" approach to justice. In 1974, crime was up 17 percent from 1973—the largest spike in forty-four years!—despite the billions of dollars that had been poured into addressing the problem. Analyzed over time, it was even worse; from 1968 to 1974, there had been a 122 percent jump in forcible rape, 67 percent increase in murder, and 43 percent boost in robberies.[46] Whether or not Martinson's "nothing works" catchphrase was true, it was clear that *some* things hadn't been working.

Douglas Lipton was beside himself with rage. How dare Martinson make such grandiose statements, draw such broad conclusions from the research project *Lipton* had directed? His own conclusions left the question open-ended: correctional treatments as a whole had not managed to significantly curb recidivism. But that didn't mean they hadn't helped! Just because they hadn't seen massive drops in numbers in every single study didn't mean you could discard the ones that showed promise. And he objected to Martinson's cavalier comment about the Rikers Island study: not only was the man dismissing his results, he was calling Lipton's qualifications into question by challenging his data.[47]

"Martinson has a serious mental problem," Lipton told his friends and colleagues. "He's bipolar. He calls himself a criminologist, but he had no credentials other than his posturing. He hadn't gotten a degree. . . . He's silly and wrongheaded."[48]

Lipton tried to change the narrative. He wrote long op-eds and sent them to the papers and called television producers, offering the "real truth." He mailed letters to CBS and ABC and NBC. "Martinson's lying," he told them. "He's twisting our results. How about I come on your show and give you the real truth?" They politely declined. Martinson's charisma and well-written report became the dominant narrative. He was attractive to the masses on two levels: he had scientific credentials and his message was delivered in laypeople's language, a common-sense conclusion to crime.

In June 1975, after a short volunteer trip to Israel, Michael and Berta Lewin deplaned at Kennedy airport. As they cleared customs and exited onto the main concourse, they headed to bag collection. Loud young men shouted out their services, some waving pamphlets about city tours and adventures. More pamphlets were strewn on the floor, imprinted with boot prints and stabbed with kitten heels. One stood out: a stark black-and-white pamphlet with a large skull on the cover.

"Welcome to Fear City," the headline read. It was subtitled "A Survival Guide for Visitors to the City of New York." Inside, it provided a list of guidelines

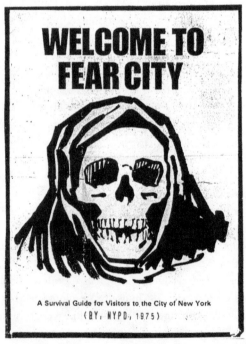

"Fear City: A Survival Guide for Visitors to the City of New York," published by the New York City Council for Public Safety in 1975. *Scan courtesy of John Landers, Brooklyn, New York*

to help guests get out of the city alive and unscathed: hunker down after 6:00 p.m., stay away from the subways, sleep near a fire exit. These suggestions, the pamphlet stated, were courtesy of the city's police and corrections officers. The pamphlets weren't a joke. They were printed in protest of the impending layoffs suggested by the mayor. More than a million pamphlets were distributed.

The pamphlet's hysteria was founded on the very real problem of New York City crime. It was a precarious, paranoid time. Unemployment was high, a million jobs had been lost since 1945 thanks to the industrial revolution and the rise of personal computing. The subways were filthy, late, and filled with pickpockets. The city's population had swelled, but its federal funding had not. The governor reached out to Washington for help. The state was heading toward bankruptcy unless the president did something soon. The city—and state!—teetered on the edge of collapse. President Ford was leery of aiding New York, blaming its budget crisis on its so-called overly generous wages, welfare system, and tuition-free colleges. Its "day of reckoning has come," he announced.

A video journalist asked New Yorkers about the city's problems.[49] "There are more kooks all the time. . . . I've been held up twice," a yellow cab driver said wearily. "New York is always broke because too much money is going to the suburbs," a well-dressed middle-aged white woman complained. "They're killing us!"

Inside Sing Sing prison, little had changed during the last decade, Lewin noted. He still held—in conjunction with surgeons from Albany Medical Center—four plastic surgery consults a month at four of the state's prisons. Noses, in particular, were always in demand; there was a backlog of five hundred patients to screen! "The primary thrust of the department's elective surgery program is to cluster patients at community hospitals, so that quality healthcare may be delivered as economically as possible," reported the Correctional Department in its annual report. "It has been heartening that the surgical staffs exhibited total professional disinterest in remunerative surgery."[50]

Lewin was unaware that his voluntary services were such an economic boon to the department, but he did know that the medical care the inmates received was far from adequate. A study of total inmate hospital admissions within the New York City jail system discovered that 30 percent of those admitted had experienced trauma to their heads, with cracked noses, broken jaws, and slashed skin[51] common. Facial scar wounds were of particular concern, the study noted. Lewin's own treatments drew some flack as well.

"There's an unwitting blindness to the real problems of prison medicine, or an undue emphasis on exotic medical problems which do not solve the problem of generally inadequate care," complained Marvin Zalman, a lawyer and professor of criminal justice from Michigan[52] in the *Journal of Criminal Law, Criminology, and Police Science.* Zalman was ambivalent toward prison plastic surgery but worried that its existence distracted from the *real* medical needs of inmates.

He was right. A year prior, criminal attorney Julie Ann Epps analyzed the expenditures of New York's maximum-security prisons. "New York budgeted one half of one percent of total prison expenditures for medical care, while Americans spend approximately six percent of disposable income after taxes on personal health care goods and services," she reported. "The per capita amount spent on medical care for all citizens is from five to eleven times the amount spent on prisoners."[53] Around 65 percent of the corrections budget was earmarked for correctional officers' salaries.

Tarred with the label "ex-con" and lacking job skills due to the decline of in-jail training programs, ex-cons had fewer choices upon release even with treatment. "It doesn't make sense," sighed parolee administrator William David Rosenberry.[54] "They go to jail in the first place because of money and then we put them back out on the street with no money and no skills, in addition to a criminal record . . . which mandates against them getting a job. Where are they going to go?"

"I don't care if an ex-convict has paid his debt to society," an industrial employer told a reporter. "I don't care if he *ever* owed a debt to society. He's spent *years* in the packed, unhealthy, plotting atmosphere of the pen and I owe too much to the workers I already have. He won't do."[55]

But there was no one speaking up for the voiceless. Mary Switzer was dead. Anna Kross had been shunted to the side. The "correctional" part of corrections had been silenced.

In August 1975, a producer from CBS News called Robert Martinson and offered him a spot on its flagship program, *60 Minutes.* "We're planning a segment on 'The Martinson Report,'" he explained. Martinson, reveling in his criminological celebrity status, happily accepted the opportunity for an even larger platform for his views.

Onscreen, he radiated benevolence, his chin-length white beard and long white locks conveying the aura of a scientific Santa. He gazed at correspondent Mike Wallace though his large round glasses.

"I looked at all the methods that we could find, vocational, educational, and a variety of other methods," he told him. "These methods simply have no fundamental effect on the recidivism rate of people who go through those prisons—the systems as a whole—probation, parole, and so forth."

"No effect at all?"

"No effect. No basic effect," Martinson replied. "Some programs did make fellas less tense, so they might be a good management program, but as far as reducing crime. . . . I didn't find any evidence."

"So, prisoners who have been exposed to no rehabilitation programs, are his chances of going back to crime better, worse, or the same as the prisoners who had the whole treatment?"

"They're the same. I know it sounds astonishing, but they're the same."

Mike Wallace quizzed Dr. Robert Carr, the prison psychologist at Marion Penitentiary in southern Illinois, the Bureau of Prison's most "cutting-edge" prison. "Two out of three prisoners wind up back in prison. Why?"

"I don't know," said Carr, a defeated look on his face, his palm pressed against his cheek. His shirt was rumpled. Carr looked away from Wallace. "We could sit here and tell you we got the answers and so on but that would be a lie."

Norman Carlson, the director of the Bureau of Prisons, provided an equally unsatisfying answer. "We don't know what causes crime," he admitted to Wallace. "We don't know what works, and what doesn't work . . . or if anything works."

"Is it conceivable that nothing works?"

"Conceivable, certainly . . . this may well be the fact," Carlson replied.

The "nothing works" doctrine became corrections' new catchphrase and Robert Martinson its poster child. *People* magazine ran a spread on him.[56] "We operate on the principle that some young fellow with a master's degree in social work can treat seventy-five or more hard-bitten cons during a half-hour interview a month," Martinson raged. "No wonder people think rehabilitation is a farce. Until my neighbors can leave their homes unafraid at 10:30 at night, I'm not satisfied." He spoke at conferences and community events and was on every correctional reporter's speed dial.

He crossed paths with Douglas Lipton at a prison conference in Philadelphia. Lipton had given up the idea that Martinson would retract his claims, but hoped they at least could be civil to one another, but when Martinson saw Lipton, he climbed onto the nearest table and began an impromptu speech about "nothing works." A crowd gathered around him. Lipton watched him rail in disbelief. The man was a colorful speaker but what he was saying was patently untrue. "Don't listen to that man," Lipton told his circle. He didn't engage with Martinson—he didn't want anything to do with him. Still, he was shocked by his behavior. Martinson was so bitter, so disillusioned, and he'd been the most hopeful of their trio!

A year after Martinson's viral article, their report, *The Effectiveness of Correctional Treatment*, was published in its full, 735-page entirety, with Lipton, Wilks, and Martinson credited as the authors. The tome provided a more nuanced overview of the rehabilitation landscape, noting that almost half of the programs surveyed lowered recidivism. They had structured their review to allow readers to draw their own conclusions, refraining from editorializing. For example, one treatment worked for one group of people but had negative results with another, which Martinson called "equivocal" but could be interpreted as specific to the population being targeted. Perhaps there was no apples-to-apples approach to comparing recidivism programs, but that didn't equate to all treatments being worthless; a focus on tailoring programs to specific communities would be a more productive takeaway. Additionally, although the report was comprehensive, it was not exhaustive, and it did not include some of the newer cognitive behavioral treatments such as methadone maintenance and work release, which had some successes (which Martinson noted in his takedown).[57] Still, it was far easier to process Martinson's synopsis than to wade through the charts and figures in the official document.

Martinson's narrative was easy to understand, and his showboating overshadowed the complexity of the real report's message. The damage was done. For years conservatives had railed against the rehabilitative-minded prison policies, and Martinson gave them the ammunition they'd been searching for. Deliberation, not desperation, was the root of all crime in their minds.

If it doesn't work, why fund it? Did America need more useless programs when inflation was spiraling out of control? Conservative politicians and the public were receptive to the "nothing works" message and pushed hard for a return to punitive treatment. They had science on their side, they argued. Coddling criminals hadn't worked. "I have not heard an intellectually respectable defense of criminal rehabilitation," James Q. Wilson, a well-known political scientist and former chairman of the White House Task Force on Crime, told *Time* magazine. The dean of the University of Chicago Law School used Martinson's report in his keynote address to compel his listeners to direct their energy away from rehabilitative solutions.[58]

Still, Lipton wasn't alone in his horror at how Martinson's message had insidiously wormed its way into policy. Academics across America vocally protested Martinson's harmful narrative. "Martinson's interpretation in *What Works?* stands in direct contradiction to the interpretation of whoever wrote *The Effectiveness of Correctional Treatment*," argued criminologist Carl B. Klockers in the *Prison Journal*.[59] "It goes far beyond what is justified by the research described in that volume."

In New York City, Sol Chaneles, Lipton's former boss and current president of the Urban Resources Corporation, penned an angry editorial for *Fortune News*.[60] Martinson is "an obscure sociologist . . . a sham," Chaneles wrote, deriding his "nothing works" mantra as "a shabby and biased incoherent charade." Martinson sniped back in the *Prison Journal*, calling Chaneles's article a "tissue of falsehoods, malicious gossip, misinformation, and bombast."[61] But it didn't seem to matter what Lipton and his peers thought—Martinson's narrative was the dominant one, and things were changing accordingly. Martinson's theories spoke to what some politicians had been working toward all along—reducing what they believed to be extraneous spending on rehabilitative programs for prisoners.

Mobilized by "The Martinson Report," the prisoner medical scandals, and a top-down tough-on-crime approach, politicians instituted sweeping changes to the system. "The use of prisoners as a subject for medical experimentation by drug companies is one of the most ethically questionable practices permitted in this country," Robert W. Kastenmeier, the House Judiciary subcommittee chairman, told the ninety-fourth Congress. "The whole coercive aspect of the institutionalized really prohibits that free choice."[62]

Although these hearings explored inmate consent, it would be a false equivalency to conflate medical experimentation and rehabilitative programs with a medical component. Consenting to cosmetic surgery, an operation designed to improve one's appearance, was far different than "consenting" to injections of typhoid or malaria or second-degree burns for a monetary fee.

"If offering one's body for medical research is such a wonderful and great contribution to humanity, then why not solicit volunteers from the free and educated population who are under more desirable circumstances, and therefore, much more capable of exercising their 'free will?'" argued Congressman Parren Mitchell. "Equally significant are the racial, social and political ramifications. It is the poor, the minorities, and the institutionalized that become the 'target populations' for risky human experimentation." Post-hearing, stringent ethical guidelines were developed. By fall 1975, only twelve state prisons still experimented on inmates.

The intensified focus on corrections did prompt some positive change. Still, the increased attention toward the incarcerated proved a double-edged sword:

even as inmates' health was protected, many of their rehabilitation programs were curtailed. Douglas Lipton was inconsolable. He'd entered the research field—first in corrections and now in drug abuse prevention—to make a difference, to help the helpless. He'd hired an oddball like Martinson to show that he respected a person's mind and that one's past behavior did not have to reflect one's future! But somehow, inadvertently, he'd helped shut the door on the notion of rehabilitation across America, the idea that a person could grow beyond their behavior and make real changes to their lives.

"For too long, law has centered its attention more on the rights of the criminal defendant than on the victim of crime," President Ford announced to Congress. "It is time for law to concern itself more with the rights of the people it exists to protect."[63]

**⑫**

# FACE-OFF

## The New Normal

Fresh Faces Help for Homely Cons—*Time*, 1980

Prisoners' Plastic Surgery Disclosed—*Los Angeles Times*, 1982[1]

The lobby of tower two was festive. As Douglas Lipton walked to the elevators, he enjoyed the spectacle. Lush green and red wreaths framed each elevator and hung from the balconies, and the walls were festooned with snowflakes and twinkling lights. Three tall Christmas trees finished the look, elegantly decorated in gold, red, and white. Christmas tunes played in the background, enhancing the holiday feel.

The sixty-seventh floor was equally uplifting, with tinsel and baubles decorating the staid desks and its steady hum of chatter. It was the Friday before Christmas, and no one could concentrate on their work. Lipton smiled at the sight and then heard the familiar peal of his office phone.

"Hello?"

"Lipton?" It was Julio Martinez, from the Division of Substance Abuse Services.

"Uh-huh."

"What can you tell me about Loony Balloony?"

"Excuse me?"

"Loony Balloony, the *drug*."

Lipton stared at the handset in confusion. He was tapped into the addict community and felt certain someone would have alerted him if a new cocktail had arisen. Martinez, even more so, considering he was five-plus years sober.

"Never heard of it," he replied.

"Well, a city councilman's got word of some new Loony Balloony drug on the street," Martinez said. "I want you to alert your field team, and get me a memo, ASAP."[2]

"I'll look into it."[3]

Loony Balloony, it turned out, was a tube of plastic cement beloved by children for its balloon-making properties; a straw and solvent mechanism was used to inflate the substance. It was possible that *some* children were inhaling acetone fumes for a high, perhaps by placing the tube in a bag and sniffing it, but it seemed improbable.

Lipton's field team mobilized, buying tubes of the stuff from candy stores across New York. One store claimed to sell one hundred tubes a week, but the team polled addicts, children, and drug counselors, and nobody had heard a whiff about it.

"This can be chalked up as a false alarm," he told Martinez. Even so, six months later, the health commission pulled the children's toy off the market.[4]

The hysteria around drugs had reached a new high across America, and New Yorkers were especially volatile. Televisions broadcasted gloomy portents, and the politicians, once so open to research and rehabilitation, looked stonily on, remaining silent, or worse, *supportive*, as punitive policies were enacted. The prisons overflowed with Black, brown, and white bodies. Lipton watched in horror as the city worked itself into a fervor, the likes of which he'd never seen before, not even in the wake of Attica.

The social shift of the 1970s had morphed into some serious changes in the criminal justice world. Martinson's emphasis that prisons did not rehabilitate was key to shaping the new policies, which idealized restoring social order and returning to "good Christian values."

The use of psychologists and social workers for inmates was sidelined, replaced by more policing and stronger sentencing.

In the 1976 election, President Jimmy Carter beat the incumbent, President Gerald Ford, by fifty-seven electoral votes, the tightest margin since 1916. Only 54 percent of registered voters turned out. Carter won the popular vote by 2.1 percent. The Carter administration talked a good game in terms of reforms, but though President Carter didn't double down on the harsh policies of presidents Nixon and Ford, he advocated in the abstract, instituting few actions that would make a noticeable difference. "Welfare, to me, is not charity. . . it is an interest in individual human beings, to let them stand on their own feet, to be proud, to have self-respect."[5]

His new stances contradicted his prior policies as governor of Georgia, where he supported the return of the death penalty and denying bail to drug dealers. As president, he emphasized that he understood American's concerns, but his changes were minimal at best.

"Crime destroys the essential fabric of our society in ways that go far beyond individual suffering and loss. In that sense, we are all victims," Carter announced at a Rose Garden event.[6] Other times, the president emphasized the accountability aspect of his policy. "Drug traffickers must understand that they face swift, certain, and severe punishment; and our law enforcement and judicial systems must have the resources to make this prospect a very real threat," President Carter told Congress.[7] "To ease the burden on the District Courts, I support widening the jurisdiction of U.S. Magistrates to include misdemeanor offenses."

Despite Carter's promises, there were numerous cutbacks due to "stagflation." Funding for Head Start, a social program for low-income youth, was severely reduced, as was the grant budget that Lipton's agency, the National Drug Research Institute, relied on. His budget cuts included a 50 percent reduction of public housing subsidies, a 10 percent reduction in Urban Development Action Grants, and a 5 percent reduction in community development grants.[8] Often, the Carter administration's social policies were more of a hindrance than a help, especially when it came to prisoner rehabilitation.

By 1977, little medical research took place inside the American prison system. This impacted sociological investigations as well; a few of Lipton's projects were killed. One that had showed particular potential was a controlled test with psychopathic inmates at Dannemora prison, where each inmate was treated with adrenaline injections.[9] "An end to the irredeemable label may be in sight when the psychopath has an organic problem," he'd proudly announced at a prison reformist meeting in Teaneck, New Jersey.[10] The new biomedical rulings put a stop to such tests. Lipton was stoic about the shuttering of his program—in the big picture, it was important, he knew—but many lacked the bandwith to take the long view. "The project is dead, d-e-a-d," a Michigan surgeon wailed to the press when his experimental brain surgeries on sex offenders were cancelled.[11]

The few rehabilitation services remaining tended to be leftovers; poorly funded services from previous reform periods. New schemes often fell on the kookier side;[12] in Cuyahoga Falls, Ohio, a probation officer made grandiose claims linking a sugar-rich diet to juvenile delinquency, and in Los Angeles County, a delinquency prevention campaign funded by Honda and the local enforcement agency supplied ten thousand Honda minibikes to young offenders.[13]

President Carter's lack of results didn't go unnoticed. "How can a president—certainly no less mentally alert than most past presidents—with many advisers of high caliber, produce such an undistinguished presidency?" commented Stephen Hess, a Brookings Institute researcher and the U.S. representative to the United Nations General Assembly in a 1978 paper. Hess blamed Carter's "lack of overriding governmental design" for creating a vacuum.[14] The president's own pollsters echoed this opinion: "More people believe you to be ineffective than effective, wishy-washy than decisive, not in control than in control," an internal report stated.[15]

All Lipton could do was hope this fallout wouldn't threaten his latest research projects: an investigation of the increasing drug use in suburban areas, the rising popularity of PCP, and Stay'n Out, a therapeutic community for imprisoned addicts. Stay'n Out was staffed by former addicts and ex-offenders and focused on helping heroin users. It was barely a year old and ran on a shoestring budget. Addicts enrolled in the program were placed in one of Stay'n Out's 186 beds[16] located on Staten Island and in Chelsea, Manhattan. They were removed from the main prison community and provided with methadone, among other treatments. Early results had been promising, but Lipton needed a long-term commitment from officials to really assess its success, and it was hard to know which way the pendulum would swing.[17]

His next problem was the new commissioner of drug abuse services, the former deputy director of the state division of budget. His attitude to research was one of suspicion. He'd called Lipton's work "self-aggrandizing" and said—to his face!—that "the only people who benefited from research was the researchers. . . . [T]hey got lines added to their resumes, and none of their research was helpful."[18] Lipton needed to win him over or face the consequences—an even *more* decimated budget.

It didn't help that Robert Martinson was still spouting his well-trodden eulogy to the rehabilitation space in every outlet conceivable. "The history of corrections is a graveyard of abandoned fads," Martinson mused in *Crime and Delinquency.* "The primary reason for the impact of 'What Works?' is the extraordinary gap between the claims of success made by proponents of various treatments and the reality revealed by good research."[19]

Lipton wasn't going to say anything about *that* again, thank you very much. He knew where he fell on the get tough versus rehabilitate spectrum. He was

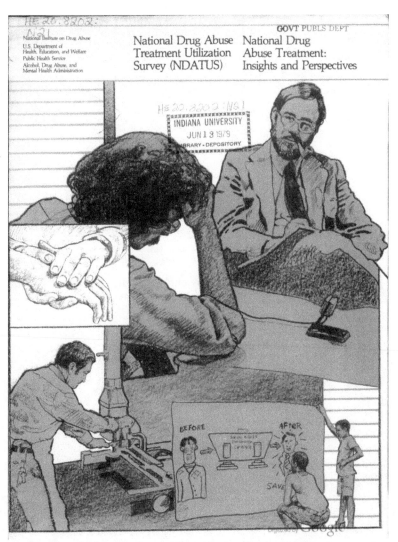

Cover page of a National Institute on Drug Abuse Survey, 1979. *Courtesy U.S. Department of Health, Education, and Welfare*

more interested in getting results than in sparring with his former assistant. Despite his troubles with the new commissioner, he found himself increasingly excited to get to the office and start work. He knew why. Work meant another chance to talk to Sherry Deren, a brilliant junior researcher with soulful brown eyes and rich brown hair. Deren specialized in drug-related illnesses and was lead investigator in researching the prevalence of HIV among New York's addicts. He'd gotten to know her on a bus ride to their Albany office. For three hours, they talked nonstop. She was nine years younger than he was, but they had so much in common! His first marriage had dissolved in 1975—after years of not quite gelling—and Deren fascinated him. She reciprocated his attention, and after a few months of dating, he shyly asked her to marry him. When you knew, you just knew. She smilingly accepted.

In most cases, changes to the criminal legislature had little effect on state-run criminal cosmetic surgery programs. The way the wardens looked at it was logical: plastic surgery wasn't an experimental corporate-funded research project, and the surgeries were purely voluntary. No one was getting horribly scarred or burned or developing cancer after their nip and tuck. After all, the rhetoric was still the same.

At Sweet Briar College in Virginia, psychology student Mary-Somers Knight explored this realm in her psychology dissertation. "Ugliness is an undefined stigma, a subtle curse. . . . [P]eople feel sorry for the ugly members of society

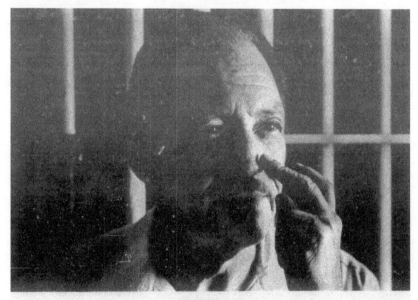

FRANK SAULTER
"I mean, I think a few improvements would help me get the kind of beautiful wife I'm visualizing."

Inmate Frank Saulter examines the result of his nose job inside Chino prison, California, 1979. *Courtesy Charles E. Young Research Library, UCLA* in the same cringing way they pity the blind or the crippled," she wrote. "Businesses capitalize on the desire to be beautiful."[20]

Over the last few decades, the sale of cosmetics had skyrocketed. In 1978, Estee Lauder's sales surpassed $300 million annually,[21] and Revlon topped the one billion mark for the first time. Beauty-related industries were booming, creating many economic opportunities, a knock-on effect of the larger attention given to appearance. In 1978 there were 542,000 registered cosmetologists across America, a 185 percent rise since 1950.[22] The number of licensed beauty shops rose from 122,000 in 1955 to more than half a million by 1978.

Much of this growth was attributed to the explosion of mass media consumption that took place in the 1970s. In 1978 households watched an average of 375 minutes of television a day, compared to 305 minutes a day in 1960.[23] Newsstands contained hundreds of magazines, with thousands more available by special order.

Over and over, these mediums trumpeted and idolized their accepted standard of attractiveness. The idealized man was tall, brawny, and clean cut, whereas heroines were slim, symmetrical, and blessed with smooth skin and sultry eyes, à la Jane Fonda and Margot Kidder, Superman's Lois Lane. And, of course, lily-white skin.

Black people and minorities had little representation, both behind the news desk and in Hollywood films and TV shows. In 1971, 6 percent of prime-time characters in comedy and dramas were Black.[24] The needle hadn't moved much by 1978. One study found that over the previous decade, Black actresses performed less than thirty starring roles. As supporting actresses, they were lumped into stereotypical categories—the funny Black friend, the sassy Black girl—which highlighted the presumed physical, intellectual, and temperamental "differences" between races. To better fit the television standard of whiteness, some Black actors used skin bleaching creams and chemically straightened their natural hair.

There were some breakout Black stars; in 1978, thirty-nine-year-old Max Cleveland Robinson became coanchor for ABC World News Tonight.[25] He was the first Black coanchor to host a primetime TV slot. In 1975, *The Jeffersons*, a sitcom about a wealthy Black family—a second spinoff of *All in the Family*—debuted on CBS. The sitcom was the first prime-time show to prominently feature an interracial couple. The hit show had a 60 percent white audience. Even so, much of the cast were light-skinned, well-groomed Black actors, emphasizing the narrative that one had to be light, wealthy, and well presented to even *think* about succeeding in America.[26] And male, of course: white men significantly outearned everyone else and Black men earned more than Black women *and* white women.

In the workforce, employee appearance had taken on a performative role, with workers required to dress and act according to their company's prescribed manner.[27] At Bartlett & Company Grain in Colorado, the dress code designated that females were not allowed to wear pantsuits. Burlington Coat Factory insisted its female employees wear dresses. Other policies included mandatory high heels and makeup as essential to the position and outlawed pantsuits and short sleeves. Even inmates were affected. In 1977, female prisoners at the Rikers Island Correctional Institution for Women brought a class action suit against the facility. One of their complaints was the institution's refusal to let them wear slacks.[28] Across the Atlantic, many British job listings requested that "attractive candidates" should apply for secretarial roles until the sex discrimination act of 1975 forced them to stop.

Unsurprisingly in this charged climate, there was a roaring trade in cosmetic surgery, the most popular procedures being face-lifts, eyelid surgery, and nose jobs. Midyear, the former First Lady Betty Ford underwent a face-lift in Palm Springs, California. "I wanted a fresh new face to go with my beautiful new life," she told *Time* magazine.[29]

The *New York Times* dedicated a full page to the popularity of plastic surgery. "People want to put their money into themselves rather than into a new car," commented plastic surgeon Dr. Peter Linden, under the subheading, "An Investment in Oneself." "It's part of the desire to make the best possible life, to get the best possible job and salary, to keep yourself as interesting a person as you can be," he added.[30]

Some patients took out loans. Others took a deep breath and spent their investments, remortgaged their houses, or dipped into their retirement. "That youth and beauty translate into dollars and cents is unquestionable," reported *D* magazine.[31] "What makes it all even more undemocratic is that in 'the melting pot,' the concept of beauty is one of the most narrowly defined. It has been homogenized, pasteurized, and predigested into factory-line uniformity: The American Beauty has a slender build, a thin, straight nose, high cheekbones, strong chin, and, most important, permanent-press skin."

Year after year, the number of surgeries performed grew approximately 5 to 10 percent reported the American Society of Plastic Surgeons.[32] Qualified cosmetic surgeons could expect to comfortably earn a six-figure salary, earning themselves a spot in the echelons of the ivory tower.

Accordingly, more surgical residents chose to specialize in this lucrative arena, and teaching hospitals stepped up their rotations to meet the demand. As the plastic surgery residency programs grew exponentially, the chance to operate on prisoners became a valuable recruiting tool for universities, especially in Texas and Utah.

Utah's program began in 1959. Surgical trainees from the Latter-Day Saints Hospital were occasionally shuttled to Utah State Prison, their time spent straightening noses, removing scars, and lifting the inmate's faces.[33] At first, a few dozen operations took place each year, but as demand increased, this rose to sixty, then eighty, then one hundred.

The inmates clamored for plastic work, and almost immediately, waiting lists were oversubscribed. "We like the program, I think it helps them," the warden told the *Deseret News*.[34] Soon, the residents were visiting twice a week, and by 1975, more than two thousand inmates had received plastic surgery. The majority of procedures were on inmates' noses.[35] One study, which assessed 487 Utah inmates, revealed a 9 percent reduction in recidivism rates among inmates paroled within five years of their surgery. The prison psychologists reported a "personality change" on the altered inmates. "We feel a person's looks are important to getting a job," the prison hospital administrator informed the press. Plastic surgery was offered to both male and female inmates, though the majority of the work went to the men—women made up around 4 percent of Utah's prison population.

"Although cosmetic surgery was once seen as an antidote for vain women, it's proving to be a rehabilitative tool for prisoners," remarked the *Deseret News*.[36]

Elaine Cohen had never liked the way she looked. Her nose was just too big for her face. It seemed that people saw it before they saw *her*. She tried to avoid mirrors, to keep her head down. She stayed away from people. Her sentence for theft and forgery put an end to that, but even locked up, she avoided social gatherings as best she could. Then, surprisingly, one of the prison matrons asked her why she didn't just get her offending proboscis fixed.[37]

"Fixed?"

"The prison's free plastic surgery program," the woman replied.

Cohen signed up immediately. The surgeon regarded her nose, lips pursed. He nodded. "Yes, I can see why you're unhappy," he told her.

Cohen looked at him hopefully. He was young for a surgeon, she thought, with spots of acne on his face and scruffs of hair at his chin. She'd been warned by the other inmates that the surgeons were trainees, that they were guinea pigs to them, but she didn't care.

The day of surgery, she was escorted from the prison to the university hospital. Smiling nurses took her pulse and slid tiny needles into her arms. The day went by in a blur. Groggy and bandaged, she returned to the prison the same day and settled into the infirmary—the rules didn't allow for public hospitals to keep prison patients overnight. The throbbing of her nose woke her up. She called the nurse for pain relief. The nurse shook her head. This wasn't something provided to inmates. Cohen begged, and the nurse gave her an aspirin, which she choked down. It did nothing.

For the next fortnight, her face felt tender and achy. Her eyes were ringed with huge black circles, like she'd battled some demon. The surgeon visited and removed her cast, and she finally got to see her revised nose.

"It's still big," she told him, turning her head side to side.

"There's residual swelling," the surgeon noted. "But yes, we didn't achieve quite the ski slope you were hoping for." He snapped a photograph.

At her next checkup, he brought her two photographs, a before and after of her face. She stared at the glossy paper. Her nose had been enormous! It was still big, but compared to that. . . . It was strange, she thought, how quickly she'd become used to her face's new proportions. Her eyes seemed bigger, her lips fuller. The male guards were friendlier.[38]

Jennifer Frei, one of the twenty-five-odd inmates at Utah's Point of the Mountain female prison, also signed up for surgery. For the last decade she'd padded her bra and coated her face with a thick layer of foundation, trying to make herself more attractive, more like the girls in the magazines.

"I want breast implants," she said during her consultation. "I'd like to be a D cup or a DD cup. Bigger is better!" She bit her lip as the surgeon cupped her breasts in his hands and pressed them this way and that. He withdrew a marker from his pocket and traced a thick black line under both of her breasts. "This is where the incision will be," he informed her. A few months later, Frei was a full D cup. She admired her new profile in the mirror: So big! So firm! She loved them!

But soon, the sutures pulled apart and the incision began weeping. Her breast felt sore all the time. That Monday, when the Avon lady turned up for her bimonthly visit, Frei listened to her talk about lipsticks and moisturizers in a daze. It was hard to focus on anything but the pain.[39]

"It aches all the time," she told a state social worker during a visit to the prison. The warden had requested the services of the social workers, looking for upgrade suggestions for the facility in general. Frei's comment was recorded in their report, which was marked "for discussion only." Utah's Department of Social Services carefully documented its findings: the prison was poorly lit and had shoddy sanitation, inadequate ventilation, and housed inmates in extremely cramped quarters. The female inmates had few opportunities for education or growth, whereas the male prisoners had many. "The men get everything," a female inmate had complained. On the medical side, the social workers noted surgical complications and inadequate record keeping and raised questions about informed consent.

In 1978, eight months after their visit, the report was leaked to the local paper. The story made the front page. "Surgeons Practice on Utah Inmates!" Reporters tracked down former and current inmates and quizzed them about the surgeries. "Breast implants are the hottest thing going out there, except maybe for nose jobs," a former inmate told the paper.[40] "It seemed like they were practicing on us, especially on the breast surgery."

Frei, whose breasts were now scarred and lumpy, felt like she'd been used. "It's not worth it," she groused. She'd take it back if she could. She recently watched a television report that discussed implant-related health problems that left her deeply frightened. "They didn't warn me there might be problems," she said.

The story caused an uproar in the community. Troubled, officials threw a press conference to explain their side of the story. Representatives from the University of Utah Medical College, Utah State Prison, and the social services department convened for a press briefing. Dr. Earl Browne, the head of plastic surgery at the college, vociferously defended their work.[41]

"There is real value in removing disfiguring things like big horrible tattoos and scars," Browne declared. "The breast implants are admittedly on the periphery of rehabilitation." And all his residents were already well qualified, he stressed. Plastic surgery training was a seven-year program, and all trainees had been pre-certified by the American Board of Surgery as ear, nose, and throat surgeons before admittance to the program.[42] Many states run similar programs, very successfully, he added. The implications that breast implants were risky is false, he said. That may have been true when they first came to market, but they've improved to a level where they aren't "dangerous to health."

Even so, the executive director of the state's social services department promised that the issue had now been resolved. "No more breast implants unless somebody can give me a good reason!" The university's media director supported this stance. "We are going to discontinue breast implants simply because the rehabilitative value of the operation has not been completely determined," they said—this kind of controversy was detrimental to the university's image.

"Breast Implants Eliminated for Women Prisoners," The *Daily Herald* dutifully reported.[43] This proved to be too little, too late. "I've had it up to the ears with the hassles caused by attempts to help prisoners with cosmetic surgery," one of the residents informed the warden. Then the prison's medical director resigned, saying he wanted to focus on his private practice. Complaints about the program persisted, and soon the University Medical Center was forced to announce that it had withdrawn this program for good.[44]

⌒

At West Virginia University, Norman Cavior's investigations into the effects of appearance bias had ramped up. He'd analyzed whether academic performance influenced interpersonal attractions (it didn't), whether adolescents ranked older adults' physical attractiveness any differently depending on their age (slightly, but by age seven there were no major differences), and whether attractiveness equated to popularity (very much so). He even analyzed whether an attractive appearance could be understood by a person's voice alone.

His results convinced him that, to a certain extent, appearance was inextricably linked with behavior. "Low physical attractiveness contributes to careers of deviancy," he reported in the journal *Criminal Justice and Behavior*.

But could one's appearance correlate to specific types of crime? And did it affect any rehabilitative treatment once institutionalized? He wasn't sure, but it seemed likely. "The physical attractiveness of a person plays a significant role in the environmental consequences that the person experiences," he wrote.[45]

Graduate student Steven Hayes volunteered to test this hypothesis with him. Hayes was intrigued by Cavior's focus on physical attractiveness; it was a demographic that most people felt was unchangeable. Everyone has prejudices, he knew, but if racism and sexism could be tackled, why wasn't appearance lumped with the other -*isms*? "Ugly" jokes were on a different level than "Black" jokes—one was socially acceptable, the other would have, hopefully, most people running for the door. Hayes applied for institutional review board approval and sourced file photographs of seventy-five Black and white female ex-cons from the Kennedy Youth Center, the majority of them Washington, D.C., kids who'd been uprooted and plopped down in West Virginia. The pair distributed these to ten white male students—because the majority of correctional workers were white men—and asked them to sort the photos into seven categories of attractiveness. The results were underwhelming. There was no statistically significant correlation between the crime committed and the women's attractiveness rating.[46]

Still, Cavior wondered if the sample size had been large enough. Only five of the seventy-five women had been sentenced for aggressive behavior. To be sure, four of the five also had been rated as "extremely unattractive," but he couldn't draw any conclusions about that—it wouldn't be scientific. On the treatment side of things, the data was more conclusive. The detention center allowed women to take unescorted "town visits"—a reward for good behavior. White women and women who achieved high beauty scores received far more of these rewards than Black women. They were paroled more, too. "Steps can be taken to avoid penalizing those female offenders with a relative lack of physical attractiveness," Cavior wrote.[47]

Cavior's body of work inspired a new generation of social scientists to examine the role of appearance in society. They assessed the behaviors and beauty responses of children as young as six, looking for antisocial tendencies, criminality, and peer hierarchy. Again and again, their research found that Americans were exceedingly undemocratic when it came to looks. Pretty people were hired more, paid better, and lived happier than their uglier peers.[48] They were healthier, spending less time in hospital, as well as less time in jail. In a mock homicide trial, the prettier the defendant, the better the treatment and sentencing, even when the crimes and guilt were identical.

But a disconnect existed between the research and a deeper public understanding of the challenges the less attractive endured. "We're the most cosmetic society on earth but we still regard vanity as a sin," a plastic surgeon who requested anonymity told the *Colorado Springs Gazette-Telegraph*.[49] "You put pressure on those conflicting values, and you realize we'd have to make an attitude change as basic as ending racism. You can't talk about ugliness because it could start a revolution."

This idea bled into a rising sociological concept called "labeling theory." Descriptions mattered, sociologists argued; when people were assigned to set groups, their behavior adjusted accordingly. One study found that children placed in "academic classes" scored higher than those placed in "opportunity classes," even when both curriculums were the same.[50] Students who were labelled early on as "deviant" experienced discrimination throughout the rest of their schooling, due to the formal and informal ways that students' reports traveled through schools. Labeling applied to physical appearance expectations as well.

One researcher tested this by asking teachers to assess various accounts of misbehavior by children, each report paired with a photograph. The attractive children were viewed more kindly, whereas the teachers noted their belief that the ugly children would reoffend, a clear case of appearance penalization, despite the children's looks bearing no relation to their offenses.[51] The research of Ray Bull, a psychologist from London, also uncovered some surprising data about children's behavior. "Until they are nine years old or older, children do not demonstrate the adult somewhat negative reaction to mildly deformed faces," he remarked in *Current Psychological Reviews*. "Our developmental study strongly suggests that the adult reaction to facial deformity is not innate but is learned by twelve years of age."[52]

Other researchers turned their attention to the current and historical body of plastic surgery work in prisons. The Rikers Island project remained the gold standard for inmate surgery studies. "It's the first and only study to use an appropriate experimental design," lauded Dr. Park Dietz, director of medical criminology research center at McLean hospital.[53] Even so, he critiqued the small sample size; after separating the participants into addict and nonaddict groups, "only for those with traumatic facial disfigurements were the numbers large enough to achieve statistical significance."

However, as more prison programs published their results and studies, a deeper picture of the benefits emerged, he reported. In 1974, Dr. Edward Lewison published an update to his 1965 report, a twenty-year assessment of nine hundred cosmetically improved inmates. His inmates had a 48 percent recidivism rate compared to 75 percent of the general prison population; ten years earlier, the numbers were 42 percent and 75 percent, respectively.

Even so, there wasn't a blanket approval for prison plastic, Dietz reported. Two studies, one of 185 federal inmates[54] in Ohio and another of a group of twenty-one Baltimore-based delinquents,[55] reported "no significant difference" in recidivism. At the Western Pennsylvania Correctional Institute, a five-year study of 388 inmates reported that re-offenses actually increased, clocking in at 34 percent, compared to 22 percent of the general prison population. In Illinois prisons, recidivism for surgically altered inmates remained low; however, a troubling trend had been noted; many of those who re-offended had given up petty thefts and moved into criminal specializations such as fraud and forgery.[56] Technically, they'd "bettered themselves," but not in the intended manner.

Despite the many successes Dietz reported, Martinson's followers seized on the instances where the surgeries had failed; for them it confirmed the narrative that current attempts at prisoner rehabilitation were a pointless endeavor. It strengthened their conviction that public funds were being wasted. Other psychologists debated just how impactful physical appearance in childhood was on adult behavior, with new research suggesting that adolescence body angst could be adjusted with therapy or vocational pursuits just as efficiently as surgery.

Many in the Carter administration pushed back on Martinson's ideology; Peter B. Edelman, the director of New York's Division for Youth, valiantly pressed for more services in a 1978 hearing before Congress.

"What disturbs me about the current fashion of saying rehabilitation has failed is that I know a significant amount of youngsters with histories of significant delinquencies who can be helped," he said. "Sometimes the breakthrough is started with a new set of teeth or plastic surgery to fix an ugly scar."[57] The senators listened politely but ultimately ignored the content of his speech. More services were cut.

From the health angle, reformers had more success. Using the press as their sounding board, they campaigned tirelessly for system-wide changes, highlighting inequities and substandard care within the incarceration complex.

In response, the New York City Board of Corrections issued the booklet "Minimum Standards for New York City Correctional Facilities," the first of its kind. Its nineteen pages detailed a new way of thinking and treating inmates, starting with nondiscriminatory care.[58] "Prisoners shall be afforded equal protection and equal opportunity in being considered for any available programs . . . and [corrections] shall provide programs, cultural activities and foods suitable for those racial and ethnic groups with significant representation in the prisoner population, including Black and Hispanic prisoners," it asserted.

The new standards emphasized prisoners' right to access basic hygiene facilities; hot and cold showers were to be made available daily, the washing facilities were to be cleaned weekly, and shaving supplies were to be made available on request and at the department's expense. Female inmates were authorized to receive free sanitary products. Laundry services were to be developed so inmates could have a twice-weekly change of clothes, and law books and access to legal clerical supplies were to be made freely available.

All written handouts needed to be available in English and Spanish, and each detention center was required to hire bilingual employees to enable inmates to access the provided programs and activities.

Whether these rules would be enforced was still in question—during her tenure as corrections commissioner, Anna Kross made similar demands—but the publication of the guidelines, which included oversight from an external board, was a step in the right direction. Many states looked first to New York when developing their own guidelines, and by officially documenting these requirements, the city set a standard for the nation.

Kross, now eighty-eight years old, was less involved in corrections—and New York policy—than she used to be. She traded her sturdy space shoes for a polished wheelchair, and her thinning hair was too sparse to anchor her beloved jaunty hats. Still, when city administrators invited her to the opening of the $23 million Anna. M. Kross Center on Rikers Island, she happily accepted. Her son-in-law, the federal judge Marvin Frankel, accompanied her return to the island.

It was an easier trip these days; her bridge project had been completed in the 1960s, and she stared out the car window as the gray brick buildings rose before her. Ideally, the need for jails would be moot, but until then, she was pleased that improvements had been made. Her namesake building would home the jail's mental health unit, drug detox unit, along with dormitories for new arrivals. As Frankel carefully wheeled her around the facility, she felt hope blossom in her chest. Her successors had stepped up. The city she loved really *was* improving. The trip was one of her last public appearances.

In August 1979, Kross's breath started coming in short, sharp bursts. Her forehead was clammy with sweat. Wheezing, she allowed her husband to drive her to Montefiore Hospital and Medical Center in the Bronx. Concerned by her breathlessness and high temperature, they kept her overnight, releasing her but cautioning her to take it easy. At home, she grew weaker and weaker, her skin paper thin, her firm jaw slackening. She died on August 27.

All the city's papers covered her death. The *New York Times* and the *Daily News* called her "the city's first woman corrections commissioner" (their fact-checkers overlooking that accolade went to Katharine Bement Davis in 1914) and devoting numerous columns to detailing her colorful life. "Kross, the daughter of a buttonhole maker from Nishwez, Russia, held the commissioner's post amid considerable publicity and controversy from 1953–1966," wrote the *Daily News*.[59]

The *New York Times* paired its obituary with a photograph of Kross looking obstreperous; as in death, so in life.[60] "For her, work was a sort of religion through which she acquired an education and overcame the hardships of poverty. Some considered Judge Kross compassionate to a fault for befriending runaway girls, peddlers, errant husbands and wives, prostitutes and petty gamblers," it wrote. A few months later, Kross's portrait took center stage at an exhibition titled *Women in New York City Government*, featured in the lobby of the surrogate court building in downtown Manhattan: "City's Women's Firsts Left Lasting Impression!"[61]

Anna Kross had not been a fan of Robert Martinson—his "nothing works" catchphrase was anathema to everything she believed in—but Robert Martinson was a fan of hers. He'd admired her straight-talking no-nonsense approach, even if their views on rehabilitation differed. Since his *60 Minutes* appearance, he'd become a regular on the corrections circuit, hopping from conference to conference, where he lectured on penology.

He'd grown increasingly bitter as the years passed; his peers accused him of everything from idiocy to scholarly malfeasance.[62] The charges were so serious that the National Academy of Sciences reexamined the validity of his 1974 opus, ultimately giving it a clean bill of health, noting it was "reasonably accurate and fair."

"Some treatment advocates have been motivated to become kinglike and shoot or at least shoot down the messengers. We have been tagged 'yellow scientists,' pessimists, and idealists in search of the magic cure for all offenders," Martinson complained in the *Federal Probation Journal.*[63]

He continued sounding off about the fallacy of rehabilitation. "The juvenile justice system today does not do an adequate job," he told CBS News in another interview. "What they really need is certainty of being caught and certainty of being punished."[64]

By 1979, however, Martinson had revised his absolutist approach to rehabilitation. He stood by his original report, but new data changed his view. He'd used software to model twenty thousand recidivism rates and found that around 25 percent of offenders recidivate, compared to the 60 or 70 percent touted in the media. "Damn it, that's not bad," he told reporters. They didn't listen. So he fell back on what had worked for him before, writing a thirteen-page polemic for the *Hofstra Law Review*, "New Findings, New Views," which published in winter 1979.[65]

In it, he recanted his "nothing works" proposition, replacing it with a more nuanced report. "Contrary to my previous position, some treatment programs do have an appreciable effect on recidivism. Some programs are indeed beneficial," he wrote. "Startling results are found again and again . . . for treatment programs as diverse as individual psychotherapy, group counseling, intensive supervision." There had been some methodological flaws in his initial assessment, he admitted.

It was too little, too late—for rehabilitation and for Martinson himself. Two weeks before Anna Kross died, he'd hurled himself out of the window of his ninth-story Manhattan apartment in a fit of pique.[66]

Kross's and Martinson's demise sounded the death knell for American rehabilitation. When Ronald Reagan was elected president in 1981, his "treat 'em tough" approach sealed the deal. Despite President Carter's good intentions, by the time he left office, illegal drugs were cheaper, easier to get, and more widely used than on the day of his inauguration.

"Choosing a career in crime is not the result of poverty or of an unhappy childhood or of a misunderstood adolescence; it is the result of a conscious, willful choice made by some who consider themselves above the law, who seek to exploit the hard work and, sometimes, the very lives of their fellow citizens," President Reagan announced.[67] The problem, as he saw it, he explained, was one of values rather than economies. Criminal behavior stemmed from moral poverty, not socioeconomic poverty. The "welfare queens" were undeserving of funds that were meant for *good* Americans. The subtext was good *white* Americans.[68]

With large numbers of Black people on welfare due to discriminatory hiring practices and educational stopgaps, it was clear what being a "good" American entailed. Some years earlier, in a conversation with then-President Richard Nixon, Reagan had mocked the delegates from Africa. "To see those, those monkeys from those African countries—damn them, they're still uncomfortable wearing shoes!" Nixon laughed at his comment and proceeded to repeat it to the secretary of state.[69] There were many other instances in which Reagan was dismissive of people of color, and many of his anticrime screeds encoded racialized warnings.

He shortly transferred the federal antidrug efforts from the Department of Health and Human Services to the Department of Justice. Almost overnight, the funding for rehabilitative services halved, with oversight generally left to the states and private organizations. This affected Lipton's agency, making his job more difficult. He reported the prevalence of drug use among college kids—"serious drug users just don't make their junior or senior year"—the rise of school-age drug users—"we're seeing it in the fifth grade, the fourth grade"— and at single-occupancy hotels. Gaming arcades were also "drug hotbeds," he reported. An analysis of 102 locations found cannabis available at sixty-six arcades, cocaine at forty, pills at twenty-seven, and heroin at twenty-five of the venues.[70] The majority of attendees were under seventeen, he added.

Reagan's "War on Drugs" set zero-tolerance policies for drug users. "We intend to do what is necessary to end the drug menace . . . and to eliminate this dark, evil enemy within," President Reagan told the world in a televised speech.[71] "Crime today is an American epidemic. In New York City, for example, less than 1 percent of felonies end in a prison term for the offender." His oration stirred the public; there should be consequences for bad behavior or everyone would act out!

Reagan's choice of words equated dark with evil, bolstering the racist narrative that Black bodies were inherently flawed, violent, and prone to criminality and drug abuse. The media ran with this portrayal and published numerous stories that linked Blacks to crime.[72] *Time* magazine's March cover story baldly laid this out: "There can be no blinking away the fact that Blacks are disproportionately involved in violent crime," it wrote; in 25 percent of violent crimes, the victims reported their assailant was Black.[73]

*Newsweek* went even further with its "crime" cover story. "One fact that can't be questioned is that a vastly disproportionate number of violent criminals are Black, an observation that until recently tended to be discreetly ignored as racist," it wrote.[74] "Although Blacks constitute only 12 percent of the U.S. population, they make up 48 percent of the prison population." In 1935, this number was 25 percent. Punitive policies and institutionalized racism had caused this divide.

By the early 1980s, cosmetic surgery was firmly established as an indicator—and pathway—to economic success. Looks were so important that a new branch of therapy was created: cosmetic behavior therapy. Psychologist W. Paul Jones described this method as "a set of procedures used by the counselor that primarily focus on increasing the client's physical attractiveness."[75] Other therapists took up the banner. Papers were published, and the practice was ironed out. "Cosmetic therapy is an effective means of minimizing visible differences using cosmetics. It mitigates psychosocial difficulties," one report stated. "Two months after learning a makeup technique to attain facial symmetry, social attitudes of patients with facial nerve paralysis were improved, making them more pro-social."

Dr. Albert Kligman, formerly a plastic surgeon at Holmesburg prison, got on the beauty bandwagon, cowriting *The Psychology of Cosmetic Treatments.* He peddled the idea that you had to be good looking to succeed and that, in some cases, skincare and makeup was every bit as effective as professional therapy. "It's wrong that people are judged on such trivial grounds but we have to live with that, we ought not to confuse what ought to be with what is," Kligman announced at the First International Symposium on the Psychology of Cosmetic Treatments.[76]

What wasn't clear was what dollar amount could be placed on beauty. Although people understood—tacitly, silently, uncomfortably—that attractive people had it easier in life, there was no easy way to measure, in dollars, one's degree of attractiveness.

Enter thirty-seven-year-old television reporter Christine Craft. In January 1981, Craft, a hearty blond California surfer girl, left her Santa Barbara TV station for an anchor role at ABC News affiliate KMBC-TV in Kansas City. KMBC-TV was owned by media conglomerate Metromedia and had wooed her with a $35,000 salary, a $15,000 pay bump from her coanchor gig in Santa Barbara. She didn't realize her male coanchor was pulling in $80,000. Still, KMBC-TV had promised her relative autonomy with her reporting[77]—and that she wouldn't have to change her appearance. Craft's background was primarily in local news, plus a stint presenting the short-lived CBS *Sports Spectacular* "Women in Sports" show from New York, whose producers insisted she bleach her hair and wear heavy eye makeup. She'd felt like a phony. KMBC-TV said it supported her; the organization recruited her, after all! The station knew what she looked like. For months before she arrived, the station publicized her appointment in the newspapers.

"Co-anchor Hired for KMBC News!"—*Kansas City Star*, 1980[78]

From day one, Craft wondered if she'd made a mistake.[79] A few minutes after finishing her first newscast, she was pulled aside by her news director, Ridge Shannon. "Do you know that your jaw is square?" She smiled thinly, unsure how to respond. A few days later, Shannon presented her with a copy of *Dress for Success*. Then an image consultant, flown in from Dallas, appeared and covered Craft in thick, heavy foundation and blusher. She gave Craft a daily fashion calendar to follow. Craft hated the attention on her looks, but she did like the story opportunities. She covered fine art, juvenile justice, sports, and so much more.[80]

Six months passed. Then, on Friday August 14, a few hours before her evening broadcast, Shannon drew Craft into his office. The feedback from our focus groups is in, he told her. "The people of Kansas City are apparently more provincial than even we had thought. They don't like you because you are too old, unattractive, and not sufficiently deferential to men. When they see your face, they turn the dial." She could work out the rest of her contract as a field reporter, but as of today, she'd been removed from the anchor chair, he told her. She quit on the spot. "I wouldn't want to scare people," she told Shannon.[81] She walked out with her head high—she wouldn't let him see her cry.

The local press was outraged. "KMBC's great mistake was in removing her as co-anchor," commented the *Kansas City Star*.[82] The station's Nielsen ratings had just been released; for the first time in years, KMBC News had achieved first place in the rankings—these numbers covering the exact period of time that Craft had coanchored.

Craft returned home to California and quickly stepped into a new on-air role. But she wasn't prepared to let this indignity go. Such outrageous behavior wasn't acceptable. What price could one place on pretty? It wasn't a required part of the job, and the ratings showed it hadn't hurt the station. But they'd hurt *her*, economically—not only did she lose the pay bump, but all promise of even larger future pay raises.

Craft filed a sex discrimination claim with the Equal Employment Opportunity Commission (EEOC); once they issued her a right-to-sue letter, she could proceed with her lawsuit. She sued Metromedia on three counts: sex discrimination, the Equal Pay Act, and fraud in hiring—the station insisted it hired her for her qualifications but fired her based on her physical appearance. Two Kansas City lawyers accepted her on a no-win, no-fee basis. The trial began mid-July 1983.[83]

It was a grueling experience. The defense played audiotapes from the focus groups that had led to Craft's dismissal. The tinny sound of the group facilitator filled the courtroom. "Is she a mutt? Let's be honest about this."

Craft cringed in her seat, the audio echoing through the courtroom. Many of the participants expressed a dislike of Craft, describing her as "cynical," "aggressive," and "not flashy."

The station manager testified; appearance was "at the top of the list" of priorities in selecting an anchor, he said.[84] The case got local and national attention. The responses varied; every "stick it to 'em, Craft," was balanced by a sexist remark. "Theoretically I dislike hiring a woman for a news job because of what she looks like. On the other hand, I don't mind watching Jane Pauley, Joan Lunden, or Diane Sawyer even when I'm not very interested in the story," reported the *Manhattan Mercury*.[85]

On August 8, 1983, the court ruled in Craft's favor on her sex discrimination and fraud claims and awarded her $500,000 in damages. It was a historic moment; this was, perhaps, the first time a court had placed a dollar value on physical attractiveness—or the lack thereof. It was clearer than ever that one's "prettiness" had a direct correlation to one's earning potential.[86]

In the wake of Craft's verdict, attention shifted to the remaining plastic surgery programs in prisons. Was it fair that inmates received taxpayer-funded treatments that many taxpayers could not afford themselves? People didn't think so and public sentiment took a downturn.

Though many of the prison programs used volunteer or trainee surgeons and cost the correctional departments little, this wasn't true across the board. In

Aiken, South Carolina, one jail revealed that it spent $1,900 on plastic surgery for two inmates. "We can't afford this," railed Aiken's city council.[87] In Pennsylvania prisons, a man who killed his wife received $5,000 in surgical treatment to rebuild his face.[88] In Virginia, plastic surgeon Jack Fisher sounded off about the lack of financial support in the *American Journal of Correction*. "There is a need to convince legislators as well as the taxpayer that such services, although at first glance an apparent luxury, are essential for total rehabilitation," he wrote. "Our own program is still without financial support. Our surgical instruments are borrowed, pharmaceutical firms donate drugs and suture material, and hospitalization costs are covered by the university."

However, California's Department of Corrections prison system paid out thousands each year in surgery-related fees. The amount of money—and surgical work—was so extreme that Senator Dan Boatwright opened an investigation into the "luxuries" on offer inside the Chino prison for men. He found that the plastic surgery was provided for free, but the medical expenses were mounting. "We shouldn't be providing them with something you can't get on the outside because you don't have money to pay for it, to wit, cosmetic plastic surgery," Boatwright told the California Department of Correction.

As complaints rolled in, more services were cut, and more rules were put in place. President Reagan increased funding to law enforcement and pushed for harsher treatment for offenders while simultaneously underfunding rehabilitative projects. His antidrug agenda primarily harmed minorities, but that was irrelevant to him; being soft on crime would hurt him in the polls. His work carried on that of Nixon and Ford, each regime building on the efforts of the last, digging a hole so large it prevented all escape. Low-level crime was targeted, whereas men who stole millions in a nursing home Medicaid fraud scheme received fines but no jail time.

Antidrug edicts targeted low-income, predominantly Black areas, despite research that found that Black and white Americans consumed similar amounts of drugs. Reagan appropriated $1.7 billion for the Anti-Drug Abuse Act of 1986, which set five-year mandatory minimum sentences for possession of five grams of crack cocaine. However, a cocaine user caught with five *hundred* grams of cocaine—one hundred times the amount of crack—received the same five-year mandatory minimum sentence. "We initially came out of committee with a 20-to-1 ratio. By the time we finished on the floor, it was 100-to-1," admitted Representative Dan Lungren to Congress at a later date. "We didn't really have an evidentiary basis for it."[89]

At $5 a gram, crack was cheaper, easier to produce and distribute, and more common among poor Black addicts than cocaine, which retailed at $50 to $75 per gram. Courts were required to enforce the new drug sentencing laws, and more money was siphoned from the existing rehabilitation programs to facilitate this. New prisons were built to handle the overflow of Black bodies. Most states switched from indeterminate sentencing (in which inmates serve a variable range of time) to determinate sentencing (a fixed amount of time), which made many parole boards obsolete. The prison population grew exponentially.

In 1984, Lipton's Stay'n Out program was evaluated. During the previous seven years, 1,500 addicts—all without histories of violence, sex crimes, or significant mental illness—had completed this in-prison inpatient program, averaging six to nine months of treatment. But how did it hold up to other drug abuse programs? His assessment focused on two things in particular: did the treatment reduce recidivism and was it more or less effective than alternative treatments—including no treatment at all?

There was a link between treatment and a decrease in recidivism, the statical analysis showed, with the defining factor being the period of immersion. "The main finding being that, as time in therapeutic community treatment increases, recidivism declines significantly," he wrote.[90] This was much more successful than drug avoidance programs like Scared Straight, which attempted to scare kids away from drugs. "Interventions based on deterrence models have shown very limited effects," he reported. Even so, he didn't know if his data would be persuasive enough to keep the program funded. "The belief that 'nothing works' still has widespread acceptance and is one of the main reasons drug treatment programs are given low priority," he complained.

Sure, there were some outliers like Jerome Miller, president of the National Center on Institutions and Alternatives. "When people say nothing works . . . it's patent nonsense, we've never tried rehabilitation in this system. Even in the so-called heyday of liberalism and mollycoddling of the sixties, you look at their budget and it's all in institutions," Miller railed on C-SPAN. "It's because we don't imagine this system as designed for our own. We were locking kids up because of race, because of class . . . we found that the greatest single predictor whether a kid would get in further trouble later on in life and whether or not they were locked up earlier in life."[91]

Lipton tried to appeal to the administration's bottom line; due to the decreased recidivism, Stay'N Out would pay for itself within two or three years of an inmate's release. He made a good case, he knew, but was anyone *really* listening? The correctional world as a whole looked bleak, and he could read the signs. America was entering a new stage of incarceration, and it didn't look good.

# 13

# PRETTY TOUGH IN TEXAS

## Investment in Prison Plastic Surgery

We have to spend money on prisons. We have to construct more of them. There's absolutely no doubt. But it's unrealistic to think that you can just create holding pens for people for five, six, seven, eight, ten years, and return them to society.—Rudolph "Rudy" Giuliani, U.S. Attorney for the Southern District of New York, 1984[1]

Jail Inmates Get a Lift, Taxpayers Get the Bill—*Fort-Worth Star Telegram*, 1989[2]

Go Directly to Jail, Collect Free Plastic Surgery!—*Pensacola News Journal*, 1989[3]

Mugging Suspect Dubbed Dumbo Offered New Ears—*Index Journal*, 1992[4]

For inmate 203981—a.k.a. Nancy Willeford, to her dwindling number of friends—January 30, 1989, began like every other day inside the Texas Department of Corrections prison system. The fluorescent lights winked on at 4:00 a.m., their electric hum a gentle backdrop to daily head count and the single-line shuffle to the showers. By 5:00 a.m.—breakfast—their whirring had faded to a distant annoyance, drowned out by the mess hall chatter.

After breakfast—half a pint of milk for coffee, one egg, two cold biscuits, and a slop of gray oatmeal—the women trudged back to the dorms for another count, and then it was on to their work assignments, where they'd fold laundry, mop floors, or, if they were lucky, take a spin in the woodshop or beauty school. Assignments like the auto shop, the print shop, the license plate factory, and pretty much everything else were reserved for the male inmates; Texas detained 44,022 inmates, of which 1,000 were women.

Instead of directing her to her work assignment, a guard conveyed Willeford to a cold white room in the medical wing. Here a white-coated doctor held a hand mirror up to her face. Willeford's watery blue eyes narrowed as she examined her reflection. Her pale skin had a gray leathery sheen to it, each line and crease exacerbated by the harsh overhead light, creating valleys and furrows in her reflection. Even her hair looked dull, its auburn tones somehow muted to mousy brown. Her hand traced the contours of her face, resting on the puffy folds under her eyes. When had these become permanent? she wondered. She couldn't remember. She looked down. In the mirror, she was old, so old. How had this happened to her? She was only forty-three.

The doctor was speaking but there was a roaring in her ears. He'd told her his name when she walked in, but she'd instantly forgotten it. She hadn't even tried to remember it—the prison doctors were all the same, after all, wide-eyed medical students shipped in from Baylor College of Medicine in Houston or the University of Texas Medical Branch in Galveston for a quick residency stint. They'd stay a while, until the thrill of prison dissipated, or their course credits were completed, or both, and then they'd leave, immediately replaced by another batch of fresh-faced students. "We could tighten that, get rid of this. . . ." The doctor gently tugged at the loose skin on her face, pulling the flesh back so the years faded away. "What do you think?" Held taut, time shrunk.

Willeford frowned. What was the catch? She wasn't some credulous fish who trusted the Department of Corrections to do the right thing. The days when she could be lured by a kind smile and shiny promises were long gone, vanished within weeks of her first go-round in 1968, on a two-year charge for murder without malice. Faces came and went, the do-gooder social workers burned out, the programs cancelled, the changes reversed—the one thing you could be certain of was that the prison always would put itself first. She was not a sucker to blindly participate in one of its games. It had enough control as it was.

Nervously, she pinched the corner of her shirt, the worn seam beginning to fray. Well, *its* shirt, really. Everything she wore was courtesy of the state, her shapeless white pullover and pants, the cheap cloth smoothed by the many bodies who wore it before her. The previous occupants of her clothes had been larger than she was; they'd stretched the elastic waistband so thin that she often had to hike up her pants to keep them from sliding down her hips. The cotton polyester blend was freezing in winter and scratchy in summer, when temperatures reached 150 degrees inside the cells. Texas prison summers were the *worst*; every few years there was a riot after one or more inmates slowly had baked to death inside the concrete blocks.

Willeford had grown old inside these walls. This was her third sentence; so far, she'd served time for murder, forgery, and possession of a firearm. Currently, she was on year four of a fifteen-year sentence for attempted murder; a heist gone wrong, she'd told her lawyer. Almost half her life had been spent behind these walls. It wasn't how she'd wanted her life to go. Not that her life had *ever* been easy.

She'd grown up in a single-parent home in Diamond Hill, Texas. Her mom never had much money, but they'd gotten by. Everything changed when she was seven years old, and her Mom moved in with Bill. Bill was loud, rude, and drank too much, and Mom always took his side. She couldn't remember when the rapes started. At sixteen, he got her pregnant, but her Mom blamed her for what happened and refused to leave Bill. They sent her to a "wayward girls" home for the birth. Her Mom reappeared when baby Sherry was a few weeks old; "You're coming home with me, and Bill and I will raise Sherry as our own," she told her. Broke and alone, Willeford returned home with her Mom. Bill's abuse continued. Sometimes she'd fight him, and sometimes she just shut her eyes and waited for it to be over. She drank whatever she could get her hands on, shot up anything that was offered to her—whatever made the pain go away.

Things were never going to change unless she did something drastic, she realized. To get free, she needed funds. It was tough to find work without an education—she'd dropped out of school due to the stress—but she was slim, charming when she wanted to be, and her glossy red-gold mane reached almost to her knees. She outlined her eyes in thick, dark kohl, mascaraed her lashes, and donned a low-cut top and her tight Wranglers; looking like this, it was easy to swing a job in the local saloon or diner. She loved getting a paycheck, but after the initial rush wore off, it became clear that this was never going to cut it. You couldn't make real money doing waitressing or shopgirl work, she realized, not the kind of money that could get her out and keep her safe. She started small; a forged check now and then, a few items pocketed at the store. Sometimes she'd exchange a blowie or more for some bills.

Then, late one Tuesday night at the Buena Vista Courts, a seedy motel in downtown Fort Worth, she was cornered by an overly handsy trucker. She panicked and shot him in the head with a 44-caliber pistol she kept in her purse.

She fled. It took two months for the police to track her down and charge her. Paroled at twenty-six years old, she found that her winning smiles didn't work as well with a criminal record hanging over her. Then she met Lathan; he was nine years older than she, with thick dark hair and a roguish smile. His family had relations to the mob, he told her, and they ran most of the scams in town. Soon enough, her mother and Bill were a horrible memory; she married Lathan, owned multiple cars, and could buy all the nice clothes and fancy dinners she desired. She wore jewelry with *everything*, hanging strings of glittering diamonds—certified by her jeweler—from her earlobes and neck. She basked in the appreciative stares she got around town. She liked looking good, feeling their admiring eyes on her. Her two-packs-a-day habit—and her heroin addiction—kept her slim.

But then she forged a check and was found with a gun (a big no-no as a felon), and things had escalated quickly. In prison, survival, rather than appearance, was the focus. How she looked became less and less important. Willeford felt disconnected from her body, her friends, her "real" life. But there were benefits to being good-looking inside the compound; attractive inmates received more leeway from the guards, better work assignments, and were paroled earlier. It was hard to maintain a beauty routine with so few resources.

The commissary sold lipstick and mascara and handle-less hairbrushes, but most inmates preferred saving their meager funds for food luxuries. Instead, they used colored pencils to line their eyes and hard candy to color their lips. Contingent on the guards, of course; break a rule or cross some invisible line, and their cells would get swept, their little palettes of humanity confiscated.

How about eye bag removal surgery? the surgeon asked her. That would really open up your face.

She silently considered his offer. She'd been vaguely aware that plastic surgery was happening inside the prison—it was around during her first go-round in 1968—but it wasn't something she'd thought very hard about. It was mostly for the men, she'd thought; there had been little outreach at the female prison. That was due, in part, to the general disregard for women in prisons, and because the surgeons were wary about accusations of improper behavior and how the women might respond to a discussion about their defects.

The majority of female prisoners in Texas was housed in women-only units in Gatesville, a small town in northeast Texas so saturated with prisoners that more than 60 percent of its residents sported state-mandated attire. Female inmates mostly had been an afterthought within the system. But during the last decade, the number of women behind bars had skyrocketed across America, from 13,258 women in state and federal prisons in 1980 to some 42,000 in 1988.[5]

This spike lit a fire under the corrections board, which ordered the department to be more inclusive, and that's why Willeford was here, drumming her feet on the plastic spindle of her severe-looking folding chair.

Cosmetic surgery seemed so extreme—but then, she wouldn't be in prison forever. She couldn't be. The very idea made something deep inside of her choke up. She couldn't blame her crimes on her fading looks, but . . . wouldn't it be nice if she left looking better than when she came in? She didn't trust the prison, but the doctor came from the outside. If he was willing to fix her face for free, well, she'd never been one to turn down free things. She told the doctor yes.

Texas's prison cosmetic surgery program began in 1954, a joint effort between university training hospitals and the prison's medical team. During its first decade of operation, 1,321 surgeries took place.[6] Residents visited twice a week, averaging forty-five hours and fifteen operations a month per student. "It's one of the finest things we have done," Texas's prison director, Oscar Byron Ellis, told reporters. "Correction of (facial defects) enhances the chance of an inmate's satisfactory adjustment to society after release."[7]

For Ellis, the proof of the program's success was evident; the attitude of his "Frankensteins" and "eagle beaks" greatly improved after their faces were lifted and their noses slimmed. They stopped getting written up for fighting. The volume of the plastic surgeries increased; hospital logs recorded 2,850 procedures in 1972.

On the experimental side, during this period the prison's administration embraced a wide variety of clinical trials that ranged from testing cholera vaccines to ingesting LSD as a treatment for psychosis to swallowing chloroquine tablets to assess visual responses. In most cases, 75 percent of all participants were Black or Hispanic.[8] Even as pushback on experimental programs grew, the Texas prison system ignored the furor as long as it could. Its argument for this was economic: sure, the results might benefit Americans as a whole, but in reality, it needed the cash. Since the first rust-red brick had been laid in 1848, the Texas correctional system had been bleeding money. Jails were horrifically overcrowded, prisons were labeled as barbaric and cruel, and despite the prison industries, they were losing fistfuls of cash every week.[9]

At the same time that the prisons were rapidly filling up, shifts in the penal code added to the overcrowding. Punishments were harsher: the sentence for drug possession increased from two to ten years to two to twenty years, and petty offenders filled the state's cells. Spending increased exponentially, far outpacing the state's expenditures in any other area. If cosmetic surgery could lower spending by slowing or stopping the revolving door, it would be a serious purse saver.

Dr. Steven Blackwell supported the concept, but he found the whole process eerie. It was a mandatory rotation for his studies, but a chill crept down his spine each time the gates clanged shut behind him. He could never relax, like some of the other residents. He was always checking behind him to assess who was around him. The prison had promised he'd be safe, but even so.[10]

The response of inmates like Tessa Diaz made it feel worthwhile. "You suffer from seeing yourself in that bad image," she told him. "The changing of my physical appearance has helped with my insides. I've got a relationship with my two sons I did not have before." Fifty-year-old Diaz received an abdominoplasty—commonly known as a tummy tuck—which involved slicing open the skin on her abdomen, trimming off the excess, and suturing the torn muscles back together. Her operation was performed under local anesthetic, with Diaz groggily aware of every snip and slice. She was sore and swollen for the following two months. Diaz didn't care. "I was freed from the bondage of my old self," she explained. "This has been a release."[11]

Abdominoplasties were rare; face-lifts and nose jobs were the big-ticket items; everyone wanted them, it seemed. Tattoo removal was also popular, and Blackwell worked hard to keep his face composed as he removed swastika after swastika. He coauthored a report about his observations. "In children's fairy tales, the prince is always handsome and good, the villain ugly and bad," he wrote—literature bore some responsibility for creating and perpetuating the concept that disfigurement equates to villainy. Three years post-op, the inmates' recidivism rate dropped to 14.7 percent compared to 36 percent of the prison's general population. The boost in their beauty led to better self-esteem, he surmised; this in turn led to better interpersonal relationships, which lowered their propensity to offend.[12]

There was another reason for Texas's big push for prison plastic surgery. The Department of Corrections had a major staffing problem, especially on the medical side, similar to what was happening on Rikers Island. Turnover was high, with prison work low on the spectrum of graduate opportunities for medical students. Salaries were low, and that, coupled with the assumptions about the quality of life in prisons, made it hard to attract junior doctors.

The Texas Department of Corrections (TDC) was in crisis. To attract new talent, it developed a medical externship program that brought in out-of-state students for a summer and rotated them between dental, general care, and plastic surgery in the prison. The TDC's summer rosters were full, but it didn't get the response it'd hoped. In exit interviews, students complained about having to cut their hair for the "ridiculous short haircut regulation" and reported they'd been "hassled" by the prison guards. The pay was also too low for them to seriously consider working there. But the students did praise their surgical experience.

"We're not in the business of making them beautiful," Dr. Armond Start, who took over the program in 1983, told the *Dallas Morning News*.[13] "Our first responsibility is to keep them incarcerated. But we ought to do anything we can to move them forward, and I believe (the surgery) can be a significant part of their rehabilitation."

Start echoed the thoughts of correctional program directors across America. By 1989, an estimated five to six thousand cosmetic surgery operations took place in prisons each year.

In New York, Douglas Lipton still plugged away at refining treatment programs for addicts. The large issue was reshaping the narrative around addicts, that they were in need of *treatment*, not punishment. A medical issue had become intertwined with a behavioral one, he posited, and it was harming everybody. "Just serving time degenerates men and their keepers inexorably," he lectured a room full of wardens and parole administrators. "Use time as an opportunity for change. It values both of them and eventually alters the quality of life for all humankind."[14] He knew that was a little overblown, but maybe that was what corrections needed—perhaps the pendulum had to swing that way in order to meet in the middle.

So far, most of his suggestions had been rejected. He'd proposed a "pre-emptive" buying scheme—for around $3 billion, he estimated, the government could purchase the entire opium and coca crops for the year from Bolivia and Peru and then destroy them. It wasn't that far-fetched, he argued. A Southeast Asian warlord had offered to sell the region's entire opium crop for the next five years to the United States for $48 million. The numbers appeared high, Lipton admitted, but when analyzed against the cost of drug treatments, they "were a steal." Lipton was only partly joking.[15]

The situation was that dire. It wasn't just the growing AIDS problem, the high school dropouts, or the high crime rates, it was the public's attitude toward drug users that was so problematic. Broadcast journalist Richard Heffner explored this conundrum on his public television talk show, *Open Mind*. "Given the cost of drugs in human suffering, it is hard to be concerned for drug addicts

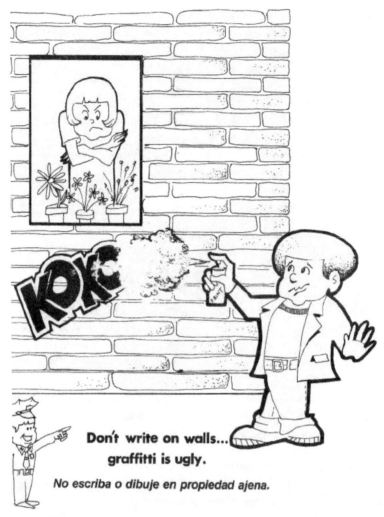

Child graffities wall. Page from New York Department of Correction coloring book for children, 1987. *Courtesy James Vann, New York Department of Correction*

rather than angry and vengeful toward them," Heffner commented to his guest, Dr. Vincent Dole, a senior physician emeritus from Rockefeller University. "It's the general problem of trying to explain prejudice. People, including the medical profession, see the addict as a frightening person, instead of a sick person," Dole replied. "If you are prepared to admit that the addict is a sick person, the question is 'what are the causes of that and what can you do most effectively to relieve it?' To blame them is not to solve the problem."[16]

⌐⌐⌐

Nancy Willeford's eye bag removal surgery took place in early February 1989. It was a big month for her and a strange month in America. Two inches of snow covered the suburbs of Los Angeles, the first GPS satellite was launched into orbit, and Paula Abdul's "Straight Up" topped the Billboard Hot 100 for three weeks. Willeford didn't pay attention; her focus was on getting through the days, one by interminable one.

Her short consultation was all that was required for her surgical work, but across the world, surgeons were collaborating with psychiatrists, and pre-plastic work was growing. "There's the fear of surgery and then there's the fear that the surgery won't make a big difference on their lives," explained Rochelle Litman, a Toronto-based psychologist who worked almost exclusively with presurgery patients.[17] "Of course, it won't—if you have your nose done, it won't make you rich or famous overnight." Plastic surgeons embraced her service and made up most of her referrals, she explained; they want their patients to have realistic expectations.

Willeford was driven to the University of Texas Medical Branch (UTMB) hospital, two hours south of the prison, and prepped for surgery. A masked nurse wheeled her into a windowless room full of men in hairnets and masks, their pale green gowns almost reaching the floor. A technician tapped her arm, once, twice, watching her veins pulse purple and blue before inserting a small needle and flooding her system with anesthetic. In the corner of the room, another man was doing something with dials and a machine. "Now count backward from ten," someone said, the voice very far away. When she was fully sedated, the surgeons got to work, pulling back the loose skin around her eyes and removing the excess fat and tissue. They neatly sutured the incisions with tiny dissolvable stitches.

Sometime later she blearily opened her eyes. She looked around—she was in a ward, somewhere, with identical beds laid out in a zebra-crossing formation. She raised one hand to her face and felt rough gauze under her fingers. She tried to sit up, woozily swayed, and settled back into her pillow. With the drugs still in her system, she felt nothing, but under the gauze, the skin around her eyes was red and raw. In a few hours, it would feel tender and itchy, and it would soon resemble a countryside patchwork of bruised browns, greens, and purples.

At her follow-up appointment a few weeks later, the swelling had faded, leaving taut pink skin behind. In the mirror, she saw the vestiges of her twenties; the carefree days she'd spent driving at top speed around town just because she could, chain-smoking Marlboros till her voice cracked and doing vodka shots as she danced to the *Rolling Stones'* "(I Can't Get No) Satisfaction." It was good to recognize herself again. When she'd left home and married Lathan, she'd felt so free, so lucky. She was luckier than she knew. Willeford was one of the last inmates to get officially beautified courtesy of the Texas Department of Corrections.

⌒⌒

The same February, Steven Long, an investigative journalist at the *Houston Chronicle*, was flipping through his latest pile of research—he was working on an investigative story about the illegal trade of rare books—when he received an anonymous tip.[18] Something weird was going down at the prison, an outraged citizen told him. The inmates—men who've done all sorts of terrible crimes—were getting beauty surgery, for free.

Long was surprised by the news. It didn't seem credible. He rang the Department of Corrections media liaison for the University of Texas Medical Branch to quickly fact-check. This won't take long, he thought, one hand lightly teasing his bushy mustache.

Most likely someone got the information mixed up. The media officer was friendly at first, but when Long explained the reason for his call, he was transferred to another department, then another, and then back to the officer he started with. "We'll look into this," he was told.

Long hung up and frowned. They were being evasive. His calls to the hospital directly followed a similar trajectory—they needed to check with so-and-so, and maybe there was surgery, but they couldn't say for sure, and they did treat inmates in general. . . . His Spidey sense was tingling. "They were embarrassed," he told his editor, making a case for pursuing this lead. "It's the dirty little secret of two state agencies!" He was given the go-ahead.

The prison's refusal to play ball spurred him on. He filed a Freedom of Information Act request along with a Texas Open Record request against the Department of Correction and UTMB, determined to get to the bottom of this. His requests were denied—medical records were strongly protected under Texas law—so Long appealed, simultaneously filing a new request with slightly tweaked language, and repeated the process, till UTMB grudgingly sent him some data, heavily redacted, eked out a document at a time. Even so, it was eye opening.

The hospital had admitted almost three thousand inmates between September 1987 and September 1988, at a total cost of $16.4 million to taxpayers. That number mostly covered the hospital's $577 daily rate and didn't include surgical or staffing costs related to the operations. He was appalled.

He bristled with every new piece of information. "We call the Texas Department of Correction hospital the TDC Hilton," a surgeon, who spoke on the promise of anonymity, informed him; inmates were two to a room with a private television and room service. Long was seething. This was how tax dollars were being spent?

Case in point: Tommy Thompson. On February 23, the craggy-faced fifty-nine-year-old was transferred to the John Sealy Hospital in Galveston to undergo a brow lift, face-lift, and liposuction. Thompson, serving a sixty-year sentence for theft and compelling prostitution, stayed there for three weeks. His recovery cost the state $12,117 in room costs alone.[19] "They treated me real well," Thompson told Long, running his hands over his face to point out the changes. "My lids drooped over my eyes so I had to strain to see," he explained. "This is the best thing yet I've done in here to make me feel better about myself." Now he could pass for fifty or even late forties. He'd like even more work, he told Long; a new set of teeth would be ideal. "They've got in terrible shape," he said. "That will make me feel 100 percent better too."

Long nodded. Later, his fingers flew across the keyboard—he kept his feelings out of his work, letting the facts speak for themselves.

Six weeks later, on April 2 (timed so as to miss April Fools' Day), the *Houston Chronicle* published his exposé on the front page. Long's report meticulously documented the number of inpatient cosmetic surgeries performed, as well as surgeries performed on an outpatient basis: 18,562 for the last fiscal year.[20] They weren't all cosmetic operations, but enough were to prompt shock and indignation.

Public outrage, already inflamed by stories of mass school shootings and terrorist attacks, boiled over. That year, on average, five Texans were murdered each day.[21] The prison administration was pulling a 180 on everything it valued. The presumption was that cosmetic surgery was some sort of twisted reward for bad behavior: murder someone then shave off ten years with a complimentary face-lift. Hold up a store, get a free nose job. "The state's not paying for this, I am," John B. Holmes Jr., the district attorney for Harris County, told Long. "I don't understand the philosophy of funding it."

Columnists and television news reports fanned the public's fury. "The big negative is that the taxpayers are stuck with the bill," wrote nationally syndicated columnist Ann Landers.[22] "I'm sure plenty of people who would like plastic surgery would be very pleased if they could get the work done with no charge."

Readers were outraged. "This is the straw that broke the camel's back," wrote Mrs. H. B. Kifsby to Texas Governor Bill Clements. "We would all like to have cosmetic surgery but we can't afford it . . . but we have to help pay for a convict? This is almost unbelievable." Kifsby signed her letter, "shocked."[23]

"We cannot afford medication for our elderly and can afford a face-lift for killers and rapists? We are taxed for everything and double taxed for some of that," complained Beverly Gowing from Friona, Texas. "I do not feel that inmate plastic surgery is helping Texas in any way."

The prison administration contested Long's claims. "While we spend many, many dollars in education teaching them a trade or vocation, sometimes we can do it much less expensively just by changing their appearance," medical director Dr. Armond Start told the press. The hospital management also protested, claiming its surgeries were of a "functional" rather than cosmetic nature—a claim that the surgeons themselves disavowed. There was "no point" to Tommy Thompson's makeover, they admitted.

The backlash was too big to control. Governor Bill Clements publicly condemned the practice and ordered Charles Terrell, chairman of the Texas Board of Corrections to look into it. "I am deeply disturbed by recent reports," Terrell told UTMB. "I am asking you to take whatever steps necessary to ensure the immediate termination of cosmetic surgery to TDC inmates."[24]

In addition to sparking disapproval, the surgeries also went against Texas law. In 1987, the Texas Department of Corrections Appropriations Bill added a rider that prohibited expending state funds to pay for an inmate's cosmetic surgery. The caveat, however, was "unless significantly disfigured and disturbed." This was passed in response to reports that some inmates had received elective breast implants.

"The cost of this gratuitous cosmetic surgery trickles down to taxpayers," complained an editorial in the *Kerville Times*.[25]

To be sure, what qualified as mental health issues related to cosmetic appearance was amorphous. The Department of Correction protested the commotion. "We definitely were aware of that rider and have not violated it," the department informed the *Houston Chronicle*, contending that it paid for only security and had no oversight as to what medical procedures were performed. Still, in response to the governor's inquiry, it instituted a policy that required all cosmetic operations to be personally approved by the prison's medical director. That would be the end of it, but the heat continued—so much so that in June, UTMB pulled out entirely, permanently nixing any and all elective cosmetic treatments, claiming it hadn't known that was prohibited. "It is our intent to limit it down so that we can stay out of trouble with everybody," the hospital spokesperson told Long.[26] The public reprisal was too much to handle.

Other states followed suit. Three days after Long's exposé was published, the governor of Louisiana discovered that $5,000 of public funds had been spent on furnishing a testicle implant to an inmate serving a twenty-five-year stretch for forcible rape. Horrified, he asked the prison if there was a medical need for the procedure. It was "strictly cosmetic," admitted the prison's medical director—there was an "unwritten rule" against inmate cosmetic surgery, he was told, but some "slip through the cracks."[27]

Legislation to prevent reoccurrences was quickly approved, sending a clear message that states would not pay for inmate beautification. The Alaska Department of Corrections updated its charter to nix this: "Elective cosmetic surgery is not to be covered by the budget." A growing raft of seemingly frivolous inmate lawsuits deepened correctional officials' belief that shuttering these programs was the right—and publicly approved—way to go. Case in point, Utah inmate Howard Shaffer's $1 million suit against the Bureau of Prisons, alleging cruel and unusual punishment and emotional suffering after his free hair transplants were discontinued.[28]

These shutdowns built on a new wave of anti-prisoner legislation, beginning with President George H. W. Bush's administration in 1989. President Bush ran on a "get tough" on crime platform, which included zero tolerance for drugs. His budget called for 70 percent of the $4.1 billion drug budget to go directly to law enforcement. "We need increased prison sentences for drug-related crimes," he explained. "Zero tolerance is not a catchword. It means, quite simply, if you do crime, you've got to do time."[29] He committed to building twenty-four thousand new beds for federal prisons and blamed "liberals" for the problems that plagued America.

"Where the liberal mind-set dominates, the net result has been the same: bad schools, dangerous streets, big deficits," he espoused. "Let me be blunt: Divided government just isn't good enough for America or for New York. It's time to ask the American people to let us show what we can do without the albatross of liberal legislatures."[30]

The Pentagon also introduced new regulations to further tighten federal laws in the realms of cosmetic surgery, specifying that governmental funds were to be used only for "the correction of birth defects, the repairing of injuries, or the

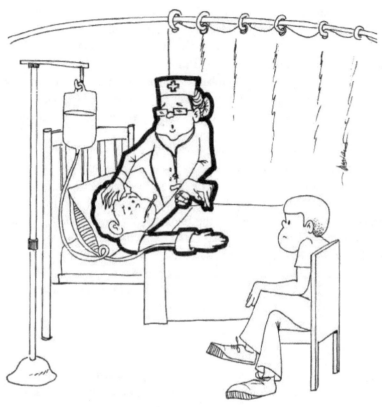

**Healthy people who take drugs become sick.**

*Personas saludables que usan drogas se enferman.*

Child sick from drugs. Page from New York Department of Correction coloring book for children, 1987. *Courtesy James Vann, New York Department of Correction, CorrectionHistory.org*

commission of breast-reconstruction procedures following mastectomies."[31] Military personnel and their families were the one exception to this rule, a left-over "morale boost" proviso from the war years. This exception was revoked the following year, but thousands of military personnel and their extended families continued to receive free breast enlargements, face-lifts, nose jobs, and liposuction treatments for the next fifteen years under the umbrella of "skills" training.[32]

Bush's first year of presidency played a pivotal role in changes to the corrections sphere. On January 18, 1989, two days before his inauguration, the Supreme Court provided him with all the ammunition needed. The justices, in an eight-to-one vote, upheld significant revisions to the federal sentencing guidelines, formally requiring the abandonment of rehabilitative practices and treatments from sentencing consideration. "The efforts of the criminal justice system to achieve rehabilitation of offenders had failed," they stated;[33] it was an "unattainable goal for most cases." Justice Harry Blackmun delivered the verdict: "The Act, as adopted, rejects imprisonment as a means of promoting rehabilitation, and it states that punishment should serve retributive, educational, deterrent, and incapacitative goals."

This wasn't the first time the Supreme Court had made this kind of sweeping, discriminatory change. News anchor Christine Craft was one of many harmed by its rulings, or lack of. After her demotion from a Kansas City news station, which didn't consider her "pretty" enough to coanchor, she sued Metromedia and won half a million dollars for appearance discrimination. Metromedia appealed, and on the second go-round, the jury ruled in Craft's favor again. This time, it awarded her $325,000, a $175,000 drop from verdict number one. Metromedia's next appeal was heard by the Eight Circuit Court of Appeals. This time, the ruling was against Craft; the court said that Metromedia had not defrauded Craft when it assured her that "no makeover or substantial changes" to her appearance were required for the job. Her $325,000—still unpaid—was revoked.

Furious, Craft appealed the verdict to the Supreme Court, a last-ditch attempt for justice, as the highest court in the land saw an average 4 to 6 percent of requested cases. She hoped the justices would see the necessity of her suit. If they found in her favor, she was home straight. The male justices demurred, with Justice Sandra Day O'Connor the only dissenting vote. "I would have accepted the case for review," O'Connor told the *New York Times*.[34] Craft's suit was declined. The justices refrained from a public comment, but the subtext was clear: they didn't want to set a precedent that protected someone from discrimination based on their level of attractiveness. In this context, it was unsurprising that so many of the prison plastic surgery programs had been recalled. Punitive measures didn't sit well with prettying up prisoners.

More scandals followed, solidifying the idea that criminal cosmetic surgery programs were a bad idea from a public relations perspective. In 1991, an inmate at the Southeastern Correctional Center at Bridgewater, Massachusetts, had his facial tattoo, a shooting star that ran from cheekbone to eye, lasered off for an estimated $2,000. "The Department of Correction should be running prisons, not beauty parlors," complained the *New York Times*.[35] "The Supreme

Court ruling that prisoners must not be subjected to 'cruel and unusual' punishment is too often interpreted as an obligation to provide questionable perks and to cater to frivolous demands. It is symbolic of the waste of public money and effort at a time when state employees are asked to take furloughs and forgo pay raises because of the fiscal bind."

Surprisingly, in most cases the benefits of a convict's cosmetic surgery—lower recidivism rates and higher employment rates when paroled—weren't in question. The issue was more individualized. The public's deep-rooted resistance to giving cons the socioeconomic benefits associated with beauty surpassed their desire to see them go straight.

Ironically, around the same time that the press wrote scathingly about inmates' frivolous treatments, they showed some support for twenty-year-old Gregory Pierre, known to New Yorkers as "the devil of the D train." Pierre was a member of the subway gangs that terrorized New Yorkers, holding passengers up at gunpoint and pistol-whipping late-night riders. Fear fluttered though the city. The police tracking the gangs had little to go on, apart from "young" and "Black"—save Pierre, whose ears poked out from the side of his head like handlebars. "We're looking for Dumbo," the cops told the press. When they finally located him in Georgia, it was easy for his victims to select him in a lineup. "He's one Black man whose penis would never be the most discussed dimension of his anatomy," joked *New York* magazine.[36]

Then the National Foundation for Facial Reconstruction (NFFR) reached out to the Department of Corrections. One of its donors was concerned that Pierre might have been psychologically scarred by his oversized ears and offered to pay for his cosmetic surgery.[37] "I don't think a criminal record should have any bearing on this, any more than if the man suffered a case of appendicitis," NFFR's president told the papers. The detective on Pierre's case agreed.[38]

Pierre's youth and notoriety bought him a pass, but across the board, all beauty surgeries were phased out. In 1994, the U.S. Bureau of Prisons edited its regulatory manual, deleting "plastic surgery significantly improves an inmate's self-image, emotional stability, and social adjustment" and adding that it does not "correct pre-existing disfigurements, including tattoos, on any part of the body."[39]

Televised coverage about crime doubled between 1992 and 1993, creating broad support for President Bill Clinton's administration in 1993 and even stronger anticrime state laws.[40] In Washington State, the senate passed the Persistent Offender Act, colloquially known as the "three strikes rule."[41] Criminals who received a third felony conviction were sentenced to life in prison without parole. California followed suit in 1994, and other states followed.

President Clinton doubled down on President Reagan and President Bush's hard-on-crime approach to policy. The House passed a $30.2 billion crime bill, $3.3 billion less than requested, with the majority of the cuts to crime prevention programs, which Republicans branded as "useless welfare spending."[42] Deeper cutbacks closed numerous therapeutic services, and without the necessary support, the numbers of addicts and mentally ill people in prisons ballooned. Once again, the prison system was in crisis, and the authorities decided that building more prisons was the answer. The revised bill eliminated a provision that would have made sixteen thousand low-level drug offenders eligible for early release.[43]

Clinton also encouraged the construction of new prisons by allocating $6 billion in the crime bill to fund this, with half going to states and the other half to federal facilities. These changes resulted in even more Black men locked up—for years, Black men had been disproportionately targeted by the police—cementing the notion that "criminal" was equivalent to Blackness in the United States,[44] a sentiment fanned by the mass media.

In 1993, *Time* magazine published its cover story "America the Violent," an in-depth analysis of President Clinton's crime bill and the political nature of the problem. The article never mentioned race, but the cover image—a huge cartoon of a devilishly grinning, red-eyed Black man wearing a hoodie, a skull hanging from a thick gold chain at his neck, his wrists handcuffed with another gold chain—made the magazine's position clear.[45] In its view, crime was an urban Black problem.

In 1994, Pell grants for prisoners were eliminated. President Clinton was well aware of the effect the crime bill had on incarceration numbers. "We have now the unfortunate distinction of having the highest percentage of our people in prison of any country in the world. Most of them are under twenty-five years of age," President Clinton admitted.[46] His solution: keep them locked up.

# AFTERWORD

## Hot Mug Shot Guy and the Future
## of Plastic Surgery in Prisons

We know what works. We know that supporting ex-offenders
and their families keeps our men out of prison. That makes a
difference in our families and can stop the cycle of poverty.—
President Barack Obama, 2007

I am not real, I am theater.—Lady Gaga, 2011

A New Look for New Life of Former Inmate—*St. Louis
Dispatch*, 2012[1]

Nancy Willeford's new look didn't provide the Cinderella ending she'd
hoped for. Two years after she was paroled, she was charged with check
forgery and possession of a firearm and returned to jail. Inside, her heroin addiction escalated, and when she was released, she turned tricks to pay for hits.
She mostly ignored her children, but when she felt gregarious, she'd let her
daughter, Sherry, comb the tangles out of her long red-gold hair.

"I thought she was beautiful," Sherry Willeford informed me via a letter that
arrived stamped with the Texas Department of Corrections seal. Sherry's on
year five of a twenty-year sentence for drug possession with intent to supply, a
first-degree felony. She hasn't spoken to her mother in a decade.

Nancy Willeford was last arrested in 2010 for concealing the whereabouts
of a wanted criminal. She was released without charge due to her age and her

chronic obstructive pulmonary disease (COPD). She can't move far from her oxygen tank, which rattles behind her as she walks. She moved into a decrepit trailer located on a scrubby piece of land in East Texas. In early 2020, a flash fire burned down her trailer and charred the left side of her face, the skin melting away and exposing bone and tendons to the air. Her meager possessions were ruined. Her granddaughter, also named Nancy, arranged for her to live in a nursing home; seventy-five-year-old Willeford's ailments include early dementia and chronic fatigue, in addition to her COPD.

The younger Nancy has mixed feelings about her grandmother. She cared for her when she was an infant but blames her for leaving her in her teens; she had to deal with her mother *and* her grandmother being imprisoned at the same time. With no adult around, she and her siblings were shuttled onto the foster care train, shunted from one big loud house to another, places she described as "abuse-filled nightmares."

"My grandmother chose a life of crime and not being a parent, and that's going to catch up to you," she said. "She told me all the time that she has regrets about prison because she wasn't there for me and my brother. I don't want to say it's karma, but . . ."

Tattooed on her right forearm in delicate italicized cursive is the phrase: "Don't judge my journey if you haven't lived my past."

By the mid-1990s, all of the "cosmetic" surgery prison programs had been shuttered. Their closure can be attributed to a mix of factors: public outrage about inmates receiving "free" beauty benefits, the Supreme Court's removal of "rehabilitation considerations" in sentencing, the scandals surrounding prisoner experimentation and the ethical violations of operating on a disenfranchised population, and a governmental directive that devalued rehabilitative solutions.

It was one thing if the increased incarceration rate actually lowered crime in general, but locking up more people had done little to change the crime rate; in fact, year on year, as harsher sentences came into play, the number of crimes actually rose despite the huge number of people that were now locked up. In 1990, after two decades of punitive policies, the FBI recorded 23,440 murders across America with New York City accounting for 2,245, a 309 percent increase since 1963.[2]

However, starting with President Barrack Obama's tenure in 2009, there's been a return to a more thoughtful discussion of rehabilitative prison practices building off the work that began in the 1950s and 1960s.

President Obama inherited a U.S. prison population of 2.3 million people—the highest ever recorded—and an incarceration complex that had become an economic driver; between private, state, and federal prisons, the number of people working corrections accounted for just 14 percent less than those employed in the auto industry.[3] A report from the Bureau of Labor Statistics published that same year reported that correctional officers and jailors had the highest employment among all occupations in state government.[4]

Between 1985 and 2000, a new state or federal prison had opened each *week*. In 2000, sixteen states abolished the use of discretionary parole. Keeping people locked up has become a profit-driven venture, the prison industrial complex—both public *and* private sector—turning the disenfranchisement of (mostly) low income and minority people into an $80 billion a year behemoth.[5]

President Obama waded in; change needed to be made to the system as a whole. He instigated lighter sentences for lower-level crimes and built a data-driven justice program to reduce arrests of the mentally ill. Government funds were redirected to pay for drug and mental health treatments, and Obama pushed for more offender reentry programs, including skills training that would provide ex-cons with work opportunities. The Fair Sentencing Act of 2010 adjusted racially targeted sentencing disparities for drug users, and the Sentencing Commission noted that it should be applied retroactively to inmates sentenced under previous regimes.

The biggest hope for change arrived with the Sentencing Reform and Corrections Act of 2015, a bill that achieved bipartisan approval. It cut excessive sentences for drug users, banned the criminal record checkbox, and freed up resources for evidence-based treatment and training programs "proven to reduce recidivism."[6]

"If we can keep on looking at the evidence, at the facts, (and) figure out what works, we can, perhaps most importantly, keep families intact and break this cycle in which young people—particularly young people of color—are so prone to end up in a criminal justice system that makes it harder for them to ever get a job and be effective citizens of this country,"[7] President Obama announced in 2015.

None of the president's plans included plastic surgery. However, as the first Black president, he was well aware of the impact that one's appearance played in one's opportunities. He also recognized this from a parent's perspective, as the father of two young daughters. "There's enormous pressure that young women are placed under in terms of looking a certain way. And being cute in a certain way. And are you wearing the right clothes? And is your hair done the right way?" he told *Time* magazine. "It's part and parcel of a broader way in which we socialize and press women to define themselves in terms of a certain appearance."[8]

⌒⌒

Throughout history, lookism—though tacitly acknowledged but rarely directly referred to—has played a large role in individuals' disenfranchisement. The term was coined in 1978 by the *Washington Post Magazine*, but it became popular in 1990, when Smith College, a liberal arts school in Northampton, Massachusetts, printed the term in a pamphlet.[9] That fall, Smith's Office of Student Affairs distributed a booklet to all incoming freshman, warning them to be on guard for ableism, classism, ethnocentrism, and lookism, which was defined as "The belief that appearance is an indicator of a person's value[10] . . . and oppression through stereotypes of those that do not fit the standard."[11]

Smith College's pamphlet was revealing—it put into words the unspoken truth that people *do* look different and that certain judgments are made about them because of it. It includes but is not limited to racism. Thirty years later, lookism initiated whole bodies of literature and analysis, building on the appearance bias research of the earlier twentieth century, of which psychologist Norman Cavior made a large contribution.

In 2021, Cavior is eighty-five years old and shows the passing of time on his face: pale age spots on his skin, a shock of white hair, and a hearing aid that loops down the back of his left ear—"It's good I never got them pinned back," he joked. He's pleased that lookism is getting more attention these days—"how a person looks underlies every experience they have," he explains, their relationships, health care, justice, education, and paychecks.

In 2011, beauty economist Daniel Hamermesh placed a dollar value on the impact of beauty on earning potential: an extra $230,000 earnings over a lifetime.[12]

The human face is a complicated piece of machinery, as cerebral as it is corporeal. Plastic surgeon Dr. Bryan Mendelson[13] sums it up nicely in his book *In Your Face*: "It can be an ally throughout life bringing great ease and opportunity, or it can be an enemy, subverting progress and sapping confidence. It may never have been right to begin with, or as with aging, it may no longer feel right."

Qualifying and quantifying this space—privately and publicly—is highly uncomfortable, even excruciating. Labeling your own or another's appearance by measures of conventional attractiveness is an admission that looks matter. Culturally, we are taught to value mind over physical matter, and such an exercise contradicts that. Then there's the awkward self-awareness that arises with the recognition of the benefits that one's skin suit has brought its wearer—and the role that age, economics, culture, and health play in that sphere.

"I think most people worry about, 'am I attractive enough?'" psychologist Steven C. Hayes said. "It's very close to something that's painful. People know these conversations are dangerous, psychologically, which is why we don't have an easy way of dealing with these deep-seated, ingrained, almost unconscious processes that are stigmatizing."[14]

People avoid things that make them uncomfortable, but this very avoidance is problematic in itself, shading the reality that others have to live with. Lack of discourse results in a lack of solutions. Ignoring the role that perceived physical attractiveness plays in society doesn't make it go away, much the same way that declaring "I don't see color" doesn't address the systemic problems of racism in society. Psychologist Nancy Etcoff wrote, "The idea that beauty is unimportant or a cultural construct is the real beauty myth. We have to understand beauty or we will always be enslaved by it,"[15]—a neat summation of this inconsistency.

There are real consequences to society's reluctance to acknowledge physical attractiveness, especially when it comes to the disenfranchised.

The Netflix-ification of incarceration presents people with more representations of inmates than ever before. Thanks to shows like *Orange Is the New Black*, *Locked Up*, and the real-life docuseries *Girls Incarcerated* and *Lock Up: County Jails*, the general public feels reasonably acquainted with the inner workings of the correctional system.

These shows don't pull any punches, as their narratives, both real and fictional, offer a grim accounting of the criminal justice system entrenched with racial biases, structural inequalities, violence, addiction, lack of rehabilitation, and officer prejudice and abuse. These broadcasts highlight the everyday indignities that inmates suffer, including lack of privacy in the restroom, lack of ownership of their belongings, and lack of control of what time they eat, sleep, and even talk to one another.

They are honest—to a point. The raw grittiness comes with a certain gloss: in *Orange Is the New Black*, the actors have clear, smooth skin, their hair artfully "disheveled" by stylists. They appear less attractive than in real life, but far more attractive than your average inmate. No makeup artists are provided in the docuseries, but the lighting and camera choices, in addition to the editing, smooth out their skin, brighten their eyes, and provide them with a healthy luster. No cosmetic surgery is necessary when you have camera magic.

Douglas Lipton, who still harbors lingering guilt about the Martinson fiasco, welcomed President Obama's shift back toward rehabilitation. He knew better than most how effective it could be. In 2000, he embarked on a new large-scale study of recidivism programs—"data collection is so much better now!"—and this time around, the results were much clearer. Many rehabilitative programs correlated positively with recidivism rates, including cosmetic surgery. This new research was never published. Lipton worked in the World Trade Center, and when the towers went down, all the data from his years of research was lost. Still, the 2009 modifications to the Rockefeller Drug Laws—ending mandatory minimum sentencing and allowing judges to consider rehabilitative paths once more—provided Lipton some satisfaction. Plastic surgery never made it to that playbook.

Almost fifty years on, remnants of Robert Martinson's "nothing works" screed have insidiously woven their way into the fabric of the incarceration world. One acolyte is criminal psychologist and researcher David Farabee, a figurehead for the anti-rehabilitation crowd; in the *Washington Post* he crowed that "prisoner recidivism is unlikely to involve workbooks, videos or talk therapy."

Today, what little plastic surgery remains in corrections is limited to medical necessity only—reconstruction in the case of breast cancer, for example—and even then often hotly contested. Recent debates around inmate plastic surgery have revolved around gender confirmation surgery for transgender inmates. In 2017, California inmate Shiloh Heavenly Quine, a trans woman, was the first U.S. inmate to receive state-funded gender confirmation surgery, and on July 10, 2019, Adree Edmo, a transgender woman in the Women's Correctional Center in Pocatello, Idaho, became the second.[16] The debate about trans surgeries, however, is about what medical procedures states should provide, and gender dysphoria is clearly a medical condition and not a cosmetic one.

Many U.S. state departments of corrections regulations still include language that gives them the discretion to provide elective surgeries. South Carolina's policy states that "Cosmetic surgery will not be authorized unless there are important considerations or possible serious psychological consequences,"[17] and Nebraska's corrections manual noted that "Elective surgery (provided for cosmetic reasons) shall not occur unless approved by the NDCS Medical Director. All expenses incurred for the elective procedure will be the responsibility of the patient unless otherwise approved." This gets muddier; some states refuse to provide inmates with abortions, insisting it's an elective surgery akin to a "nose job."[18]

In 2020, a contract between the Texas Department of Criminal Justice (TDCJ) and the University of Texas Medical Branch in Galveston contained a proviso for "elective cosmetic surgery" in its correctional care plan but required written approval from TDCJ's division director of health services.[19] I filed a public information request to see any requests or approvals filed, and TDCJ replied its records held "nothing responsive to your request."

Lindsey Linder, the former policy attorney for the Texas Criminal Justice Coalition, thinks it's shortsighted to focus the majority of rehabilitative services on reshaping offender's brains rather than their bodies. She doesn't think cosmetic surgery is the solution to the prison problem, but she does believe it can be a tool to aid vulnerable people. "We respond too quickly with a criminal justice response and we should have more public health responses," she said. "It's our responsibility to help people with high needs and build a public health response to the root causes of criminality."

Given the disenfranchisement of inmates in general and discriminatory sentencing practices, the question becomes one about whether appearance bias can be fixed, perhaps by work-based training or through legal enforcement. Appearance, as it relates to the core concept of attractiveness, is not a protected status. To some extent, historic legislation actually discriminates based on appearance, with numerous nineteenth- and twentieth-century city ordinances—colloquially known as the "ugly laws"—literally banning the unattractive from participating in society, to the extent of confining them to their homes.[20] In 1867, San Francisco designated that "any person, who is an unsightly or disgusting object, shall not expose himself or herself to public view" or face a misdemeanor or fine. Chicago, New Orleans, and many others enacted similar statutes. In the mid-twentieth century, states began repealing these laws; in 1974, Chicago was the last city to close it down.

In 2021, only the state of Michigan, Washington, D.C., and a handful of cities including Santa Cruz, California, and Binghamton, New York, have enacted laws that explicitly protect their residents from appearance discrimination.[21] In general, this is not an area of law that has been challenged, and aside from protection under disability legislation, people lack legal recourse. To be fair, it's no easy feat to protect the "unattractive," in part because attractiveness can be such a subjective concept; beauty isn't a trait that can be uniformly measured, unlike other protected classes (under Title VII) such as race, age, and nationality.

Despite cosmetic surgery's exodus from prisons, many still see cosmetic improvements—of a less extreme kind—as vital to reforming offenders. Charities such as Dress for Success, Sharp Men, and Jackets for Jobs provide free grooming, styling, and clothing to ex-cons to help them present themselves professionally in order to get a job. Chicago's Grace House takes this even further, with an annual three-day "extreme makeover" social, in which it gifts free makeup, hair, and fashion styling to ease the reintegration of female ex-cons.

In Dallas, Texas, Attitudes & Attire takes a two-pronged approach, providing free interview attire in conjunction with the Hopeful Smiles program, which provides free dental work (such as bridges and veneers) to help former offenders create the best first impression. Sometimes the prisons themselves take on this role. At the beauty salon inside the Coffee Creek Correctional Facility in Oregon, female inmates receive free services, including balayage, Brazilian blowouts, eyelash extensions, and gel manicures and pedicures[22] the week before they're released.

"I wear makeup every day," said Joyce Pequeno, an inmate serving twenty years inside the Coffee Creek Correctional Facility. "I do it because it makes me feel good, like a real human being not just a number in the system. To me it's like putting my shield on." At the prison salon, Pequeno has had her hair dyed, pedicures, and her gang-related tattoos lasered off—"that's not who I am anymore."

Still, some outside organizations still view cosmetic surgery as a solution. In 2010, Vicky Williams was released from Chillicothe Correctional Center prison in Missouri after serving thirty-two years of a fifty-year sentence for arranging the murder of her allegedly abusive husband. Williams was twenty-four years old when she entered the prison's stark gray confines and fifty-five years old when she left. She stepped out into a new world and immediately discovered that it was a world that didn't want her. No one would hire her. Was her gray mullet and grooved skin to blame? she wondered.

Connections for Success, a nonprofit that helps former inmates and abuse victims, stepped in. It provided work training and a referral to a local collective that approached it about providing a surgical and salon makeover to someone in need. In 2012, her benefactors gave Williams $18,000 of free services, which included a face-lift, a brow lift, liposuction, and color treatment, dying her hair a pleasant toffee brown. I no longer "look like a criminal," she told reporters.[23]

Today, the idea that someone "looks like a criminal" has been well and truly debunked, but an awareness of the science doesn't deter unconscious

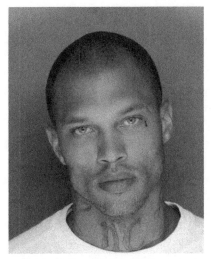

Mug shot of Jeremy Meeks, the "hot mug shot guy." *Courtesy the Stockton Police Department*

associations that stem from popular culture exemplified by villain tropes in movies like *Scarface*.

There can be a flip side to this, however, when attention is drawn to a highly attractive felon that upends society's unconscious understanding of criminality. In 2014, thirty-year-old Jeremy Meeks, a former Crips gang member from Stockton, California, was arrested in a gang sweep, his mug shot posted to Stockton Police Department's Facebook page. In it, Meeks's pale blue eyes stare sultrily, his chiseled cheekbones and Raphaelite jaw perfectly framing his full lips. Below his left eye is a small tattoo of a tear.

His photo went viral, and pictures of the "hot mug shot guy" were plastered all over the national and international press. This notoriety culminated into a modeling contract with White Cross Management, and Meeks now struts the runways in New York and London during fashion week.[24] For a period, he even dated British heiress Chloe Green, daughter of the billionaire retail emperor Philip Green.

"A criminal record is not something to be glamorized—but a reformed ex-con who happens to be criminally good-looking? That's one way to shake up a model casting moment," wrote *Vogue* magazine, who described Meeks as "a buff bad boy."[25]

Meeks is far from the only "fit felon." His peers include "Prison Bae," a.k.a Mekhi Alante Lucky, arrested for speeding and theft in North Carolina, whose chiseled jaw, luminous black skin, and blue and brown heterochromic eyes landed him a modeling contract with St. Claire Modeling and a string of profitable gigs. Each "cover-worthy" felon goes some way toward moving the needle on the "criminal type" but simultaneously exemplifies how, in many cases, redemption is reserved for the ravishing.

Researchers who explore this space are often subject to ridicule or, in the case of appearance research as it relates to crime, often denounced as racists, their work labeled controversial. A 2010 study by professors from Louisiana State University and Georgia State University reported that attractiveness "reduces a young adult's propensity for criminal activity and being unattractive increases it."[26] Further studies reported that attractive children receive better grades in school, and in 2017, researchers at the Metropolitan State University of Denver reported that attractive college students received significantly higher grades[27] from their professors. Of course, "pretty privilege" in and of itself doesn't account for the issues a conventionally pretty person with invisible disabilities such as chronic pain or mobility problems might face or the dismissal of their pain as "pretty people problems."

In 2019, a study by Bonnie Berry, director of the Social Problems Research Group in Washington State further underscored the power physical appearance still holds in the justice system: "the less attractive the subjects, the more likely they are to be arrested, holding constant offending behavior," she wrote.[28] Her findings frustrate her. "What you look like is beyond your control—it doesn't say anything about how good or bad the person is," she said. "It's a matter of genetics and economics. It's an inequality that hasn't been studied very much."[29]

Today, the focus is on changing people's unconscious biases through education, literature, and sensitivity bias training for schools, prisons, and advocates. Berry thinks that's a good start but said that changing the shape of society's underlying prejudices is a long-term project—decades or more—even then experts may never be successful in fully eliminating appearance-related stigmas and stereotypes. There is no shame in a person opting for a more immediate solution, she said, an outlook echoed by many of the experts consulted. "If we need to change our appearance to gain employment or for other social advantages, there is nothing 'wrong' with doing so in the sense that this endeavor levels the playing field," she explained. "Appearance bias, like homophobia, racism, sexism, disablism, classism, and all the other 'isms' are forms of social inequality that needlessly lead to individual and social harm."

The majority of psychologists and criminologists I interviewed acknowledged that providing someone with cosmetic surgery is a far quicker and more effective way of improving their lot than waiting for a cultural attitude shift. The many plastic surgeons I spoke with also maintained that cosmetic surgery can change a person's life. "There's an incredible metamorphosis that occurs," said plastic surgeon Dr. Steven Blackwell, the director of a cleft lip and palate program at Shriners Hospitals for Children in Houston and former plastic surgeon for Texas State prisons. "It's common sense to do something to improve self-worth. It won't turn a sociopath into a non-sociopathic personality, but it may help those who are marginal."

For a multitude of reasons, cosmetic surgery treatments in prisons are no more, and although the knee-jerk reaction to public displeasure is understandable, in the long term it has proved a shortsighted approach. Crime rates have continued to rise, especially among female offenders, and studies as recent as 2020 continue to link unattractiveness with perceived criminality, some even using computer vision technology to draw these conclusions.

An analysis of the different prison surgery programs found that the majority of them lowered recidivism, in some cases dropping it from 75 percent to between 14 percent and 50 percent. Although it's true that many of these reports lacked controls and some of the data was flawed, time after time, the results were replicated. It worked, and it was cost effective.

Of course, people's looks don't tell the whole story; they don't confer intelligence, generosity, or propensity for good or bad behavior. But the intersectionality of an individual's appearance and society's response to it can't be dismissed. Unattractiveness might equate with biased treatment, but so too does socioeconomic status or racist, homophobic, sizeist, and sexist attitudes—and more—in conjunction with other prejudices.

However unfairly, research has proved that more conventionally attractive people have higher earning potential and that improving offenders' appearances boosts their earning ability and lowers their likelihood of future crimes. But it takes money to achieve this, and the majority of criminals live in poverty. The public's knee-jerk reaction was understandable, but therein lies the crux of the problem: cosmetic surgery programs were canceled not because they failed, but because they *succeeded*. Hence the reaction to their success; the currency of beauty is valued so highly by society that people would rather have criminals re-offend than bless them with a physical advantage, an advantage *over them*.

The public's outrage and instantaneous renunciation reflects a culture that prioritizes the pretty over everyone else. However, society's Pavlovian reaction doesn't allow for the intersectional experiences of unattractive people living in a world where their face, race, economic status, and skin tone means they're inordinately criminalized and treated as second class by employers, teachers, and the justice system. Colorism bias runs parallel to the beauty bias, resulting in 25 percent pay disparities among different shades of Black skin.[30] By recognizing this bias and treating it—whether through plastic surgery, a shift in societal attitudes, or more—society isn't giving offenders a leg up, it's just leveling the field.

Barring that, there are some interesting projects tackling the idea of representation. In November 2018, the British Film Institute (BFI), a nonprofit dedicated to expanding British film production and distribution, announced that it would no longer provide funding for movies that featured stereotypically "scarred" villains, a change prompted by the "I Am Not Your Villain" campaign run by Changing Faces, a U.K. charity that challenges discrimination and campaigns for face equality.[31] "Film is a catalyst for change and we are committing to not having negative representations depicted through scars or facial difference in the films we fund," the BFI announced. "BFI diversity standards call for meaningful representations on-screen. We urge the rest of the film industry to do the same."[32]

Depictions of albinism in movies as a criminal trait (for example, the sociopathic twins in *Matrix Reloaded* and Silas in *The Da Vinci Code*) has also declined, thanks to the concerted media efforts by the National Organization for Albinism and Hypopigmentation to reclaim the condition. "Dermatologic disease does not equate to moral degeneracy in reality," wrote San Francisco dermatologist Dr. Vail Reese in a paper published by the *Journal of the American Medical Association*. "However, typically, if you see a scar in a film, usually done with prosthetic makeup, that's gonna be the bad guy."[33]

Not everyone has welcomed these changes—"Are they going to cancel *The Lion King* now?" complained one reader—but these cultural media shifts help shape a world where the less attractive aren't automatically tarred with criminality.

Larger shifts are happening in the correctional sphere right now. President Obama's Sentencing Reform and Corrections Act of 2015 never made it through Congress, but in 2018, cherry-picked parts were subsumed into the First Step Act, which was signed into law by President Trump. Under the First Step umbrella, mandatory minimum sentences for nonviolent drug users were shortened, the federal three-strikes rule switched from a life sentence to twenty-five years for offenders with three or more felony convictions, and judges were given more discretion when sentencing.

States have stepped up as well. New Jersey's prison population dropped 33 percent from 2010 to 2020, and California's inmate population fell 40 percent during that same period.[34] Due to concerted efforts in New York City, there's been a sharp decrease in incarceration in the city; in 2019 the city's jails housed 7,000 inmates compared to 11,000 five years earlier. Statewide, the number of prisoners dropped from 62,559 in 2008 to 47,476 in 2019.[35]

In October 2019, New York's city council voted to close Rikers Island, plus an additional three jails. In their place, the city would build new, more rehabilitative facilities, and the island itself would potentially become a public park. The pandemic, a terrible tragedy that's caused untold horror and suffering throughout the world, proved a surprising boon for decarceration. Concerned about inmates' safety—someone serving time for petty theft didn't deserve a death sentence—there was a large uptick in early releases. By February 2020, the New York City jail population stood at 5,447. As of January 7, 2021, it was 5,063.

However, the pandemic also has slowed Rikers' shutdown; originally planned for 2026, it's been pushed back to 2027. It's possible more delays will occur.

"Rikers Island is a symbol of brutality and inhumanity," Councilman Corey Johnson announced[36] during the hearing about the fate of Rikers. All of America's prisons and jails have sordid histories, but Rikers Island, built on sewage and sorrow, is a moral stain on the city. Its race riots, murders, overdoses, and abuses shame the city. Closing Rikers, an especially significant symbol, sends a message. After all, if this book has proved anything, it's that appearance *and* action matter.

# ACKNOWLEDGMENTS

This book could not have been written without the help and support of numerous people: friends, archivists, and experts all kind enough to grant me their time and provide me with detailed information or complex carbohydrates. Thank you to my wonderful agent Eliza Rothstein for seeing the potential in the book and my publisher Jake Bonar for trusting my vision and championing my manuscript.

I extend my heartfelt thanks to Douglas Lipton—who was unfailingly patient and always willing to explain things to me—and his incredible recall of events long ago, which made my work so much easier. Getting to meet and chat with Norman Cavior was another great pleasure; he welcomed me into his home and was completely transparent about his work—thank you. And thanks to Richard Kurtzberg and Carol Brodsky, who were kind enough to sift through their memory banks for me and illuminate this period.

I can't say enough good things about Barbara Lewin, who was kind enough to discuss the work of her father, Dr. Michael Lewin, and dig into her childhood recollections of home life and his habits; you made the book so much richer by sharing these details. I want to share so much appreciation for the input of Dr. Richard Bloomenstein and Dr. Morton Goldstein, who willingly shared their tales of their plastic surgery residencies at Montefiore Medical Center and their experiences of visiting Rikers Island and Sing Sing Correctional Facility.

Again, more thanks to the many plastic surgeons with whom I consulted for this work whose many insights (if not their own stories) helped shape the book:

the now deceased Dr. Melvin Spira, Dr. Harry Glassman of Los Angeles, Dr. Leo Munick, Dr. Steven Blackwell, Dr. Daniel B. Tuerk, Dr. Elliot Jacobs, Dr. Jack Fisher, and Dr. Sam Most.

Thanks to journalist Steven Long for digging through the case files of his mind and to Lindsey Linder for patiently explaining the ins and outs of the criminal justice system. Much appreciation to Wallace Mandell, our discussion really opened my eyes, and much thanks to Steven C. Hayes, Bonnie Berry, Robert Agnew, Daniel Hamermesh, and Autumn Whitefield-Madrano for their generosity with their time and their patience in explaining psychological concepts and historic precedents to me.

Thank you to Chris Eskridge for connecting me to the wonderful Ed Latessa, and Latessa for being a font of knowledge and insight, and criminologist Kevin Thompson, whose data was heaven-sent.

Thank you for the kindness of the many inmates and former offenders interviewed; your willingness to discuss difficult events and experiences was gratefully received; thank you in particular to Sherry Willeford, Joyce Pequeno, Claudia S., and Melissa Hutchison.

My San Francisco #writerpod provided invaluable support and occasional outdoor picnics during the process; the amazing Daniela Blei, Ellen Airhart, and Larissa Zimberoff rock, and my book is so much better for your thoughtful reads. Also, Nathan Hurst, you rock—I so appreciate you for taking the time to give me feedback and line edits; your editorial eye was really helpful. Thank you to Zach St. George for believing in my vision and for poor quality vodka. Brad Balukjian and Carla Walter, thank you for being some of the earliest readers of this work and for your encouragement when the work felt like an unwieldy mess. Extra props to the wonderful folks at the San Francisco Writers Grotto for letting me take a backseat as board member during the intensive writing part and for championing my work; in particular, members of the pub committee: Kevin Smokler, Kathy Seligman, Jenny Bitner, Connie Hale, and many, many more. Your cheer, encouragement, and generosity with your time and experience was deeply appreciated.

Writing is a frustrating, lonely process, and I am grateful for the support and encouragement of my friends and family, whose memes, calls, Zooms, and Amazon deliveries from both sides of the pond kept me going: Nicole Reamey, Arlo Reamey-Brindle, Juliette Jardim (see, I *do* know how to spell your name), Lillian Rafii, Kulsum Vakharia, Sonia Paul, Katia Savchuk, Becky Dixon, Bryony Hewer, Debra Peters, Sebastian Bird, Dr. Harman Boparai, Alex Roumbas-Goldstein, Ali-Heriyanto Lambo, Alissa Figueora, Gemma Cartwright, the wonderful Thad Eirich, Lisa Shaverin, Adina Ben-Ari, Simon Rabinowicz,

Jack Rabinowicz, Danielle Rabinowicz, Margie Woodring, Tim Woodring, Jodi Eirich, Toby Eirich, Laura Ellison, Meg Waltner, and Carly Holmes.

Thank you to the crew at #2040Sutter, your companionship and friendship has been an unexpected joy amid all of this: Roberta Rosen, Alex St. John, Miki St. John, and the indomitable Kaley St. John.

Thank you to the Rockefeller Archive Center, which awarded me a grant to travel to and conduct research at its archives and to Joan Berry and Collin Anthony from the Stanford McCoy School of Ethics, who saw the potential in my proposal and invited me to share it with a cohort of undergraduates via a Zoom lecture.

So many librarians and archivists went out of their way to help me collect the information needed, even amid the coronavirus pandemic. This work could not have been completed without their kindness and patience: Elisa Ho, researcher extraordinaire at the American Jewish Archives, supported this project and patiently answered all my questions, even when they were repeats due to my Gmail chains; Adam Leverone at Getty Images for his helpfulness in providing access to a much-needed file; Traca Wolfe from the Max Chambers Library at the University of Central Oklahoma, who went above and beyond to provide me vital documents; Gayle Martinson of the Library, Archives, and Museum Collections of Wisconsin Historical Society; Melissa Dorsten of Ohio Library Services; Sandra E. Yates from the McGovern Historical Center, who patiently and quickly processed several requests for scans; Thomas C. McCarthy of the New York Correction History Society Archives for his willingness to discuss all things Anna Kross; thank you to James Vann, formerly of the New York Department of Correction for humoring my questions; Jessica Murphy at the Center for the History of Medicine, Harvard Medical School, was a font of knowledge and access; Ken Cobb from the New York Municipal Archives; and the California Historical Society.

To Laurie Thompson and Carol Acquaviva from the Anne T. Kent room at the Marin County Free Library, I so appreciate your patience and turnaround when I was throwing unreasonable deadlines at you; Don Chaddock of the California Department of Corrections and Rehabilitation; Connie Delhanty and Sheila Smalling from Montefiore Medical Center archives; Aryn Glazier from the Dolph Briscoe Center for American History, Austin, Texas; Ellen Belcher, special collections librarian at John Jay; Drew Bourn, the historical curator at the Lane Medical Library at Stanford Medical History. Thank you to Shawn Dellis and Mark Torees of the Pacifica Radio Archives for their speedy responses, Jeff Thompson, librarian and archivist from the Church History Library in Utah, the awesome Erin McGarvey for her copyediting chops, the wonderful people at the Rowman & Littlefield Publishing group, and many, many more.

# NOTES

## INTRODUCTION

1. Anna Kross, *Progress through Crisis* (New York: New York City Department of Correction, 1955–1963).

2. Sander L. Gilman, *Making the Body Beautiful: A Cultural History of Aesthetic Surgery* (Princeton, NJ: Princeton University Press, 1999), 16.

3. Henry Solomon, "Sing Sing Report: For Better Surgery," *New York Tribune,* January 10, 1910.

4. Newswire, "Surgery on Criminals: New York Official's Plan to Remove Bad Streaks," *Chattanooga (TN) Daily Times,* January 10, 1910.

5. Newswire, "Surgery to Help Convicts," *Baltimore Sun,* January 10, 1910.

6. Naci Mocan and Erdal Tekin, "Ugly Criminals," *National Bureau of Economic Research,* 2006; B. W. Darby and D. Jeffers, "The Effects of Defendant and Juror Attractiveness on Simulated Courtroom Trial Decisions," *Social Behavior and Personality: An International Journal* 16, no. 1 (1988): 39–50; Rachel A. Gordon, Robert Crosnoe, Xue Wang, and Patricia J. Bauer, "Physical Attractiveness and the Accumulation of Social and Human Capital in Adolescents and Young Adulthood: Assets and Distractions," *Monographs of the Society for Research in Child Development* 78, no. 6 (2013): 1–137, accessed February 3, 2021, www.jstor.org/stable/43772912; Ray Bull, "Physical Appearance and Criminality," *Current Psychological Reviews* 2 (1982): 262–81; A. Chris Down and Phillip M. Lyons, "Natural Observations of the Links between Attractiveness and Initial Legal Judgments," *Personality and Social Psychology Bulletin* 17, no. 5 (1991): 541–47.

7. Alan Slater, Gavin Bremner, Scott P. Johnson, Penny Sherwood, Rachel Hayes, and Elizabeth Brown, "Newborn Infants' Preference for Attractive Faces: The Role of Internal and External Facial Features," *Psychology, Medicine Infancy* (2000): 265–74.

8. Maria Sosa and Erika Carillo, "A Dangerous Cosmetic Surgery Killed 14 Women in Five Years," USC Annenberg, Center for Health Journalism, 2019; and American Society of Plastic Surgeons, "Press Release: Plastic Surgery Societies Issue Urgent Warning about the Risks Associated with Brazilian Butt Lifts," plasticsurgery .org, August 6, 2018.

9. American Society of Plastic Surgeons, "2019 Plastic Surgery Statistics Report," ASPS National Clearinghouse of Plastic Surgery Procedural Statistics, 2019. For the salary disparities, see Stephen Miller, "Black Workers Still Earn Less Than Their White Counterparts," Shrm.org, June 11, 2020.

10. Adam Looney and Nicholas Turner, "Work and Opportunity before and after Incarceration," The Brookings Institution, March 14, 2018.

11. Authors Bruce Western and Becky Pettit, "Incarceration and Social Inequality," American Academy of Arts and Sciences, June 2010, www.amacad.org/publication/ incarceration-social-inequality.

12. Keri Blakinger, "Toothless Texas Inmates Denied Dentures in State Prison," *Houston Chronicle*, September 23, 2018, www.chron.com/news/houston-texas/hous ton/article/Toothless-Texas-inmates-denied-dentures-in-state-13245169.php.

13. Josh Saul, "An Inmate Had Skin Cancer and Needed Radiation. This Prison Gave Him Tylenol," *Newsweek*, December 21, 2017.

14. Mark Siegler and Selwyn O. Rogers Jr., *Violence, Trauma, and Trauma Surgery: Ethical Issues, Interventions, and Innovations*, (Cham, Switzerland: Springer, 2020).

15. U.S. Department of Health and Human Services, Centers for Disease Control and Prevention, National Center for Health Statistics, "National Hospital Ambulatory Medical Care Survey: 2017 Emergency Department Summary Tables," 2017, www.cdc.gov/nchs/data/nhamcs/web_tables/2017_ed_web_tables-508.pdf and www .cdc.gov/nchs/hus/contents2018.htm?search=Emergency_department_visits; Charles Dodge Rees, Adam Blancher, Paige Bundrick, Mickie Hamiter, Tara Moore-Medlin, and Cherie-Ann O. Nathan, "Assessment of Facial Injury by 'Slock' in Incarcerated Patients," *Otorhinolaryngology Hypersensitivity Treatment* 1, no. 2 (2020): 1–4, DOI: 10.31038/OHT.2020121.

16. Mariel Alper, Matthew R. Durose, and Joshua Markman, "2018 Update on Prisoner Recidivism: A 9-Year Follow-Up Period," Bureau of Justice Statistics, 2018, www .bjs.gov/index.cfm?ty=pbdetail&iid=6266.

17. Douglas C. McDonald, "Medical Care in Prisons," *Crime and Justice* 26 (1999): 427–78, DOI: 10.1086/449301.

18. Melvin Delgado and Denise Humm-Delgado, *Health and Health Care in the Nation's Prisons* (Lanham, MD: Rowman & Littlefield, 2008), 4–24.

19. Ames Grawer, "What Is the First Step Act—And What's Happening with It?" Brennan Center for Justice, June 23, 2020; and Federal Bureau of Prisons, "An Overview of the First Step Act," n.d., www.bop.gov/inmates/fsa/overview.jsp.

20. Joe Biden, "The Biden Plan for Strengthening America's Commitment to Justice," n.d., https://joebiden.com/justice.

21. Dave Davies, "Former Physician at Rikers Island Exposes Health Risks of Incarceration," NPR Radio, March 18, 2019.

22. The Sentencing Project, "Criminal Justice Facts," n.d., www.sentencingproject.org/criminal-justice-facts.

## CHAPTER 1. BABY BLUES AND THE BAD MEN BIRTHRIGHT

1. Michael L. Lewin, "Subtotal Nasal Reconstruction in Infants and Children for the Correction of Acquired Defects," in *Transactions of the 5th International Congress of Plastic and Reconstructive Surgery*, ed. J. T. Hueston (Melbourne: Butterworths, 1971), 1029; Michael L. Lewin, "Total Rhinoplasty in Infants, Reports of a Case of Waterhouse-Friederichsen Syndrome," *The Plastic and Reconstructive Surgery Journal* (1955): 131–42.

2. "Weather History for Paterson, NJ," Old Farmer's Almanac, accessed August 31, 2020, www.almanac.com/weather/history/NJ/Paterson/1953-01-23.

3. Carolyn Moehling and Anne Morrison Piehl, "Immigration, Crime, and Incarceration in Early Twentieth-Century America," *Demography* 46, no. 4 (November 2009): 739–63.

4. Helen Stapinski, "When America Barred Italians," *New York Times*, June 2, 2017.

5. Lewin, "Total Rhinoplasty in Infants."

6. Virginia Lambert, "Child Abuse Is Hard to Prove," *(Paterson, NJ) Morning Call*, July 17, 1968.

7. Diane Pham, "New Year's Eve in Numbers: Fun Facts about the Times Square Ball Drop," 6sqft, December 30, 2019, www.6sqft.com/new-years-eve-in-numbers-fun-facts-about-the-times-square-ball-drop.

8. "The New Year," *The (MT) Missoulian*, January 1, 1950; "Number of Televisions in the US," The Physics Factbook, https://hypertextbook.com/facts/2007/Tamara Tamazashvili.shtml.

9. Zoe Mitchell, "Mr. Potato Head," PBS, July 20, 2018, www.pbs.org/wgbh/americanexperience/features/mr-potato-head.

10. Michelle Parnett-Dwyer, "Mr. Potato Head: He's a Real Spud," *ToyTales*, February 11, 2019, https://toytales.ca/mr-potato-head-hes-a-real-spud/; "New Toys Just Arrived in Honolulu!" *Honolulu Star Bulletin*, October 1, 1953; "History of Children's Games and Toys," The People History, www.thepeoplehistory.com/toys.html.

11. "Harry S. Truman," History.com, February 5, 2020, www.history.com/topics/us-presidents/harry-truman; "Executive Orders," Harry S. Truman Library and Museum, The National Archives, www.trumanlibrary.gov/library/executive-orders.

12. Robert F. Zeidel, "A 1911 Report Set America on a Path of Screening out 'Undesirable' Immigrants," *Smithsonian Magazine*, July 16, 2018.

13. Diana Bretherick, "The 'Born Criminal'? Lombroso and the Origins of Modern Criminology," History Extra, 2015, www.historyextra.com/period/victorian/the-born-criminal-lombroso-and-the-origins-of-modern-criminology.

14. Cody Jorgensen and Anthony Walsh, *Criminology: The Essentials* (London: Sage, 2019); David G. Horn, *The Criminal Body: Lombroso and the Anatomy of Deviance* (London: Routledge, 2003).

15. Matt Simon, "Fantastically Wrong: The Scientist Who Seriously Believed Criminals Were Part Ape," *Wired*, July 19, 2018, www.wired.com/2014/11/fantastically-wrong-criminal-anthropology/.

16. Christopher Woolf, "A Brief History of America's Hostility to a Previous Generation of Mediterranean Migrants—Italians," The World from PRX, November 26, 2015, www.pri.org/stories/2015-11-26/brief-history-america-s-hostility-previous-generation-mediterranean-migrants.

17. Woolf, "A Brief History of America's Hostility"; Bretherick, "The 'Born Criminal.'"

18. Simonetta Conti, "La Donna Delinquente' Di Cesare Lombroso," Lastampa. it, 2016, www.lastampa.it/2016/05/22/cronaca/la-donna-delinquente-di-cesare-lombroso-ibSJny8QdxahDFBnkuRFxJ/pagina.html.

19. Claire Wang, "Stanford's History with Eugenics," *Stanford Daily*, December 7, 2016, www.stanforddaily.com/2016/12/07/stanfords-history-with-eugenics/.

20. E. Lucile Dessery, "A Study of the Mental Inferiority of the Italian Immigrant" (master's thesis, University of California, 1922); I. A. Hourwich, *Immigration and Labor: The Economic Aspects of European Immigration to the United States* (New York: B. W. Huebsch, 1922); W. P. Dillingham, *Reports of the Immigration Commission* (Washington, DC: Government Printing Office, 1907–1910).

21. Dessery, "A Study of the Mental Inferiority of the Italian Immigrant"; I. A. Hourwich, *Immigration and Labor*.

22. Michael L. Lewin, Countway Medical Library Archives, Harvard University, Boston, folders 5–8.

23. Lewin, Countway Medical Library Archives.

24. Time Nash, "The 1930s Hairstyles Let a Girl Be a Girl," The Finer Times, November 22, 2009, www.thefinertimes.com/The-1930s/1930s-hairstyles-let-a-girl-be-a-girl.html.

25. "State Industrial School Chief Calls for Help," *Billings Gazette*, March 20, 1952.

26. Velva Hulen, Poet's Corner, *(Escondido, CA) Times-Advocate*, 1953.

27. J. E. Joy, Poet's Corner, *(Escondido, CA) Times-Advocate*, August 22, 1953.

28. Open Forum, *Chatham Press*, January 2, 1953.

29. "College President to Talk at YMCA," *Asbury (NJ) Park Press,* January 12, 1953.

30. W. K., "New Noses for Old in Pakistan," *New York Times,* October 31, 1954.

31. Lewin, "Subtotal Nasal Reconstruction," 1029; Lewin, "Total Rhinoplasty in Infants," 131–42.

32. "Surgeon Gives Tiny Baby New Nose," *Boston Globe,* October 31, 1954.

33. "Baby's Lost Nose Replaced by Long One," *Miami News,* October 27, 1954.

34. "Baby Given New Nose So Parents Will Accept Him," *(NJ) Record,* November 4, 1954.

35. "Baby Given New Nose"; Lewin, "Subtotal Nasal Reconstruction."

## CHAPTER 2. SING SING PRISON AND PLASTIC SURGERY SOCIAL WORK

1. "Census of Population and Housing," Census.gov, accessed June 4, 2015.

2. Joseph Louderback, "Famous First Due: Sing Sing," *FireHouse,* January 31, 2005, www.firehouse.com/home/news/10508226/famous-first-due-sing-sing; H. H. Hart, *Plans and Illustrations of Prisons and Reformatories* (New York: Russell Sage Foundation, 1922).

3. Martin Kivel, "Lonely Hearts Killers Go Stoically to Doom," *Daily News,* March 9, 1951.

4. Dick Owen, "Inside Sing Sing," *Daily News,* February 11, 1962.

5. *Annual Report of the New York State Commission of Correction 1961* (Albany, NY: State Commission of Correction, 1961), 120.

6. New York Department of Correction, "Population Ups and Downs," *Correction* 18, no. 1 (September 1, 1953): 15.

7. "Dr. Morris Smith, Surgeon, Educator; Halloran Surgical Chief, Long at St. Luke's, Dies at 64—On Cornell Medical Staff," *New York Times,* July 3, 1950, www.nytimes.com/1950/07/03/archives/drmorris-smith-surgeoneducator-halloran-surgical-chief-long-at-st.html.

8. James Dawson, *Sing Sing Prison: Its History, Purpose, Makeup and Program* (New York: State Department of Correction, 1953), https://nysl.ptfs.com/data/Library1/Library1/pdf/11937788.pdf.

9. "New York Police Record Three Violent Deaths during First Hours of New Year," *(NY) Post-Star,* January 2, 1953.

10. Richard Dolsky, "Cosmetic Surgery in the United States: Its Past and Present," *American Journal of Cosmetic Surgery* 16, no. 2, (1999): 109–14.

11. City of New York, *Report of the Department of Correction for the Year 1921* (New York: Press of Clarence S. Nathan, 1921), https://babel.hathitrust.org/cgi/pt?id=mdp.39015074707251&view=2up&seq=192&size=400.

12. Lewis E. Lawes, *Twenty Thousand Years in Sing Sing* (Philadelphia: Blakiston, 1932).

13. Amos Osborne Squire, *Sing Sing Doctor* (Garden City, NY: Doubleday, Doran, 1937).

14. "New York to Beautify Prisoners," *Hartford Daily Courant*, December 20, 1934.

15. Maxwell Maltz, *New Faces, New Futures: Rebuilding Character with Plastic Surgery* (New York: Smith, 1936), 259.

16. "Making Angel Faces?" *Lancaster Era*, December 24, 1934.

17. "Shall We Remodel Criminals or Remodel Prison?" *Courier*, January 22, 1953.

18. "NY May Beautify City Jail Inmates," *Daily Capital News*, December 21, 1934; "Beauty Clinic for Thugs!" *Charleston Daily Mail*, April 30, 1936; "The Place of Beauty Shops in a Reign of Law and Order," *Arizona Republic*, November 11, 1936.

19. "Shall We Remodel Criminals or Remodel Prison?" *Courier*, January 22, 1935.

20. "Ugly Burglar Is Given New Face; Vista of Law-Abiding Life Opens," *Arizona Republic*, August 12, 1949; "Surgeons to Work on Nose and Dentist on Teeth Blamed for Crimes," *Cincinnati Enquirer*, July 17, 1948.

21. "Ugly Duckling Felon Pondered," *Circleville (OH) Herald*, June 19, 1948.

22. "Burglar Called Misfit in Society Gets New Face and Second Chance," *Pittsburgh (PA) Press*, July 17, 1948; Richard McLaughlin, "New Face Turns 'Ugly Thief' Honest," *Akron (OH) Beacon Journal*, March 27, 1949.

23. Willian Engle, "Ugly Ducklings Need Not Be Ugly," *Pittsburgh (PA) Sun-Telegraph*, August 7, 1949; "The Case of the Ugly Thief," *Time*, November 4, 1949.

24. Engle, "Ugly Ducklings."

25. "Ugly Burglars New Face May Bring Him New Life," *Pampa (TX) Daily News*, April 21, 1949.

26. "Ugly Burglar Becomes Smiling Man in Love," *Pittsburgh (PA) Press*, September 16, 1950.

27. "Nuptials of Once Ugly Burglar Delayed by Rain," *Newark (OH) Advocate*, October 26, 1950; "Ugly Crook's Face to Get New Look," *New Journal (OH)*, July 17, 1948.

28. "The Case of the Ugly Thief," *Time*, April 11, 1949.

29. "Wedding Bells Ring for Ugly Burglar," *Cincinnati Enquirer*, November 11, 1950.

30. "Ugly Burglar Married," *New York Times*, November 11, 1950.

31. "Ugly Burglar and Beauty Wed," *(OH) Tribune*, November 26, 1950.

32. Letter from Sing Sing patient to Dr. Michael L. Lewin, 1955, Michael L. Lewin Papers, 1927–1994, National Archives of Plastic Surgery, PS 16, Countway Library of Medicine Archives, Harvard University, Boston, box 1.

33. Michael L. Lewin Papers, 1927–1994, National Archives of Plastic Surgery, PS 16, Countway Library of Medicine, Harvard.

34. Michael L. Lewin, "Plastic Surgery in Rehabilitation of the Prison Inmate," *Aorn Journal* 7, no. 1 (April 1968): 64–68, https://aornjournal.onlinelibrary.wiley.com/doi/abs/10.1016/S0001-2092(08)70265-5.

35. American Correctional Association, *A Manual of Correctional Standards: Prepared by the Committee to Revise the 1946 Manual of Suggested Standards for a State Correctional System* (New York: American Correctional Association, 1954).

36. Albert W. Alschuler, "The Changing Purposes of Criminal Punishment: A Retrospective on the Past Century and Some Thoughts about the Next," *University of Chicago Law Review* 70, no. 1 (2003): 1–22, DOI: 10.2307/1600541.

37. W. Averell Harriman, *Public Papers of Averell Harriman: Fifty-Second Governor of the State of New York, 1955–58* (Albany, NY: n.p., 1958), 1286.

## CHAPTER 3. CRIME'S CINDERELLA COMPLEX

1. "Facelifting Helps Criminals," *Bedford (IN) Daily-Times Mail*, January 14, 1958.

2. Michael Lewin, Michael L. Lewin Papers, 1927–1994, National Archives of Plastic Surgery, PS 16, Countway Library of Medicine, Harvard, Boston, box 1, folder 3.

3. "History and Milestones," Montefiore Medical Center, accessed September 2, 2020, www.montefiore.org/about-history-and-milestones.

4. D. Russell, *Black Genius* (New York: Skyhorse Publishing, 2009), 381–85; W. Douglas Fisher and Joann H. Buckley, *African American Doctors of World War I* (Jefferson, NC: McFarland, 2015), 155–274; R. Watkins, "On Becoming a Black Doctor," *Black Enterprise* (1975): 20–21; H. Washington, *Medical Apartheid: The Dark History of Medical Experimentation on Black Americans from Colonial Times to the Present* (New York: Doubleday, 2006).

5. Michael L. Lewin Papers.

6. Michael L. Lewin Papers, folder 4.

7. Michael L. Lewin Papers, box 1, folder 8.

8. Michael L. Lewin Papers.

9. Christopher Effgen, "New York Crime Rates 1960–2018," www.disastercenter.com/crime/nycrime.htm; Kevin Baker, "'Welcome to Fear City'—The Inside Story of New York's Civil War, 40 Years On," *Guardian*, May 18, 2015, www.theguardian.com/cities/2015/may/18/welcome-to-fear-city-the-inside-story-of-new-yorks-civil-war-40-years-on; "Lindsay's Legacy," *Daily News*, November 15, 1965; "Nightly New York Crime Drama," *Tallahassee Democrat*, May 9, 1965.

10. "Racial Demonstrations and Crime," *(Shreveport, LA) Times*, March 21, 1965; "New York Crime Fight Moves to Street," *Orlando Evening Star*, April 23, 1965; Douglas Sefton, "Host of Problems to Ring Him in New Years Day," *Daily News*, November 15, 1965; "Big Problems Face Mayor in New Year," *Daily News*, November 15, 1965; NYPR Archive Collection, "Safety in the Street," WNYC, April 21, 1965, www.wnyc.org/story/safety-in-the-street/.

11. "Hijacking of Trucks Is Up 200%," *Anderson Daily Bulletin*, April 1, 1953.

12. Yasmeen Khan, "Demand for School Integration Leads to Massive 1964 Boycott—In New York City," WNYC, February 3, 2016, www.wnyc.org/story/school-boycott-1964/.

13. "Higher Unemployment Rates 1957–60: Structural Transformation or Inadequate Demand," Subcommittee on Economic Statistics of the Joint Committee on Economic Committee, Congress of the United States, 1961.

14. Hal Boyle, "Inside the U.S. . . . Judge Anna Kross Says Women May Solve Crime," *(Lockhaven, PA) Express,* July 14, 1951.

15. American Jewish Archives, Kross-Wagner Memos, Reports 1950–1968, MS-176, box 33, folder 3.

16. "9 Prisoners Saw Their Way out of Jail," *Battle Creek (MI) Enquirer,* January 3, 1947.

17. Anna Kross, *Progress through Crisis* (New York: New York City Department of Correction, 1955–1963), 11.

18. Eleanor Roosevelt, "My Day: September 11, 1961," Eleanor Roosevelt Papers Digital Edition, accessed September 2, 2020, www2.gwu.edu/~erpapers/myday/displaydoc.cfm?_y=1961&_f=md005001.

19. Joseph P. Lyford, *The Airtight Cage: A Study of New York's West Side* (New York: Harper & Row, 1966).

20. Anna Kross, *Annual Report* (New York: New York City Department of Correction, 1954).

21. Kross, *Progress through Crisis*, 30.

22. U.S. Congress, Committee on the Judiciary, *Juvenile Delinquency (Exploitation of Minors in Interstate Confidence Racket): Hearings before the Subcommittee to Investigate Juvenile Delinquency of the Committee on the Judiciary, United States Senate, Eighty-fourth Congress, Second Session, Pursuant to S. Res. 173, and S. Res. 303, Eighty-fourth Congress, Investigation of Juvenile Delinquency in the United States, December 11, 12, and 17, 1956* (Washington: U.S. Government Printing Office, 1956).

23. Kitty Hanson and Sydney Merkin, "House of Detention Serves as a Crime Finishing School," *Daily News,* February 10, 1955.

24. *Studies in American Humor* 1 (1994).

25. Gary Susman, "Disney's 'Cinderella': 25 Things You Didn't Know about the Beloved Fairy Tale Classic," Moviefone, February 15, 2015.

26. Special Collections, Claremont Colleges Library, "Richard III," Interpretations of Shakespeare, or, What You Will, 2016, https://shakespeareatclaremont.omeka.net/exhibits/show/interpretations-of-shakespeare/richard-iii.

27. 2 Samuel 14:25–33, www.biblegateway.com/passage/?search=2+Samuel+14%3A25-33&version=NIV.

28. Daniel 1:4.

29. Jessica Pallingston, *Lipstick: A Celebration of a Girl's Best Friend* (London: Simon & Schuster, 1999); Geoffrey Jones, *Beauty Imagined: A History of the Global*

*Beauty Industry* (Oxford: Oxford University Press, 2015); Sarah Schaffer, "Reading Our Lips: The History of Lipstick Regulation in Western Seats of Power" (2006 third year paper, Harvard), http://nrs.harvard.edu/urn-3:HUL.InstRepos:10018966.

30. Stevie McGlinchey, "The History of 1940s Makeup—1940 to 1949," *Glamour Daze*, May 29, 2013, https://glamourdaze.com/history-of-makeup/1940s.

31. "Plastic Surgery: It's No Longer Reserved for the Vain," *New York Times*, September 27, 1971, www.nytimes.com/1971/09/27/archives/its-no-longer-reserved -for-the-vain-and-rich.html.

32. British Pathé, "1950s Nose Job, Early Plastic Surgery Scenes," YouTube, August 10, 2011, www.youtube.com/watch?v=eBp0fy7viRo.

33. Harry Kalven Jr. and Hans Zeisel, "The American Jury," *Washington & Lee Law Review* 158 (1967), https://scholarlycommons.law.wlu.edu/wlulr/vol24/iss1/18.

34. "Plastic Surgery: It's No Longer Reserved for the Vain"; Kathleen A. Cairns, *The Enigma Woman: The Death Sentence of Nellie May Madison* (Lincoln: University of Nebraska Press, 2009); F. Monahan, *Women in Crime* (New York: I. Washburn, 1941); "Veteran Warden Writes of Women Prisoners," *Minneapolis Star*, December 27, 1941.

35. Angela S. Ahola, Sven Å. Christianson, and Å. Hellström, "Justice Needs a Blindfold: Effects of Gender and Attractiveness on Prison Sentences and Attributions of Personal Characteristics in a Judicial Process," *Psychiatry, Psychology and Law* 16 (2009): S90–S100, DOI: 10.1080/13218710802242011.

36. Kalven and Zeisel, "The American Jury."

37. G. R. Thornton, "The Ability to Judge Crimes from Photographs of Criminals: A Contribution to Technique," *Journal of Abnormal and Social Psychology* 3 (1939).

38. "Specialists Go 'Up' the River," *Medical World News*, September 15, 1961, 44–45.

39. Michael L. Lewin Papers, box 1, folder 8.

40. Ralph. S. Banay, "Physical Disfigurement and Crime," *Federal Probation* (1943).

41. Ralph S. Banay, *We Call Them Criminals* (New York: Appleton Century, 1957).

42. Jeff Quitney, "Coast Guard Officer United States Coast Guard (USCG) Recruiting Film," Vimeo, 1955, https://vimeo.com/339737680.

43. Despo Kritsotaki, Vicky Long, and Matthew Smith, eds., *Preventing Mental Illness: Past, Present and Future* (n.p.: Palgrave Macmillan, 2019); Ralph S. Banay, "Physical Disfigurement as a Factor in Delinquency and Crime," *Federal Probation Journal* 7, no. 1 (June 1943): 21.

44. Doris Reno, "Bare Strides in Plastic War Surgery," *Miami Herald*, March 10, 1943.

45. Morton Goldstein, personal communication, 2019.

46. Richard Bloomenstein, personal communication, 2018.

47. New York State Commission of Correction. *Annual Report of the New York State Commission of Correction* (Albany, NY: State Commission of Correction), 1964.

48. D. Owens, "Inside Sing Sing," *Daily News*, February 18, 1962.
49. Richard Bloomenstein, personal communication, 2019.
50. John Jay Rouse, *Firm but Fair: The Life of Sing Sing Warden Lewis Lawes* (n.p.: Xlibris, 2000).
51. Owens, "Inside Sing Sing."

## CHAPTER 4. LIGHTS, CAMERA, VIOLINS! THE SPECTACLE OF PRISON SURGERY

1. "Japanese Beauty Akiko Kojima Named Miss Universe 1959 Film Direct," You-Tube, July 17, 2017, www.youtube.com/watch?v=poDwEsxEYaw.
2. Ed Herlihy, "Universal-International News, Miss Universe. Miss Japan Wins '59 Crown," YouTube, 1959, www.youtube.com/watch?v=poDwEsxEYaw.
3. Patrick McNulty, "Miss Universe Title Goes to Japanese Girl," *La Crosse (WI) Tribune*, July 24, 1959.
4. Associated Press, "Not True Says Miss Universe: Injections of Bust Denied," *Amarillo (TX) Globe Times*, August 13, 1959; Akiko Kojima, "'Oh My Gosh,' Says Surprised Miss Japan," *La Crosse (WI) Tribune*, July 24, 1959; Garber Davidson, "A Crown and a Faraway Smile: Miss Universe Floating on Cloud," *Tennessean*, July 26, 1959.
5. Shirley Jennifer Lim, *A Feeling of Belonging: Asian American Women's Public Culture, 1930–1960* (New York: New York University Press, 2006), 176.
6. Associated Press, "International Battle Rages—Was Beauty Puffed by Plastic?" *Greenville (SC) News*, August 14, 1959.
7. Associated Press, "Did Miss Universe Have Surgery Job?" *Orlando Sentinel*, August 14, 1959.
8. Staff writers, "Plastic Surgery Given Parolees," *(Hackensack, NJ) Record*, November 10, 1964; Deborah A. Sullivan, "Advertising Cosmetic Surgery," *AMA Journal of Ethics, Illuminating the Art of Medicine* (2010), https://journalofethics.ama-assn.org/article/advertising-cosmetic-surgery/2010-05.
9. "Dr. Brady's Health Quiz: The Unsatisfactory Noses and the Funny Face Surgeons," *Nebraska State Journal*, October 19, 1930; Lana Thompson, *Plastic Surgery* (Santa Barbara, CA: Greenwood, ABC-CLIO, 2011), 64.
10. J. Howard Crum, "Historical Health Fraud and Alternative Medicine Collection," American Medical Association Archives, Chicago.
11. Lillian. G. Genn, "Why Beauty Treatments May Cure America's Crime," *Detroit Free Press*, October 4, 1936.
12. Associated Press, "Miracle of Surgery Gives Ex-Convict New Start," *Marysville (OH) Journal Tribune*, March 28, 1932.
13. Associated Press, "Gangsters Go in for Face Lifting, Hardened Mugs May Emerge from Ether Resembling Great Screen Lovers," (Jackson, MI) *Clarion Ledger*, March 26, 1932.

14. Dorothy Killagen, "Operation on Face Changes Woman Slayer," *(Wilkes-Barre, PA) Evening News*, March 18, 1932.

15. Lillian G. Genn, "Why Beauty Treatments May Cure America's Crime," *Detroit Free Press*, October 4, 1936.

16. Maxwell Maltz, *New Faces, New Futures: Rebuilding Character with Plastic Surgery* (New York: R. R. Smith, 1936).

17. Associated Press, "N.Y. May Give New Faces to Its Criminals," *(Binghamton, NY) Press and Sun-Bulletin*, December 20, 1934.

18. John Howard Crum, *The Truth about Beauty: How to Acquire a Beautiful Face and Figure* (New York: Blue Ribbon Books, 1936).

19. John Kobler, "New Personalities Are for Sale through Latter-Day Surgery and Operations Can Be Performed in Public," *Pittsburgh (PA) Post-Gazette*, April 20, 1934.

20. William Weer, "Miss X Is Now Miss Y as Knife Fools the Eye," *Brooklyn (NY) Eagle*, March 18, 1932.

21. "Do You Like the Bizarre?" *Montgomery (AL) Advertiser*, March 22, 1932.

22. Lillian G. Genn, "Every Woman Has the Right to Beauty," *Public Ledger*, 1932.

23. Kobler, "New Personalities Are for Sale."

24. Crum, *The Truth about Beauty*.

25. Killagen, "Operation on Face Changes Woman Slayer"; Genn, "Every Woman Has the Right to Beauty"; "Retoucher," *New Yorker*, July 23, 1932.

26. John Howard Crum, *The Making of a Beautiful Face: Or, Face Lifting Unveiled* (New York: Walton, 1928).

27. Genn, "Every Woman Has the Right to Beauty."

28. John Howard Crum, *The Truth about Beauty: How to Acquire a Beautiful Face and Figure*, (New York: Blue Ribbon Books), 1936.

29. Associated Press, "Gangsters Go in for Face Lifting."

30. Kilgallen, "Operation on Face Changes Woman Slayer."

31. United Press, "Miracle of Surgery Gives Ex-Convict Fresh Start," *Marshall (TX) News Messenger*, March 25, 1932.

32. Kilgallen, "Operation on Face Changes Woman Slayer."

33. Thyra Samter Winslow, "Beauty for Sale," *New Republic*, November 25, 1931.

34. Kobler, "New Personalities Are for Sale."

35. "Do You Like the Bizarre?" *Montgomery (AL) Advertiser*, March 22, 1932.

36. "Do You Like the Bizarre?"; Weer, "Miss X Is Now Miss Y."

37. Dorothy Roe, "500 Women Watch as Surgeon Remodels Lips, Ears," *Tampa Bay Times*, March 23, 1933.

38. "1937 Beauty Type Defined as Exotic," *New York Times*, March 24, 1936.

39. "Six Faint Watching Operations on Noses," *New York Times*, March 11, 1937; Sam Brewer, "3 Nose Operations Conventions Stunt: Six Persons Faint," *Chicago Tribune*, March 11, 1937.

40. Richard L. Dolsky, "Cosmetic Surgery in the United States: Its Past and Present," *The American Journal of Cosmetic Surgery* 16, no. 2 (1999): 109.

41. "Dr. J. Howard Crum's Famous Donut Reducing Diet," Sally L. Steinberg Collection of Doughnut Ephemera, 1920s–1987, Archives Center, National Museum of American History; "That Dunking Diet," *Lebanon (PA) Daily News*, March 20, 1941.

42. "Dr. J. Howard Crum's Famous Donut Reducing Diet"; "That Dunking Diet"; Michael L. Lewin Papers, Center of History of Medicine, Harvard University, Boston, box 1, folder 1–3.

43. "Plastic Surgeon's Help Wanted at Oahu Prison," *Honolulu Advertiser*, April 2, 1961; Tomi Knaeffler, "Tattoo Removal Helps Inmate," *Honolulu Star-Bulletin*, March 30, 1963.

44. "Specialists Go 'Up' the River," *Medical World News*, September 15, 1961.

45. Personal communication, Barbara Lewin-Tankel, 2018–2021.

46. David Anderson and Robert Cromie, "New Faces, New Lives," *Des Moines (IA) Register*, May 22, 1949.

47. John F. Pick, "Plastic Surgery as a Complement to Correctional Therapy," *Proceedings of the 79th Annual Congress of Correction of the American Prison Association* (1949): 58.

48. United Press International, "Convicted Killer Gets New Face," *Indianapolis (IN) Star*, June 24, 1961.

49. Michael L. Lewin, "Autobiography, Including Photos and Tributes," Michael L. Lewin Papers, 1927–1994, National Archives of Plastic Surgery, PS 16, Countway Library of Medicine, Harvard, Boston, box 1, folder 1.

50. D. A. Ogden, "Use of Surgical Rehabilitation in Young Delinquents," *British Medical Journal*, February 14, 1959, 432.

51. D. A. Ogden, "A Borstal Typological Survey," *British Journal of Delinquency* 5, no. 2 (1954): 99–111, www.jstor.org/stable/23639847.

52. Dr. A. A. Bartholomew, "Correspondence," *British Medical Journal*, March 7, 1959, 650.

53. D. A. Ogden, "Correspondence," *The British Medical Journal*, April 4, 1959, 924.

54. Associated Press, "Should Men or Women Judge Beauty Contests?" *Hartford (CT) Courant*, August 30, 1959.

55. Michael L. Lewin, "Plastic Surgery in Rehabilitation of the Prison Inmate," *AORN Journal* 7, no. 4 (1968): 64–69, https://doi.org/10.1016/s0001-2092(08)70265-5.

56. Associated Press, "Erase Scars, Reduce Crime," *(Sioux Falls, SD) Argus-Leader*, November 5, 1963.

57. William Skirving, "Surgery Offers Convicts Hope: Life to Have New Face," *(Albany, NY) Knickerbocker News*, September 15, 1962.

## CHAPTER 5. THE RIKERS ISLAND EXPERIMENT, A.K.A. THE SURGICAL AND SOCIAL REHABILITATION OF ADULT OFFENDERS

1. "Surgeon at Prison Helps Remove Scars That Fosters Crime," *New York Times*, October 24, 1963.

2. Paul Allen, "Prisoner's Life Scarred by Crime and Confidence," *Raleigh (NC) Times*, June 14, 1963.

3. Personal communication, Douglas Lipton, 2018–2021.

4. Personal communication, Barbara-Lewin Tankel, 2019–2021.

5. Michael L. Lewin, *The Surgical and Social Rehabilitation of Adult Offenders* (Bronx, NY: Montefiore Hospital and Medical Center, 1968), preface.

6. Michael L. Lewin, Autobiography, including photos and tributes, Michael L. Lewin Papers, 1927–1994, National Archives of Plastic Surgery, PS 16, Countway Library of Medicine, Harvard, Boston, box 1, folder 1.

7. Personal communication, Douglas Lipton, 2019.

8. Dorie E. Apollonio and Stanton A. Glantz, "Minimum Ages of Legal Access for Tobacco in the United States from 1863 to 2015," *American Journal of Public Health* 106, no. 7 (2016): 1200–1207, https://doi.org/10.2105/ajph.2016.303172.

9. Jack Roth, "Death of a Junkie in Prison Stirs Plea for Treatment in Hospitals," *New York Times*, February 13, 1964.

10. "Swim from Rikers Island Fatal for Escaping Youth," *New York Times*, September 7, 1963.

11. Associated Press, "Diphtheria Case Reported at Women's Prison Here," *New York Times*, July 16, 1964.

12. Anna Kross, *Progress through Crisis* (New York: New York City Department of Correction, 1955–1963), 41.

13. Warren Hall, "Kim and the Crowded Cells," *Daily News*, January 5, 1964.

14. Noga Shalev, "From Public to Private Care: The Historical Trajectory of Medical Services in a New York City Jail," *American Journal of Public Health* 99, no. 6 (2009): 988–95, https://doi.org/10.2105/ajph.2007.123265.

15. James F. Howard, "Treatment Facilities Existing in U.S. Penal Institutions," *American Journal of Correction* 25, no. 2 (March–April 1963): 18.

16. Anna M. Kross Papers, The American Jewish Archives Radio, Box 21, Folder 1–6.5, http://collections.americanjewisharchives.org/ms/ms0176/ms0176.html.

17. Max Wylie, *400 Miles from Harlem: Courts, Crime, and Correction* (New York: Macmillan, 1972), 66.

18. Edward O'Neill, "City Hall," *Daily News*, August 7, 1955.

19. Elizabeth Carpenter, "Contrasting Careers of 2 Successful Women Show Cross Section of New York," *Abilene (TX) Reporter News*, October 1, 1954.

20. Virginia Irwin, "Annie: The Poor Man's Judge," *St. Louis Dispatch*, September 7, 1947.

21. Melissa Block, "Yes, Women Could Vote after the 19th Amendment—But Not All Women. Or Men," NPR, August 26, 2020.

22. G. Richard Bacon et al., *Struggle for Justice: A Report on Crime and Punishment in America*, (New York: Hill and Wang, 1971), 114.

23. Lawrence O'Kane, "Jail Doctors Ask Apology by Chief," *New York Times*, January 27, 1962.

24. United Press, "Warm Walls," *Orlando Sentinel*, December 13, 1963.

25. Phyllis Batelle, "Chic Dinner Table Regarde Strong Influence on Husband," *Fort Worth (TX) Star Telegram*, November 4, 1953.

26. American Correctional Association, *American Journal of Correction* 31 (November–December):1965.

27. Calvin C. Jillson, *Lone Star Tarnished: A Critical Look at Texas Politics and Public Policy* (London: Routledge, 2020).

28. Anonymous male, Letter, May 25, 1961, Mayor's Information Center, Mobile Unit, Police Dept. Departmental Correspondence, Robert F. Wagner Labor Archives, Tamiment Institute Library, New York University.

29. "1961 Events & Facts," accessed September 23, 2020, www.babyboomers .com/1961.

30. New York State Department of Labor, Division of Research and Statistics, "History of Unemployment Insurance Legislation in the United States and New York State, 1935–2007," Publication #RS16 (2/09), May 1978; Paul Healy, "Border Cops Riding Shotgun on Airlines," *Daily News*, August 11, 1961.

31. "The Hot 100 Chart 1962," *Billboard*, accessed September 23, 2020, www .billboard.com/charts/hot-100/1962-10-19.

32. Paul Vitello, "George Whitmore Jr., Who Falsely Confessed to 3 Murders in 1964, Dies at 68," *New York Times*, October 15, 2012.

33. Jacob Rader Marcus, *The American Jewish Woman, 1654–1980* (New York: Ktav Publishing House, 1981).

34. Virginia Irwin, "Annie, the Poor Man's Judge," *St. Louis Post-Dispatch*, September 7, 1947.

35. Vernon Fox, "Toward an Understanding of Criminal Behavior," *American Journal of Economics and Sociology* 21, no. 2 (April 1962): 145–58.

36. Elizabeth Chen, "Old Ferry Stations Seek Protected Status," *Mott Haven Herald*, January 21, 2012, www.motthavenherald.com/2012/01/21/old-ferry-stations-seek -protected-status/.

37. Tom McCarthy, "Labor Holiday Remembrance: 72 Killed While En Route to Rikers Island Penitentiary Construction Site in 1932," New York Correction History Society, accessed September 21, 2020, www.correctionhistory.org/html/chronicl/ rikersbell/1932-Rikers-Penitentiary-Laborers-Steamer-Disaster.html.

38. Daniel Glaser, *Preparing Convicts for Law-Abiding Lives: The Pioneering Penology of Richard A. McGee* (Albany: State University of New York Press, 1995); New York (State) Legislature, *Legislative Document*, vol. 22 (New York: J. B. Lyon, 1923); New York (State) Legislature, *Annual Report of the State Commission of Prisons*, vol. 29 (New York: State Commission of Prisons, 1923).

39. Tracy Evans, "Deconstructing Race: Eugenics in the United States," Lumen Learning (Cultural Anthropology, Santa Ana College), accessed September 24, 2020, https://courses.lumenlearning.com/culturalanthropology/chapter/eugenics-in -the-united-states/.

40. John Doyle, "Measuring 'Problems of Human Behavior': The Eugenic Origins of Yale's Institute of Psychology, 1921–1929," *MSSA Kaplan Prize for Yale History* 3 (2014), https://elischolar.library.yale.edu/mssa_yale_history/3; Claire Wang, "Stanford's History with Eugenics," *Stanford Daily*, December 8, 2016, www.stanforddaily .com/2016/12/07/stanfords-history-with-eugenics.

41. Paul A. Lombardo, "When Harvard Said No to Eugenics: The J. Ewing Mears Bequest, 1927," *Perspectives in Biology and Medicine* 57, no. 3 (2014): 374–92, https:// doi.org/10.1353/pbm.2014.0023.

42. "Harvard Refuses Eugenics Bequest," *Boston Globe*, May 9, 1927.

43. E. Kozeny, "Experimentelle Untersuchungen zur dusdruckskunde mittel photographisch-statistischer Methode" ("Experimental Investigation of Physiognomy Utilising a Photographic-Statistical Method"), *Archiv für die gesemate Psychologie* 114 (1962): 55–71.

44. Noga Shalev, "From Public to Private Care: The Historical Trajectory of Medical Services in a New York City Jail," *American Journal of Public Health* 99, no. 6 (2009): 988–95, https://doi.org/10.2105/ajph.2007.123265.

45. "Tree Moving Set on Rikers Island, 15,000 in Nursery to Be Replaced by Buildings," *New York Times*, September 17, 1964, www.nytimes.com/1964/09/17/archives/ treemoving-set-on-rikers-island-15000-in-nursery-to-be-replaced-by.html.

46. Tom McCarthy, "Overview of DOC," Correction History, accessed September 21, 2020, www.correctionhistory.org/html/chronicl/nycdoc/html/overview.html.

47. "Rikers Island Timeline: Jail's Origins and Controversies," *Daily News*, March 18, 2017, www.nydailynews.com/news/crime/rikers-island-timeline-jail-origins-contro versies-article-1.3001976.

48. Jarod Shanahan and Jack Norton, "A Jail to End All Jails," Urban Omnibus, February 2, 2018, https://urbanomnibus.net/2017/12/jail-end-jails/.

49. Richard M. Silberstein, Wallace Mandell, and John D Dalack, "Avoiding Institutionalization of Psychotic Children," *Archives of General Psychiatry* 19, no. 1 (January 1968): 17, https://doi.org/10.1001/archpsyc.1968.01740070019003.

50. Clyde E. Sullivan and Wallace Mandell, *Restoration of Youth through Training: A Final Report* (Staten Island, NY: Wakoff Research Center, 1967).

51. Personal communication, Wallace Mandell, 2019.

52. Signe Hald Andersen, Lars Højsgaard Andersen, and Peer Ebbesen Skov, "Effect of Marriage and Spousal Criminality on Recidivism," *Journal of Marriage and Family* 77, no. 2 (April 2015): 496–509, https://doi.org/10.1111/jomf.12176.

53. Claire W. Herbert, Jeffrey D. Morenoff, and David J. Harding, "Homelessness and Housing Insecurity among Former Prisoners," *RSF: The Russell Sage Foundation Journal of the Social Sciences* 1, no. 2 (2015): 44, https://doi.org/10.7758/ rsf.2015.1.2.04.

54. Don Whitehead, "Rebellion against Crime," *Orlando Sentinel*, February 10, 1957.

55. Alison Martin, "John Dillinger's Escape from a Crown Point Jail Cell Made Headlines 86 Years Ago This Week," *Chicago Sun-Times*, March 4, 2020.

56. "Dillinger's Plastic Surgery on Pulaski Rd. (or Crawford Ave.?)," Chicago Crime Scenes Project, accessed September 21, 2020, http://chicagocrimescenes.blogspot.com/2009/10/dillingers-plastic-surgery-on-pulaski.html.

57. "John Dillinger," History.com, November 9, 2009, www.history.com/topics/crime/john-dillinger.

58. Osgood Nichols, "Sleuths Track Their Man Even When Criminals Disguise by Face Lifting," *Washington Post Magazine*, September 16, 1934.

59. Marian Murray, "Improving on Acts of Gods," *American Mercury*, 1935.

60. Murray, "Improving on Acts of Gods"; Nichols, "Sleuths Track Their Man."

61. Jacques W. Maliniac, "Plastic Surgeon and Crime," *Journal of Criminal Law and Criminology* (winter): 1935.

62. United Press, "Surgery Has Become Fad for Criminals," *(North Tonawanda, NY) Evening News*, September 20, 1934.

63. "Plastic Surgery Used by Criminals," *Los Angeles Evening Post Record*, January 9, 1934.

64. "Facelifting for Criminals Now Fine Art," *(Wilmington, DE) News Journal*, July 27, 1934.

65. "Can't Conceal Identity from Uncle Sam," *Philadelphia Inquirer*, July 26, 1942.

66. "The Man Who Lived Twice, Plot Summary," IMDb, www.imdb.com/title/tt0027939/plotsummary?ref_=kw_pl.

67. "Gaol's Facial Cures," *Sydney (Australia) Morning Herald*, February 21, 1960.

68. Ralph Moncrieff, "Convicts Receive Plastic Surgery for Improvement Inside and Out," *The Santa Cruz (CA) Sentinel*, June 2, 1961.

69. "Is Ugliness the Root of Crime?" *Miami News*, September 16, 1962.

70. James Keller, "3 Minutes A Day: Doctor's Skill Deters Crime," *(Glen Falls, NY) Post-Star* July 9, 1964.

## CHAPTER 6. JAIL HOUSE PSYCH OUT

1. David Halberstam, "Prisoners to Get Plastic Surgery," *New York Times*, October 22, 1964.

2. Dr. Michael L. Lewin, "Of Children and Convicts," public affairs pamphlet distributed by Montefiore Medical Center, 1963.

3. "City Jail Population at Record; Mrs. Kross Repeats Warnings," *New York Times*, February 24, 1964.

4. "City Population at Record," February 24, 1964.

5. Anna Kross, *Progress through Crisis: 1954–1965* (New York: New York Department of Correction, 1965), 24.

6. *Rikers Review*, spring 1964.

7. Jeremiah Moss, "Klein's Fat Men's Shop," Jeremiah's Vanishing New York, June 21, 2010, http://vanishingnewyork.blogspot.com/2010/06/kleins-fat-mens-shop.html.

8. Photograph of American civilians standing at counter in store to buy horse meat. Official caption: "Rome, 7/21/45—Americans buy horse meat—Acme Photo through Rome OWI—Approved by appropriate military authority (List A but) 7166." Detroit, Michigan, July 21, 1945, www.ww2online.org/image/americans-buying-horse-meat-detroit-michigan-circa-1945.

9. Personal communication, Norman Cavior, 2018–2021. Questions about penis enlargement were the most common questions the plastic surgeons received.

10. Personal communication, Wallace Mandell, 2019.

11. "Mrs Kross Sure Her Job Is Safe," *New York Times*, June 20, 1956.

12. "Juror Criticizes Correction Head," *New York Times*, May 16, 1956.

13. "City Investigates Jail Money Loss," *New York Times*, September 6, 1962.

14. "Prison Cook Held in Narcotics Case; Accused of Smuggling to Rikers Island Inmates," *New York Times*, March 7, 1964, www.nytimes.com/1964/03/07/archives/prison-cook-held-in-narcotics-case-accused-of-smuggling-to-rikers.html.

15. Sumner Waddell, "Her Cross Is Heavy," *Rikers Review*, spring 1964.

16. "President Gives Jobs to Ten Women—Mrs. Kross Gets Award," *New York Times*, March 5, 1964.

17. Audio diary and annotated transcript, Lady Bird Johnson, March 4, 1964, Lady Bird Johnson's White House Diary.

18. Jack Roth, "Death of 'Junkie' in Prison Stirs Plea for Treatment in Hospitals," *New York Times*, February 13, 1964.

19. "Jail Guard Found Dead," *New York Times*, July 8, 1964.

20. New York State Appellate Division, *Records and Briefs*, vol. 99, www.google.com/books/edition/Records_Briefs_New_York_State_Appellate/QUXtKBvsqAcC?hl=en&gbpv=1&bsq=826; "Prison Reform," in *Nomination of Nelson A. Rockefeller of New York to Be Vice President of the United States: Hearings before the Committee on Rules and Administration, United States Senate, Ninety-Third Congress, Second Session* (Washington: U.S. Government Printing Office, 1974), 109–14.

21. Committee on Education and Labor, Special Subcommittee on Education, *Correctional Rehabilitation Study Act of 1965: Hearing, Eighty-Ninth Congress, First Session, April 7, 1965* (Washington, DC: U.S. Government Printing Office, 1965).

22. American Correctional Association, *A Manual of Correctional Standards Prepared by the Committee to Revise the 1946 Manual of Suggested Standards for a State Correctional System*, (New York: American Correctional Association, 1957), 234.

23. "Mrs. Kross Seeks Stay of July Retirement Date," *New York Times*, June 7, 1963.

24. "Model City Prison Given a Preview," *New York Times*, February 14, 1964.

25. Sydney Schaenberg, "Surgery to Remove Deformities Found to Reduce Repeaters amongst Ex-Convicts Here," *New York Times*, August 22, 1966.

26. Srinivas Konda, "U.S. Correctional Officers Killed or Injured on the Job," *Correct Today* 75, no. 5 (2013): 122–23.

27. Richard Kurtzberg, Norman Cavior, and Howard Safar, "Plastic Surgery and the Public Offender," *Rehabilitation Record* (March–April 1967).

28. National Council on Crime and Delinquency, *Current Projects in the Prevention, Control, and Treatment of Crime and Delinquency* (New York: National Research and Information Center on Crime and Delinquency, 1962), 326.

29. National Council on Crime and Delinquency, *Current Projects in the Prevention, Control, and Treatment of Crime and Delinquency*, 3–8.

30. National Council on Crime and Delinquency, *Current Projects in the Prevention, Control, and Treatment of Crime and Delinquency*, 3–8; Kross, *Progress through Crisis*.

31. Kross, *Progress through Crisis*; Anna M. Kross, The American Jewish Archives Records, American Jewish Archives, Cincinnati, Ohio.

32. Harry Schlegel, "All His Yak-Yak on Salary Cuts Was Just That, Lindsay Says," *Daily News*, April 11, 1966.

33. Peter T. White, "The World in New York City," *National Geographic* (1964): 50–106.

34. "Atlanta Metro Area Population 1950–2020," MacroTrends, accessed December 13, 2020, www.macrotrends.net/cities/22922/atlanta/population.

35. Associated Press, "Which Technology the 1964 World's Fair Got Right," *New York Post*, April 12, 2014.

36. "Beauty/Beast? Surgeons to Life Crooks Tattoos," *Sydney Morning Herald*, October 25, 1964.

37. Associated Press, "Surgeons to Remove Tattoos, Scars in Prisoner Rehabilitation Experiment," *(York, PA) Gazette and Daily*, October 14, 1964.

38. Sol Chaneles and Jerome Snyder, *Santa Makes a Change* (New York: Parents' Magazine Press, 1970).

39. Committee on Education and Labor, *A Prospectus of Working Women's Concerns, Hearings before the Subcommittee on Employment Opportunities of the Committee on Education and Labor, House of Representatives, One Hundredth Congress, First Session, Hearings Held in Washington, DC, July 21 and 22, 1987* (Washington, DC: U.S. Government Printing Office, 1987).

40. Plastic surgery, *Social Service Outlook*, New York State Department of Social Services, April 1967.

41. Anna Kross, Department of Health, Education and Welfare, 1964, American Jewish Archives, MS-176, box 14, folder 8.

42. Clyde E. Sullivan, *MDTA Experimental and Demonstration Findings: Job Development and Placement of the Ex-offender* (Washington, DC: United States Department of Labor, 1968), 49.

## CHAPTER 7. BEAUTY BEHIND BARS

1. Mary C. Bounds, "Texas Penitentiary Lets Inmates Put on a New Face before Leaving," *Dallas Morning News*, March 10, 1965.

2. Joseph Hixson, "Surgeon's Scalpels Fight Crime," *Democrat and Rochester (NY) Chronicle*, January 16, 1965.

3. "Dock Jobs Sold for $1,000 Each. Kickbacks to Loan Sharks," *New York Daily News*, January 2, 1965.

4. Joseph R. Hixson, "Surgery Tested on Twisted Lives," *Philadelphia Inquirer*, January 14, 1965.

5. Hixson, "Surgeon's Scalpels Fight Crime."

6. Corrections Letters and Complaints, Robert F. Wagner Archives, New York, 1965.

7. Judson Hand, "Face Charges in Jail Suicide," *Daily News*, December 24, 1969.

8. Sidney Fileds, "Is Jail the Answer?" *Daily News*, September 9, 1966.

9. Sylvia Kronstadt, "The Absolute Rulers of Society's Garbage Can," December 1975, http://kronstantinople.blogspot.com/2012/02/absolute-rulers-of-societys-garbage-can.html.

10. Lyndon B. Johnson, "Special Message to the Congress on Law Enforcement and the Administration of Justice," American Presidency Project, March 8, 1965, www.presidency.ucsb.edu/node/242223.

11. Lyndon B. Johnson, "Special Message to the Congress: Toward Full Educational Opportunity," American Presidency Project, January 12, 1965, www.presidency.ucsb.edu/documents/special-message-the-congress-toward-full-educational-opportunity.

12. Johnson, "Special Message to the Congress on Law Enforcement and the Administration of Justice."

13. Anna M. Kross, The American Jewish Archives, MS-176, box 35, folder 12.

14. Patrick A. Langan, *Race of Prisoners Admitted to State and Federal Institutions, 1926-86* (Washington, DC: U.S. Department of Justice, Office of Justice Programs, Bureau of Justice Statistics, 1991).

15. Elizabeth Hinton, *From the War on Poverty to the War on Crime: The Making of Mass Incarceration in America* (Cambridge, MA: Harvard University Press, 2016).

16. In many instances, the New York Department of Correction and the New York Police Department used "Puerto Rican" as a catchall descriptor for people of Hispanic origin.

17. *The Surgical and Social Rehabilitation of Adult Offenders* (Bronx, NY: Montefiore Hospital and Medical Center, 1968), appendix 1.

18. Richard Kurtzberg, Norman Cavior, and Howard Safar, "Plastic Surgery and the Public Offender," *Rehabilitation Record* (March–April 1967).

19. *The Surgical and Social Rehabilitation of Adult Offenders* (Bronx, NY: Montefiore Hospital and Medical Center, 1968). His behavior was also cited in interdepartmental correctional memos.

20. Steven V. Roberts, "Crime Rate of Women up Sharply over Men's," *New York Times*, June 13, 1971.

21. Douglas Sefton, "Host of Problems to Ring Him in New Year's Day," *Daily News*, November 15, 1965.

22. Meda Chesney-Lind and Lisa Pasko, *Girls, Women, and Crime: Selected Readings* (Los Angeles: Sage, 2013), 187.

23. Paul Harvey, Part 6 of 9, FBI Records: The Vault, https://vault.fbi.gov/paul -harvey/Paul%20Harvey%20Part%2006%20of%2009%20/view.

24. Kathrin Perutz, *Beyond the Looking Glass: America's Beauty Culture* (New York: William Morrow, 1970).

25. Perutz, *Beyond the Looking Glass*; Anna Kross, *Progress through Crisis* (New York: New York City Department of Correction, 1955–1963), 16.

26. LaMar Taylor Empey, *Alternatives to Incarceration* (Washington, DC: U.S. Department of Health, Education, and Welfare, 1967), 17–18.

27. Women's News Service, *Calgary Herald*, April 13, 1964.

28. "Women Gets Wish, State Prison Term," *New York Times*, December 17, 1963.

29. Gertrude Samuels, "Rescue for the Wayward Girls," *New York Times Magazine*, July 23, 1961.

30. Sara Harris, *Cast the First Stone* (New York: McGraw-Hill, 1957).

31. Perutz, *Beyond the Looking Glass*.

32. Perutz, *Beyond the Looking Glass*; Harris, *Cast the First Stone*.

33. Dick Nolan, "Face of a Crook," *San Francisco Examiner*, May 2, 1965.

34. Hans Abeles, 1966 Medical Division Reports, American Jewish Archives.

35. "Japanese Women Gain Beauty by Losing Face," *Des Moines (IA) Tribune*, March 12, 1964.

36. Robbie Mantooth, "People Take Beauty Dreams to Plastic Surgeons," *Daily Oklahoman*, September 6, 1964.

37. Beverly Mindrum, "Fountain of Youth Still Untapped," *Minneapolis (MN) Star*, May 21, 1964.

38. Alexander Edmonds, "The Poor Have the Right to Be Beautiful: Cosmetic Surgery in Neoliberal Brazil," *Journal of the Royal Anthropological Institute* 13, no. 2 (2007): 363–81.

39. Perutz, *Beyond the Looking Glass*.

40. Joseph P. Lyford, *The Airtight Cage: A Study of New York's West Side* (New York: Harper & Row, 1966).

41. Lyford, *The Airtight Cage*; Perutz, *Beyond the Looking Glass*, 137.

42. Ann Clausmeyer, "Elimination of Fear Is Boast of Warden," *(Hackensack, NJ) Record*, October 1, 1965.

43. Ann Clausmeyer, "Mothers and Children behind Bars," *(New York) Press and Sun Bulletin*, October 4, 1965.

44. N. Marion, *Federal Government and Criminal Justice* (n.p.: Springer, 2011).

45. James McWilliams, "Restoring Prisoners' Access to Education Reduces Re- cidivism," *Pacific Standard*, April 16, 2019, https://psmag.com/education/restoring -prisoners-access-to-education-reduces-recidivism.

46. Elizabeth Kai Hinton, "From Social Welfare to Social Control: Federal War in American Cities, 1968–1988" (PhD diss., Columbia University, 2013).

47. United States Congress, *Hearings Cong. 89 sess. 1, Labor & Public Welfare, vol. 2, 1965.* (Washington, DC: U.S. Government Printing Office, 1965).

48. United States Congress & Senate, *Hearings Cong. 89 sess. 1, Education & Labor, v. 5, 1965.* (Washington, DC: U.S. Government Printing Office, 1965).

49. Adam Bernstein, "Florida Democrat Sam Gibbons, 92, Helped Push War on Poverty Legislation through Congress," *Washington Post*, Oct. 10, 2012.

## CHAPTER 8. THE MANY FACES OF PRISON PLASTIC

1. Associated Press, "Elimination of Scars Aids Criminal Reform," *Boston Globe*, August 22, 1966.

2. *The Scar Beneath*, directed by James Lieberman (1964; Atlanta: Communicable Disease Center, U.S. Public Health Service), courtesy National Archives and Records Administration.

3. *The Scar Beneath.*

4. Melvin S. Heller, "The Private Reflections of a Prison Psychiatrist," *The Prison Journal* 54, no. 2 (1974): 15–33.

5. "Statewide Listings for Thursday," *Tampa Bay Times*, February 19, 1967.

6. Newswire, "Danville B&PW Unit Tours Penitentiary," *(Sunbury, PA) Daily Item*, April 28, 1966. Reviews can be found in California Nurses Association, *CNA Bulletin* 62 (1966); *The American Journal of Correction*, 26–30 (1964); and elsewhere.

7. Anna M. Kross Papers. Series F. Folder 26–29, American Jewish Archives, Cincinnati, Ohio.

8. Sydney Schaenberg, "Surgery to Remove Deformities Found to Reduce Repeaters amongst Ex-Convicts Here," *New York Times*, August 22, 1966.

9. "Rehabilitated Inmates Lose Their Tattoos," *Detroit Free Press*, October 29, 1964.

10. Norman Cavior, personal communication, 2018–2020.

11. Press release, "Remarks by Mrs. Lyndon B. Johnson, 12th Annual Meeting of Keep America Beautiful, Inc., New York, New York, 10/7/1965," "Mrs. Johnson—Speeches," Reference File, LBJ Presidential Library, accessed October 10, 2020, www .discoverlbj.org/item/ref-ctjspeeches-19651007-1200.

12. Melitta Schmideberg, address to Third World Congress of Psychiatry, Montreal, June 1961.

13. The New York Herald Tribune wire, "The Rot in New York," *Montgomery (AL) Advertiser*, March 15, 1965.

14. Anna Kross, *Progress through Crisis* (New York: New York City Department of Correction, 1955–1963), 51; Anna M. Kross Papers. Series D. Folder 11, American Jewish Archives, Cincinnati, Ohio.

15. "290,000 Sought to Help Addicts," *New York Times*, May 8, 1964.

16. Walter Cronkite, *The Addicted*, Columbia Broadcasting System, aired January 1, 1958, https://licensing.screenocean.com/record/217435.

17. United States Bureau of Prisons, United States Probation System, United States Administrative Office of the United States Courts, *Federal Probation. v. 27, 1963* (Washington, DC: Administrative Office of the United States Courts, 2005).

18. Associated Press, "Whip Juvenile Delinquents," *Petaluma (CA) Argus-Courier*, February 14, 1964.

19. Dr. Joyce Brothers, "Plastic Surgery Has Many Facets," *(Baltimore) Evening Sun*, August 8, 1967.

20. Brennan Williams, "Jennifer Jackson, First Black Playmate, on Life after Baring It All and 'The Playboy Club,'" *The Huffington Post*, November 25, 2011. Letters from "Reader's Letters," *Playboy*, June 1965.

21. Matt Schudel, "Hugh Hefner, Visionary Editor Who Founded Playboy Magazine, Dies at 91," *Washington Post*, September 27, 2017.

22. Thomas O. Echewa, "A Reply to an American Negro," *Negro Digest*, September 1965.

23. Edward Lewison, "An Experiment in Facial Reconstructive Surgery in a Prison Population," *Canadian Medical Association Journal* 92 (1965): 251–54.

24. International News Service, "Prison Inmate Promised Face," *Arizona Republic*, June 9, 1949.

25. *Corrections: Hearings, Ninety-second Congress, First Session* (Washington, DC: U.S. Government Printing Office, 1972), 251.

26. Jay Jenkins, "Prisoners Get a Lift by Surgery," *Charlotte (NC) Observer*, July 6, 1966.

27. United Press International, "Juvenile Escapees Being Sought," *Bucyrus (OH) Telegraph-Forum*, December 28, 1964.

28. Associated Press, "Priest's Auto Stolen by Pair of Juveniles," *Washington (OH) Record-Herald*, December 28, 1964.

29. United Press International, "Youth Sentenced to Life, for Rape, Murder, of a Nurse," *Sandusky (OH) Register*, February 22, 1966.

30. Associated Press, "Boy Faces Adult's Charges," *Newark (OH) Advocate*, May 26, 1965.

31. Associated Press, "Youth, 16, Quizzed in Second Killing," *Cincinnati Enquirer*, May 1, 1965.

32. Associated Press, "Judge Continues Hearing in Nurse's Death," *(East Liverpool, OH) Evening Review*, May 1, 1965.

33. Associated Press, "Youth Indicted in Murder of Nurse," *Salem (OH) News*, June 10, 1965.

34. United Press International, "Plastic Surgery Failed Its Task, Youth Convicted," *Lancaster (OH) Eagle Gazette*, February 22, 1966.

35. Newswire, "Man with a Big Nose Was Spurned," *Daily Mail*, June 13, 1964.

36. "Donald Smelley on FBI's Ten Most Wanted List," *Carlsbad (NM) Current-Argus*, July 3, 1966.

37. Arthur Mann, "New York Helps Offenders . . . Place Now, Talk Later," *Employment Service Review* 2 (1965).

38. Woody Klein, *Lindsay's Promise: The Dream That Failed; a Personal Account* (New York: Macmillan, 1970).

39. Peter Osnos, "New York Mayor John Lindsay. Remember Him?" *The Atlantic*, January 30, 2019, www.theatlantic.com/entertainment/archive/2010/05/new-york-mayor-john-lindsay-remember-him/57215/.

40. *Fun City Revisited: The Lindsay Years*, PBS documentary, https://vimeo.com/53560997.

41. Harry Schlegel, "All His Yik Yak on Salary Cuts Was Just That," *Daily News*, April 11, 1966.

42. Associated Press, "Goes More in Sorrow Than Anger—McGrath," *Boston Globe*, February 25, 1965.

43. United Press International, "Convicts Nabbed in Tunnel Escape Try," *Bennington (VT) Banner*, May 5, 1964.

44. Edward O'Neil, "19 City Aides Will Get 38G in Raises," *Daily News*, September 15, 1966.

45. "10 City Biggies Face a Stop on Paychecks," *Daily News*, June 11, 1966.

46. Wallace Mandell, Michael Lewin, Richard Kurtzberg, Marvin Shuster, and Howard Safar, "S.S.R. Follow-up Interview, appendix 3," in *Surgical and Social Rehabilitation of Adult Offenders* (New York: Staten Island Mental Health Society, 1967).

47. Personal Communication, Carole Ferguson, 2019.

48. Marvin Shuster and Michael Lewin, "Needle Tracks in Narcotic Addicts," *New York State Journal of Medicine* (1968): 34.

49. Michael L. Lewin Archives, PS16, box 1, folders 30–36; Shuster and Lewin, "Needle Tracks in Narcotic Addicts."

50. Personal communication, Douglas Lipton, 2018–2021.

51. Application for Continuation Research or Demonstration Grant, U.S. Department of Health, Education, and Welfare, Washington, DC, July 1, 1966.

52. *Supplemental Appropriations for 1966: Hearings, Eighty-ninth Congress, First Session, United States. Congress. Senate. Committee on Appropriations* (Washington, DC: Government Printing Office, 1965).

53. *Welfare in Review* 8–9 (1971): 2.

54. Thomas E. Backer, *Drug Abuse Technology Transfer* (Washington, DC: Department of Health and Human Services, Public Health Service, Alcohol, Drug Abuse, and Mental Health Administration, 1991).

55. Annual Report of the Surgeon General, U.S. Public Health Service, 1966.

## CHAPTER 9. CHANGING PLACES AND FACES

1. New York Times News Service, "Beautified Ex-Convicts Repeat Less," *New York Times*, August 22, 1966.

2. Christine Doyle, "Does the Face Make the Criminal?" *Observer Sun*, June 18, 1967.

3. Richard Kurtzberg, Norman Cavior, and Howard Safar, "Plastic Surgery and the Public Offender," *Rehabilitation Record* (March–April 1967).

4. "Sociologist's Topic Is Problem Youth," *(Hackensack, NJ) Record*, April 27, 1965.

5. "Talk Scheduled by Drug Expert," *(Hackensack, NJ) Record*, April 15, 1965.

6. "Police Board's Value Debated," *(Hackensack, NJ) Record*, November 17, 1966; "Narcotics Panel Speakers Named," *(Hackensack, NJ) Record*, January 16, 1967.

7. Personal communication, Douglas Lipton, 2018–2021.

8. Joseph F. Spillane, *Coxsackie: The Life and Death of Prison Reform* (Baltimore: Johns Hopkins University Press, 2014).

9. Sydney Schanberg, "Scar Removal Found to Reduce Repeaters among Ex-Convicts; Surgery to Remove Deformities Found to Reduce Repeaters among Ex-Convicts Here," *New York Times*, August 22, 1966.

10. Schanberg, "Scar Removal Found to Reduce Repeaters."

11. John D. Harris, "The Junkie Priest," *Pageant Magazine* 20, no. 1 (1965): 167.

12. Personal communication, Douglas Lipton. 2018–2021.

13. Kenneth R. Donecker, "Result of Coddling," *Fort-Worth Star Telegram*, December 14, 1966.

14. "Coddling the Criminal," *(Syracuse, NY) Post-Standard*, May 6, 1965.

15. Joseph Zullo, "New York City Crime Rises 6.5 Pct. In '66," *Chicago Tribune*, February 21, 1967.

16. Judith Axler, "U.S. Crime Rises 5%, Too Easy Guns, Says FBI," *Daily News*, March 8, 1966.

17. Mae C. Quinn, "Revisiting Anna Moscowitz's Kross's Critique of New York City Women's Court: The Continued Problem of Solving the 'Problem' of Prostitution with Specialized Criminal Courts," *Fordham Law Journal* 33, no. 2 (2006) for vagrancy, and "Mayor, Rocky, Sign Pact for Addict Cure," *Daily News*, May 5, 1967, for compulsory rehabilitation.

18. Personal communication, Norman Cavior, 2018–2021.

19. Anna M. Kross papers, American Jewish Archives, Cincinnati, Ohio.

20. Abbey Lincoln, "Who Will Revere the Black Woman?" *Negro Digest*, September 1966, 16–19. The full quote in its entirety: "A good job has been done on the black people in this country, as far as convincing them of their inferiority is concerned. The general white community has told us in a million different ways and in no uncertain terms that 'God' and 'nature' made a mistake when it came to the fashioning of us and ours. The whole society, having been thoroughly convinced of the stained, threaten-

ing, and evil nature of anything unfortunate enough to be, or referred to as black, as an intended matter of courtesy refers to those of African extraction as 'colored' or 'Negro.'"

21. Rick Rojas and Khorri Atkinson, "Five Days of Unrest That Shaped and Haunted, Newark," *New York Times*, July 11, 2017.

22. D. Apfelberg, F. Masters, and D. Robinson, "Pathophysiology and Treatment of Lightning Injuries," *Journal of Trauma—Injury, Infection and Critical Care* 14, no. 6 (1974): 453–60.

23. F. Masters, J. W. Alexander, and J. A. Moncrief, "In Vitro Determination of Tetanus Immunity," *Plastic and Reconstructive Surgery* 40, no. 2 (1967):199.

24. Frank W. Masters, "Cosmetic Surgery. Correcting Emotional, Rather Than Functional, Defects," *Journal of the Kansas Medical Society* 67, no. 3 (1966): 128–33.

25. Frank Masters and D. C. Greaves, "The Quasimodo Complex," *British Journal of Plastic Surgery* (1967).

26. *Abstracts on Criminology and Penology* 8 (1968): 151.

27. *The New Scientist* 34, nos. 539–51 (1967): 632.

28. Dr. E. Anthony, "Cheek by Jowl," *Justice of the Peace and Local Government Review* 132 (1968).

29. Christine Doyle, "Does the Face Make the Criminal?" *(London) Observer*, June 18, 1967.

30. Wallace Mandell, "Plastic Surgery Program for Rehabilitation of Offenders," (report presented at Research in Correctional Rehabilitation seminar, Washington, DC, July 6–7, 1967).

31. Personal communication, Wallace Mandell, 2019.

32. William Wirtz, *Manpower Development and Training in Correctional Programs, MDTA Experimental and Demonstration Findings No. 3* (Washington, DC: U.S. Department of Labor, 1968).

33. W. Mandell, "Making Correction a Community Agency," *Crime & Delinquency* 17, no. 3 (1971): 281–88, DOI: 10.1177/001112877101700305.

34. Hearings Cong. 90 Sess. 1 Appropriations v. 7 (Washington, DC: Government Printing Office, 1967), 629–31.

35. Hearings Cong. 90 Sess. 1 Appropriations v. 7, 629–31; Michael L. Lewin, *The Surgical and Social Rehabilitation of Adult Offenders* (Bronx, NY: Montefiore Hospital and Medical Center, 1968), preface and chapters 1–2.

36. Lewin, *Surgical and Social Rehabilitation*, preface and chapters 1–2.

37. Hearings Cong. 90 Sess. 1 Appropriations v. 7, 629–31. Lewin, *Surgical and Social Rehabilitation*, chapter 2. Wirtz, *Manpower Development and Training in Correctional Programs*.

38. Hearings Cong. 90 Sess. 1 Appropriations v. 7, 629–31. Lewin, *Surgical and Social Rehabilitation*, chapter 2. Wirtz, *Manpower Development and Training in Correctional Programs*.

39. Lewin, *Surgical and Social Rehabilitation*, chapter 2.

40. U.S. Bureau of Prisons, "Guidelines for Plastic Surgery Program in Corrections," pamphlet, 1968.

41. Tom Tiede, "Surgeons Change Crime's Face," *Herald Journal*, April 28, 1969.

42. Michael L. Lewin, "Plastic Surgery in Rehabilitation of the Prison Inmate," *Aorn Journal* (1968).

## CHAPTER 10. TEENAGE DIRTBAGS OR PROM QUEENS IN THE MAKING?

1. "World Bids Adieu to a Violent Year; City Gets Snowfall," *New York Times*, January 1, 1968.

2. Associated Press, "State Convicts Receiving Plastic Surgery New Look," *(Grand Junction, CO) Daily Sentinel*, April 24, 1968.

3. Pat Leisner, "Her Facelift: Medicaid Surgery Transforms Mrs. Douglas into Cachita," *(Yonkers, NY) Herald Statesman*, January 22, 1968.

4. "Doctors Ask Study," *(Syracuse, NY) Post Standard*, May 24, 1966.

5. Editorial comment, *Herald Statesman*, May 16, 1967.

6. W. D. Maxwell, "Correcting a Billion Dollar Boner," *Chicago Tribune*, July 31, 1967.

7. Mary K. Somers, "Physical Appearance and Personality" (Sweet Briar College, 1975).

8. Bruce Biossat and John Troan, *What You've Got Coming from Medicare and Social Security* (New York: Pocket Books, 1968), 33.

9. Bruce Biossat, "Doctor Bill Rules Change Makes Payment Easier," *Asbury Park (NJ) Press*, January 14, 1968.

10. Biossat, "Doctor Bill Rules Change."

11. Personal communication, Leo Munick, 2020.

12. Acme Streaming, "The Beatles Are a Threat to Our Children, Especially Girls. A Warning from Cincinnati," August 1964, YouTube, www.youtube.com/watch?v=R0nY33UgHmo.

13. Wendy Beckman, "Supreme Court Justice Sharon Kennedy Serves the Community by Changing One Mind at a Time," *Counselor* (2013).

14. John W. Saffell, "Plastic Surgery, Is It One of the Answers in Rehabilitation?" *Motive* 15, no. 2 (May–June 1969).

15. Leo Munick, "Adolescents and Plastic Surgery, Some Case Reports," *Ohio Medical Journal* (1980).

16. Bill Bozeman, "Plastic Surgery Solving Juvenile's Problems," *Cincinnati Enquirer*, August 26, 1968.

17. Associated Press, "Cosmetic Surgery for Children Sees Upswing," *Austin (TX) American*, August 29, 1968.

18. Ruth Winter, "Plastic Surgery Aids Ego," *(Louisville, KY) Courier-Journal*, October 17, 1965.

19. Norman J. Knorr, J. E. Hoopes, and Milton Edgerton, "Psychiatric Approach to Adolescent Disturbance in Self Image," *Plastic and Reconstructive Surgery* 41, no. 3 (1968): 258–43.

20. Julie Bryne, "Philanthropist Slotkin Offers New Noses, Faces, and Ears," *Los Angeles Times*, July 4, 1972.

21. "Local Jaycettes Plan Christmas Ornament Sale," *Lead (SD) Daily Call*, October 18, 1979.

22. "October Claimed Cosmetic Surgery Month," *Rapid City (SD) Journal*, October 6, 1974.

23. "Boy Declare Nat'l Cos Surgery Week," *(Mitchell, SD) Daily Republic*, October 14, 1967.

24. Associated Press, "Cosmetic Surgery for Children Sees Upswing," *Austin (TX) American*, August 29, 1968.

25. Ronald Yogman, "Experts Say Crime Can Be Skin Deep," *Evening Independent*, October 7, 1966.

26. "Start Program to Help Cons upon Release," *Daily News*, May 4, 1967.

27. Gertrude Samuels, "Help Wanted: The Hard-Core Unemployed," *New York Times Magazine*, January 28, 1968.

28. "Island of the Damned," *New York Times*, April 26, 1970.

29. Gertrude Samuels, "Youths Who Don't Make Headlines," *New York Times Magazine*, June 23, 1957.

30. William J. Waters, "Burglars Crude and Professional," *Ithaca (NY) Journal*, July 13, 1968.

31. Robert E. Dallos, "The Burglar Protection Racket Business Is a Big Business Now," *Ithaca (NY) Journal*, December 24, 1968.

32. Associated Press, "List Area Men Killed in Viet," *Daily News*, February 7, 1968.

33. State Commission of Correction, *Annual Report of the New York State Commission of Correction* (Albany, NY: Albany State Commission of Correction, 1968), 26–44.

34. "Now Sold for Looks, the Foot Sufferers Status Symbol," *Austin (TX) American*, December 8, 1968.

35. "Adult School Plans Series," *(Bridgewater, NJ) Courier-News*, September 11, 1968.

36. "Looking Around," *(Shepherd, TX) San Jacinto News-Times*, October 24, 1968.

37. "Island of the Damned," *New York Times*, April 26, 1970.

38. Janos Marton, "Today in NYC History: The Great Garbage Strike of 1968," Untapped New York, March 9, 2020, https://untappedcities.com/2015/02/11/today-in-nyc-history-the-great-garbage-strike-of-1968/.

39. "Recalling the City's Garbage Strike of 1968," Bowery Boogie, January 21, 2013, www.boweryboogie.com/2013/01/recalling-the-citys-garbage-strike-of-1968-video/.

40. Joseph D'Adamo, "Voice of the People," *Daily News*, March 30, 1968.

41. "Murder in Central Park," *Daily News*, July 7, 1968.

42. Daniel O'Grady, "Takes Plea in Fire That Hurt 19," *Daily News*, March 15, 1968.

43. Paul N. Marker, "Should It Be Told Like It Is in Juvenile Cases?" *(Elmira, NY) Star-Gazette*, November 28, 1968.

44. Michael K. Corey, "A Problem for Society," *Miami News*, December 5, 1968.

45. *Juvenile Delinquency Prevention Act of 1967: Hearings before the General Subcommittee on Education of the Committee on Education and Labor House of Representatives*, Ninetieth Congress (1967): 433.

46. United Press International, "Junior Delinquents," *(Provo, UT) Daily Herald*, June 22, 1966.

47. Juvenile Delinquency Prevention and Control Act of 1968, Public Law 90-445 (1968), 462, www.govinfo.gov/content/pkg/STATUTE-82/pdf/STATUTE-82 -Pg462.pdf.

48. United State Congress, Proposed Juvenile Delinquency Prevention and Control Act, *Journal of the Senate of the United States of America* (1967).

49. President Lyndon Johnson, "Remarks in Morgantown at a Dinner Honoring Representative Harley O. Staggers of West Virginia," October 26, 1968.

50. United Press International, "Hoover Said to Miss Point on Criminal Rehabilitation," *(Binghamton, NY) Press and Sun Bulletin*, May 21, 1967.

51. "Jersey City Gets a 'Moms Squad' for Delinquents," *New York Times*, March 28, 1969.

52. Eleanor T. Glueck, "A More Discriminative Instrument for the Identification of Potential Delinquents at School Entrance," *Journal of Criminal Law, Criminology, and Police Science* 57, no. 1 (1966): 27–30, www.jstor.org/stable/1140950?seq=1.

53. Bob Teague, "A Black Man Says, Charlie Doesn't Even Know His Daily Racism Is a Sick Joke," *New York Times*, September 15, 1968.

54. Robin Morgan, "I Was There: The 1968 Miss America Pageant Protest," History.com, October 19, 2018; Susan Faludi, "A Note on the New York Radical Feminists," *The New Yorker*, April 15, 2013; New York Radical Feminists Records, 1969–2011, Archives and Manuscript Collection, Duke University.

55. Eleanor Fischer, "First Protests at Miss America Pageant," WNYC, September 8, 1968, www.wnyc.org/story/first-protest-miss-america-pageant-1968/.

56. Judy Klemesrud, "There's Now Miss Black America," *New York Times*, September 9, 1968.

57. Molly Vorwerk, "Groundbreaking 1968 Pageant Proved Black Is Beautiful," *USA Today*, February 15, 2018.

58. Fischer, "First Protests at the Miss America Pageant."

59. Associated Press, "Crime Soars 16% in a Year," *Daily News*, March 15, 1968.

60. *The Public Looks at Crime and Correction* (Washington, DC: The Joint Commission on Correctional Manpower and Training, 1968).

61. Walter Rugaber, "2 Negro Children Held as Delinquents," *New York Times*, December 12, 1968.

62. "U.S. Says Alabama Beats Delinquents, *New York Times*, November 9, 1969.

63. Harvey Swados, "The City's Island of the Damned," *New York Times*, February 21, 1970.

64. United Press International, "Rikers Probe Seek Causes after 12 Are Injured in a Riot," *(Hackensack, NJ) Record*, July 11, 1968.

65. Associated Press, "White Prisoners Indicted for Attack on Black Inmates," *(Greenwood, SC) Index Journal*, August 13, 1968.

66. Norman Cavior, "The Relationship of Physical Attractiveness to Physical Attractiveness Self Concept and Popularity" (unpublished manuscript, University of Houston, 1968).

67. Norman Cavior and Paul Dokecki, "Physical Attractiveness and Popularity among Fifth Grade Boys" (paper presented at the meeting of the Southwestern Psychological Association, Austin, Texas, April 18, 1969); personal communication, Norman Cavior, 2018–2021.

68. Pamela A. Roby, "Politics and Prostitution—A Case Study of the Revision, Enforcement, and Administration of the New York State Penal Laws on Prostitution," *Criminology* 9, 425 (1971–1972); Herman Schwartz, Richard Denzer, and Jerome Skolnick, "Drafting a New Penal Law for New York," *Buffalo Law Review* 18, no. 2 (1969).

69. Robert Martinson, "Prison Notes of a Freedom Rider," *The Nation*, 1962, 4–6.

70. Members of the Governor's Special Committee on Criminal Offenders, *Preliminary Report of the Governor's Special Committee on Criminal Offenders* (New York: State of New York, 1968).

71. Research Utilizations Branch, *Plastic Surgery for Public Offenders, One of the Many Special Programs in Corrections* (Washington, DC: Division of Research and Demonstrations, 1969).

72. Martha Lentz Walker, *Beyond Bureaucracy: Mary Elizabeth Switzer and Rehabilitation,* (Lanham, MD: University Press of America, 1985).

73. Walker, *Beyond Bureaucracy.*

74. Walker, *Beyond Bureaucracy.*

75. Douglas Lipton, Robert Martinson, and Judith Wilks, *The Effectiveness of Correctional Treatment: A Survey of Treatment Evaluation Studies* (New York: Praeger, 1975), 282–95.

76. Lipton, Martinson, and Wilks, *The Effectiveness of Correctional Treatment.*

77. National Institute of Law Enforcement and Criminal Justice, *New Approaches to Diversion and Treatment of Juvenile Offenders* (Washington, DC: U.S. Government Printing Office, 1972), 13.

78. Committee on Labor and Public Welfare, Subcommittee on Employment, Manpower, and Poverty, *Emergency Employment Act, Background* (Washington, DC: U.S. Government Printing Office, 1967), 17.

79. David Hoffman, "1968—Street People in New York City," YouTube, April 3, 2013. www.youtube.com/watch?v=_d4P8xdrmvQ.

80. Elizabeth Kai Hinton, "From Social Welfare to Social Control, Federal Warfare in American Cities, 1968-1988" (PhD diss., Columbia University, 2013).

81. Personal communication, Norman Cavior, 2018-2021; personal communication, Steven C. Hayes, 2020.

82. Norman Cavior and Ramona L. Howard, "Facial Attractiveness and Juvenile Delinquency among Black and White Offenders," *Journal of Abnormal Psychology* 1 (1973): 202-13.

83. Cavior and Howard, "Facial Attractiveness and Juvenile Delinquency."

84. National Criminal Justice Information and Statistics Service, *Census of Prisoners in State Correctional Facilities, 1973* (Washington, DC: U.S. Department of Justice, Law Enforcement Assistance Administration, 1977), 207.

85. "Proposes Plastic Surgery Choice for Blacks," *Jet*, April 8, 1971, 22.

86. National Institute of Law Enforcement and Criminal Justice, *New Approaches to Diversion and Treatment of Juvenile Offenders.*

87. U.S. Social and Rehabilitation Service, Division of Research and Demonstration, *An Annotated List of SRS Research and Demonstration Grants* (Washington, DC: National Technical Information Service, 1971), 139.

88. National Institute of Law Enforcement and Criminal Justice, *New Approaches to Diversion and Treatment of Juvenile Offenders.*

89. Jon K. Meyer, John E. Hoopes, Michael E. Jabaley, and Richard Allen, "Is Plastic Surgery Effective in the Rehabilitation of Deformed Delinquent Adolescents?" *Plastic and Reconstructive Surgery* 51 (1973): 53-85.

90. Sally Thran, "Doctors' Study Link between Appearance and Behavior," *St. Louis Post-Dispatch*, October 10, 1969.

## CHAPTER 11. HARD PASS: THE "NOTHING WORKS" PROBLEM

1. "Plastic Surgery Made Us Better Teachers," *Instructor*, December 1969.

2. Lester L. Coleman, "Plastic Surgery Now as Acceptable as Wigs," *(Santa Rosa, CA) Press Democrat*, November 15, 1970.

3. Kevin Baker, "Welcome to Fear City—The Inside Story of New York's Civil War, 40 Years On," *Guardian*, May 18, 2015.

4. "Women in Prison, Part 2," WNED (Boston: American Archive of Public Broadcasting, 1975), http://americanarchive.org/catalog/cpb-aacip-81-558czgg5.

5. Jessica Mitford, *Kind and Usual Punishment: The Prison Business* (New York: Knopf, 1975).

6. "Reformatory on Rikers Island Scored by Social Work Students," *New York Times*, December 21, 1969.

7. "City's Jail Population Rated 183% above Capacity," *New York Times*, October 4, 1970.

8. Thom Akeman, "Many Inmates Are Young," *Ithaca (NY) Journal*, September 16, 1971.

9. Heather Ann Thompson, *Blood in the Water: The Attica Prison Uprising of 1971 and Its Legacy* (New York: Pantheon Books, 2016).

10. For Clinton prison: New York State Department of Efficiency and Economy, *Annual Report*, vol. 4 (Albany, NY: J. B. Lyon, 1915). For Texas: Executive Budget, Texas, Office of the Governor, 1972. For federal prisons: Subcommittee on the Constitution of the Committee on the Judiciary, "Civil Rights of Institutionalized Persons Hearings before the Subcommittee on the Constitution of the Committee on the Judiciary," United States Senate, Ninety-fifth Congress, First Session, on S. 1393 (Washington, DC: U.S. Government Printing Office, 1977). For Attica: House. Select Committee on Crime, "American Prisons in Turmoil Hearings," Ninety-second Congress, First and Second Sessions (Washington, DC: U.S. Government Printing Office), 1972.

11. Johanna Simis Kunigonde, "Adolescents and Plastic Surgery: Psychosocial and Medical-Ethical Issues" (Erasmus University Rotterdam, 2001).

12. "Plastic Surgery Made Us Better Teachers."

13. Dean C. Miller, "Executives Getting Face Lifts," *New York Times*, September 1, 1972.

14. Harriet Van Horne, "Sen. Proxmire's Facelift," *Lowell (MA) Sun*, February 22, 1972.

15. Van Horne, "Sen. Proxmire's Facelift."

16. Lynn Norment, "Plastic Surgeons: Artists," *Ebony*, September 1980.

17. David A. Jones, *The Health Risks of Imprisonment* (Lexington, MA: Lexington Books, 1976).

18. University of Pennsylvania Law School, "Healthcare and Conditions in Pennsylvania's State Prisons," August 1972.

19. University of Pennsylvania, "News Notes," *Law Alumni Journal* (Fall 1971): 39.

20. Otolaryngology is the study of diseases of the ear and throat. Sometimes referred to as a head and neck surgeon or ENT.

21. "Prisons Assailed in Pennsylvania," *New York Times*, October 29, 1972.

22. "Study Finds Fault with Healthcare in State Prisons," *(Chambersburg, PA) Public Opinion*, October 26, 1972.

23. "Prison Task Force Created Following Law Group's Study," *Daily Pennsylvanian*, October 26, 1972.

24. "Inmates Rent Bodies for Research, Panels Told," *(Decatur, IL) Herald and Review*, March 9, 1973.

25. "Blacklisted Specialist Reinstated by the FDA," *Philadelphia Inquirer*, August 25, 1966.

26. Marvin Zalman, "Prisoners' Rights to Medical Care," *Journal of Criminal Law, Criminology and Police Science* 185 (1972): 63.

27. Kitty Caparella, "Noses Go Straight," *Philadelphia Daily News*, October 24, 1972.

28. Zalman, "Prisoners' Rights to Medical Care."

29. Harrison Weber, "Federal Court Mulls Suit over Inmate Medical Care," *(Waterloo, IA) Courier*, December 10, 1973.

30. United Press International, "Prisoner Sues Government," *(Dover, OH) Daily Reporter*, March 21, 1973.

31. Jessica Mitford, "Kind and Unusual Punishment in California," *Atlantic*, March 1971.

32. Jessica Mitford Papers, box 28, Harry Ransom Center, University of Texas at Austin, PO Box 7219, Austin, Texas.

33. Jessica Mitford, "Experiments behind Bars," *Atlantic*, January 1973.

34. "The Mail," *Atlantic*, April 1973.

35. U.S. Congress, *Quality of Health Care—Human Experimentation, 1973: Hearings, Ninety-third Congress, First Session* (Washington, DC: U.S. Government Printing Office, 1973).

36. U.S. Congress. *Quality of Health Care*. Mitford spoke on March 7, 1973, at 9:20 a.m.

37. Lesley Oelsner, "U.S. Bars Crime Fund Use on Behavior Modification," *New York Times*, February 15, 1974.

38. Nathaniel J. Pallone, *Rehabilitating Criminal Sexual Psychopaths: Legislative Mandates, Clinical Quandaries* (New Brunswick: Transaction Publishers, 1990); Richard Singer, "Consent of the Unfree: Medical Experimentation and Behavior Modification in the Closed Institution, Part II," *Law and Human Behavior* (1977): 101–62; Ralph K. Scwitchgebel, *Legal Aspects of the Enforced Treatment of Offenders* (Washington, DC: U.S. Government Printing Office, 1979).

39. "It Doesn't Work," *60 Minutes*, CBS, August 24, 1975.

40. Robert Martinson, "Collective Behavior at Attica," *Federal Probation* 36, no. 3 (1972).

41. Associated Press, "Sociologist Says Public Is Cool to Prison Reform," *Daily News*, May 8, 1972.

42. Ben H. Bagdikian, "A Human Wasteland in the Name of Justice: Prisons Have Various—Some Contradictory," *Washington Post*, January 30, 1972.

43. Lucia Mouat, "Penal Refomers Come—But Too Slowly," *Christian Science Monitor*, January 19, 1973.

44. Robert Martinson, "Paradox of Prison Reform," *New Republic*, April 1, 6, 15 and 29, 1972.

45. National Advisory Commissions on Criminal Justice Standards and Goals, *Proceedings of the National Conference on Criminal Justice* (Washington, DC: National Advisory Commission on Criminal Justice Standards and Goals, 1973). Also mentions his allusion to the report with a footnote: "Robert Martinson and others, *The Treatment Evaluation Survey* (State of New York, Office of Crime Control Planning, as yet unpublished)." The full quote is "It would be folly for planning agencies, correctional officials, and policymakers to ignore a body of studies of this kind."

46. Robert Fishman, "An Evaluation of Criminal Recidivism in Projects Providing Rehabilitation and Diversion Services in New York City," *Journal of Criminal Law and Criminology* 68, no. 2 (1977): 283, DOI: 10.2307/1142851. The changes in reporting and sentencing influenced the growth—the impact from statewide, mandated Uniform Crime Reporting programs, for example, was felt—but this alone does not account for the upward trajectory of crime.

47. Personal communication, Douglas Lipton, 2018–2021.

48. Personal communication, Douglas Lipton, 2018–2021.

49. "1970s Grime and Crime in New York—Public Transportation Issues," YouTube, April 11, 2011, www.youtube.com/watch?v=EdDUmvPK2OM.

50. New York State Correctional Services, *Annual Report* (1974).

51. Lloyd F. Novick and Mohamed S. Al-Ibrahim, *Health Problems in the Prison Setting* (Springfield, IL: Thomas, 1977).

52. Zalman, "Prisoners' Rights to Medical Care."

53. Julie Ann Epps, "Constitutional Limitations of Prisoners' Right to Medical Treatment," *Mississippi Law Journal* 44, no. 3 (1973): 525–36.

54. Kitsi Burkhart, "Why Prisons Aren't the Answer," *(Philadelphia, PA) Bulletin*, 1971.

55. "I Won't Hire Ex-Convicts," *Penal Press*, Fall 1971.

56. Lee Wolfhert, "Criminologist Bob Martinson Offers a Crime-Stopper: Put a Cop on Each Ex-Con," *People*, February 23, 1976.

57. Francis T. Cullen and Paul Gendreau, "Assessing Correctional Rehabilitation: Policy, Practice, and Prospects," *Criminal Justice 3* (2000).

58. Norval Morris, keynote address (105th Congress of Corrections, Louisville, August 18, 1975).

59. S. Adams, "Evaluation: A Way out of Rhetoric" (paper presented at the conference of the Evaluation of Community-Based Corrections, University of Washington, Seattle, December 18, 1975).

60. Sol Chaneles, "A Look at Martinson's Report," *Fortune News*, November 1975.

61. Robert Martinson, "Letters to the Editor," *Prison Journal* 55, no. 1 (1975): 65–66, DOI: 10.1177/003288557505500106.

62. Subcommittee on Courts, Civil Liberties, *Prison Inmates in Medical Research, 94th Congress, 1st Session* (Washington, DC: U.S. Government Printing Office, 1975).

63. Gerald Ford, "Special Message to the Congress on Crime," American Presidency Project, June 9, 1975, www.presidency.ucsb.edu/node/257109.

## CHAPTER 12. FACE-OFF: THE NEW NORMAL

1. Michael Seiler, "Prisoners' Plastic Surgery Disclosed," *Los Angeles Times*, May 22, 1982.

2. Associated Press, "Loony Ballooney," *(East Liverpool, OH) Evening Review*, May 23, 1977.

3. Bruce D. Johnson and Douglas Lipton, "Creative Tensions: Issues in Utilizing Ethnographic Research within a Single State Agency," in *Ethnography: A Research Tool for Policymakers in the Drug and Alcohol Fields* (Rockville, MD: U.S. Department of Health, Education, and Welfare, 1980), 43.

4. Russel Skelton, "Health Commission Bans Balloons," *(Melbourne, Australia) Age*, June 1, 1979.

5. Jimmy Carter, "Department of Health, Education, and Welfare Remarks and a Question-and-Answer Session with Department Employees," The American Presidency Project, February 16, 1977, www.presidency.ucsb.edu/node/243981.

6. Jimmy Carter, "Federal Law Enforcement Assistance Programs Remarks Announcing Reorganization Legislation and a Department of Housing and Urban Development Program," The American Presidency Project, July 10, 1978, www.presidency.ucsb.edu/node/247736.

7. Jimmy Carter, "Drug Abuse Message to the Congress," August 2, 1977, The American Presidency Project, August 2, 1977, www.presidency.ucsb.edu/node/243653.

8. David H. Feinberg, "Urbanity," *Harvard Crimson*, February 23, 1980, www.thecrimson.com/article/1980/2/23/carter-to-cities-drop-dead-pblbast/.

9. Beryl Menon," Hope for the Hard-Core Convict," *(New Jersey) Record*, January 20, 1972.

10. Johnson and Lipton, "Creative Tensions," 43.

11. Associated Press, "Funds for Brain Surgery Experiment Are Cut Off," *(Benton, Michigan) News-Palladium*, March 14, 1973.

12. CBS Evening News, "Barbara Reed," aired June 1977 on CBS, www.youtube.com/watch?v=E2cJopeQPAw.

13. Carol Osmon, "Mini-Bikes Help 'Rescue' Juvenile Offenders," *Christian Science Monitor*, February 25, 1976.

14. Stephen Hess, "Jimmy Carter: Why He Failed," Brookings, January 21, 2000, https://www.brookings.edu/opinions/jimmy-carter-why-he-failed/.

15. Robert A. Strong, "Jimmy Carter: The American Franchise," UVA Miller Center, https://millercenter.org/president/carter/the-american-franchise.

16. Gregory P. Fallin, Harry K. Wexler, and Douglas S. Lipton, "Drug Treatment in State Prisons," in *Treating Drug Problems: Volume 2: Commissioned Papers on Historical, Institutional, and Economic Contexts of Drug Treatment* (n.p.: National Academies Press, 1992).

17. Fallin, Wexler, and Lipton, "Drug Treatment in State Prisons."

18. National Institute on Drug Abuse Forecasting Branch, "Substance Abuse and Ethnographic Research in New York," *Proceedings* 2 (1979).

19. Robert Martinson, "California Research at the Crossroad, *Crime and Delinquency* (1976).

20. Mary-Somers Knight, "Physical Appearance and Personality" (master's thesis, Sweet Briar College, 1975).

21. Jams Tarmy, "The Inside Story of Estée Lauder's $89 Billion Success," *Bloomberg News*, November 10, 2020.

22. United States Bureau of Labor Statistics, *Occupational Outlook Handbook, 1980–81 Edition* (Washington, DC: U.S. Government Printing Office, 1980), 149.

23. Alexis Madrigal, "When Did TV Watching Peak?" *Atlantic*, May 30, 2018.

24. Amunoo Mohamed, "African Americans in Primetime Broadcast TV and BET," (master's thesis, University of Delaware, 2013).

25. Laura M. Holson, "Max Robinson, a Largely Forgotten Trailblazer for Black Anchors," *New York Times*, June 21, 2015.

26. Naima Cochrane, "How Norman Lear's Historic Black Sitcoms Changed American Television," *Vibe*, May 22, 2019, www.vibe.com/2019/05/norman-lear-black-families-on-american-television.

27. Peter W. Kerman, "Sex Discrimination in Help Wanted Advertising," *Santa Clara Law Review* 15, no.1 (1974): 183–209.

28. Forts v. Malcom, 426 F. Supp. 464 (S.D. New York, 1977).

29. Associated Press, "The Unveiling of a New Ford," *Time* (October 23, 1978).

30. Nadine Brozan, "Cosmetic Surgery's New Image: No Longer Only for the Rich," *New York Times*, December 12, 1978.

31. A. J. Love, "The Rewards and Perils of Plastic Surgery," *D*, July 1978.

32. Brozan, "Cosmetic Surgery's New Image."

33. Jose Garcia Velasco, R. M. Woolf, and T. R. Broadbent, "Plastic and Reconstructive Surgery in a State Prison," *Rocky Mountain Medical Journal* 64, no. 1 (1967): 40–43.

34. Steve Hale, "Utah Inmates Anxious for Plastic Surgery," *(Salt Lake City, UT) Deseret News*, July 6, 1963.

35. Sue Thurman, "Cosmetic Surgery Aids Rehabilitation," *(Salt Lake City, UT) Deseret News*, April 10, 1975.

36. Thurman, "Cosmetic Surgery Aids Rehabilitation."

37. Personal communication, former inmate Claudia S. Cohen (name has been changed for privacy), 2020.

38. Personal communication, Claudia S. Cohen.

39. Personal communication, Claudia S. Cohen.

40. Robert D. Mullins and Joe Costanzo, "Surgeons Practice on Utah Inmates," *(Salt Lake City, UT) Deseret News*, May 15, 1978.

41. Angelyn Nelson, "Report Notes Faculty Prison Data," *Salt Lake Tribune*, May 17, 1978.

42. United Press International, "Two Doctors Defend Surgical Procedures at Prison," *Salt Lake Tribune*, May 16, 1978.

43. United Press International, "Breast Implants Eliminated for Women Prisoners," *(Provo, UT) Daily Herald*, May 19, 1978.

44. United Press International, "Cosmetic Surgery Out at Utah Prison," *(Salt Lake City, UT) Daily Herald*, March 22, 1979.

45. Helene Enid Cavior, Steven C. Hayes, and Norman Cavior, "Physical Attractiveness of Female Offenders: Effects on Institutional Performance," *Correctional Psychologist* 1, no. 4 (1974): 321–31.

46. Personal communication, Steven C. Hayes, 2020.

47. Cavior, Hayes, and Cavior, "Physical Attractiveness of Female Offenders."

48. Frank Greve, "Ugly: It's a Dirty Four-Letter Word That's More Than Skin Deep," *Colorado Springs Gazette-Telegraph*, March 26, 1978.

49. Greve, "Ugly."

50. Brian R. Mitchell, "Labelling, Physical Attractiveness and Correctional Decision-Making," (master's thesis, University of Ottawa, 1979).

51. J. Rich, "Effects of Children's Physical Attractiveness on Teachers' Evaluations," *Journal of Educational Psychology* 67 (1975): 599–609.

52. Ray Bull, "Physical Appearance and Criminality," *Current Psychological Reviews* (1982): 269–72.

53. Park Elliot Dietz, "Cosmetic Surgical Treatment of Offenders," *Medical Criminology Notes #2, The Bulletin* (1977): 465–69.

54. Arnold G. Schuring and R. Edward Dodge, "The Role of Cosmetic Surgery in Criminal Rehabilitation," *Plastic and Reconstructive Surgery* 40, no. 3 (1967): 268–70.

55. Jon K. Meyer, John E. Hoopes, Michael E. Jabaley, and Richard Allen, "Is Plastic Surgery Effective in the Rehabilitation of Deformed Delinquent Adolescents?" *Plastic and Reconstructive Surgery* 51 (1973): 53–58.

56. Associated Press, "New Face for Convict," *St. Joseph (MO) News-Press*, June 23, 1961.

57. Peter B. Edelman, *Serious Youth Crime: Hearings before the Subcommittee to Investigate Juvenile Delinquency of the Committee on the Judiciary, United States Senate, Ninety-fifth Congress, Second Session, April 10 and 12, 1978* (Washington, DC: U.S. Government Printing Office, 1978), 316–20.

58. New York City Board of Correction, "Minimum Standards," www1.nyc.gov/site/boc/jail-regulations/minimum-standards.page.

59. Obituary, *Daily News*, August 30, 1979.

60. Joan Cook, "Anna M. Kross Dies; An Ex-City Official," *New York Times*, August 27, 1979.

61. David Medina, "City's Women's Firsts Left Lasting Impression," *Daily News*, November 5, 1979.

62. Communicating with Prisoners Collective, "Robert Martinson, Freedom Rider," www.acrosswalls.org/section/communicative-walls/economic-analysis/robert-martinson/.

63. Robert Martinson and Judith Wilks, "Is the Treatment of Criminal Offenders Really Necessary?" *Federal Probation* 40 (1976): 3–9.

64. "Robert Martinson Appears on CBS Evening News in 1977," YouTube, July 29, 2016, www.youtube.com/watch?v=io__Rz61ZBM.

65. Robert Martinson, "New Findings, New Views: A Note of Caution Regarding Sentencing Reform," *Hofstra Law Review* 7, no. 2 (1979): 243–58.

66. Jerome Miller, "The Debate on Rehabilitating Criminals: Is It True That Nothing Works?" *Washington Post*, March 1989.

67. Ronald Reagan, "Remarks at the Annual Conference of the National Sheriff's Association in Hartford, Connecticut," The American Presidency Project, June 20, 1984, www.presidency.ucsb.edu/node/260831.

68. Rima L. Vesely-Flad, *Racial Purity and Dangerous Bodies* (n.p.: Fortress Press, 2017).

69. Tim Naftali, "Ronald Reagan's Long-Hidden Racist Conversation with Richard Nixon," *Atlantic*, July 30, 2019.

70. Associated Press, "Arcades Are Dug Hotbeds," *Pittsburgh Post-Gazette*, March 16, 1982.

71. Ronald Reagan, "Remarks Announcing Federal Initiatives against Drug Trafficking and Organized Crime," October 14, 1982, www.reaganlibrary.gov/archives/speech/remarks-announcing-federal-initiatives-against-drug-trafficking-and-organized-crime.

72. Melissa Hickman Barlow, "Race and the Problem of Crime in *Time* and *Newsweek* Cover Stories, 1946 to 1995," *Social Justice* 25, no. 2 (1998):149–83.

73. "The Curse of Violent Crime," *Time*, March 23, 1981.

74. "The Epidemic of Violent Crime," *Newsweek*, March 1981, 50.

75. W. Paul Jones, "Cosmetic Behavior Therapy," *American Mental Health Counselors Association Journal* 2, no. 2 (1980): 53–58.

76. Fawn Vrazo, "To Make It in Society, You've 'Gotta' Look Nice," *Bismarck (ND) Tribune*, September 28, 1983.

77. Sally Wilkins, "Judging the News by Appearance," *(Melbourne, Australia) Age*, May 12, 1982.

78. "Co-anchor Hired for KMBC News!" *Kansas City Star*, December 3, 1980.

79. Barry Garron, "Channel 9 Drops Craft as Anchor," *Kansas City Star*, August 16, 1981.

80. Christine Craft, *Christine Craft: An Anchorwoman's Story* (Santa Barbara, CA: Capra Press, 1986).

81. Barry Garron, "Anchors Shocked by Firing of Christine Craft," *Kansas City Star*, August 25, 1981.

82. Barry Garron, "KMBC's Co-anchor a Casualty of Public Whim," *Kansas City Star*, August 17, 1981.

83. Craft v. Metromedia, Inc., 572 F. Supp. 868, 876 (W.D. Mo. 1983), aff'd in part, rev'd in part, 766 F.2d 1205 (8th Cir. 1985), cert. denied, io6 S. Ct. 1285 (1986).

84. Frank Prial, "Christine Craft: Reporter or Symbol or Both?" *New York Times*, September 7, 1983.

85. Andy Rooney, "Diane Swayer Gets Offer Cronkite Never Had," *Salina (KS) Journal*, August 6, 1983.

86. Doreen Kays, "Christine Craft: Older, Wiser, Still Not Deferring to Men," *(Montreal, Quebec) Gazette*, April 2, 1988.

87. Associated Press, "County Seeks Advice on Jail," *Aiken (SC) Standard*, October 23, 1981.

88. Associated Press, "Convict Wants Taxpayers to Pay for His Face" *(Owosso, MI) Argus Press*, June 6, 1978.

89. *Congressional Record*, 156, no. 112 (2010).

90. Fallin, Wexler, and Lipton, "Drug Treatment in State Prisons."

91. "Alternatives to Prison," C-SPAN, January 7, 1988, www.c-span.org/video/?1124-1/alternatives-prison.

## CHAPTER 13. PRETTY TOUGH IN TEXAS: INVESTMENT IN PRISON PLASTIC SURGERY

1. "Rudolph Giuliani: American Justice, Part II," Richard Heffner's Open Mind, December 1, 1984.

2. Ann Landers, "Jail Inmates Get a Lift, Taxpayers Get the Bill," *Fort-Worth (TX) Star Telegram*, July 13, 1989.

3. Ann Landers, "Go Directly to Jail, Collect Free Plastic Surgery," *Pensacola (FL) News Journal*, July 13, 1989.

4. Associated Press, "Mugging Suspect Dubbed Dumbo Offered New Ears," *(Greenwood, SC) Index Journal*, March 1992.

5. Texas Criminal Justice Coalition, "The Surge of Women into Texas' Criminal Justice System," 2018, https://texascjc.org/; The Sentencing Project, "Incarcerated Women and Girls," November 24, 2018.

6. Melvin Spira, John H. Chizen, Frank J. Gerow, and S. Barom Hardy, "Plastic Surgery in the Texas Prison System," *British Journal of Plastic Surgery* 19, no. 4 (1966): 364–71.

7. Associated Press, "Plastic Surgery Prison Gives Men New Outlook," *Corpus Christi (TX) Caller Times*, January 13, 1958.

8. Texas Department of Corrections Treatment Directorate, *Impact of the New Penal Code, Special Study No.10* (Huntsville, TX: Research and Development Divisions, 1975).

9. Robert Perkinson, "Texas Tough: The Rise of America's Prison Empire" (New York: Metropolitan Books, 2010).

10. Personal communication, Dr. Steven Blackwell, 2019.

11. A. M. Freedman, M. M. Warren, L. W. Cunningham, and S. J. Blackwell, "Cosmetic Surgery and Criminal Rehabilitation," *Southern Medical Journal* 81, no. 9 (1988): 113–16.

12. Freedman, Warren, Cunningham, and Blackwell, "Cosmetic surgery and criminal rehabilitation."

13. "Changing the Face of Convicts' Futures," *Dallas Morning News*, January 19, 1986.

14. National Institute on Drug Abuse, *Drug Abuse Treatment in Prisons and Jails* (Rockville, MD: U.S. Dept of Health and Human Services, 1992).

15. Victor Malarek, *Merchants of Misery* (Toronto: Macmillan, 1989).

16. "Dr. Vincent P. Dole: Addiction: A Medical Rather Than a Moral Issue," Richard Heffner's Open Mind, September 11, 1988.

17. "Counselling prior to Cosmetic Surgery," *Edmonton Journal*, November 11, 1989.

18. Personal communication, Steven Long, 2019.

19. Landers, "Jail Inmates Get a Lift."

20. Steven Long, "Free Cosmetic Surgery Done on Prisoners," *Houston Chronicle*, April 2, 1989.

21. Texas Department of Public Safety, "Crime in Texas, Calendar Year 1989."

22. Ann Landers, "Just Another Pretty Face," *Austin (TX) American Statesman*, July 13, 1989.

23. Governor William P. Clements Jr. Official State Papers, First Term, 1979–1983, 12/C000047, Cushing Manuscript Collection Database, Cushing Memorial Library and Archives, Texas A&M University Libraries, College Station, Texas.

24. Governor William P. Clements Jr. Official State Papers, Second Term, 1987–1991, Texas State Library and Archives Commission.

25. "Prisoner Facelifts Unfair to Taxpayers," editorial, *Kerrvile (TX) Times*, April 4, 1989.

26. Steven Long, "UTMB to Halt Cosmetic Surgery for TDC Inmates," *Houston Chronicle*, June 6, 1989.

27. Associated Press, "Legislative Briefs: Cosmetic Surgery," *(Alexandria, LA) Town Talk*, May 28, 1989.

28. Associated Press, "Inmate Files Hairy Suit," *Deseret (UT) News*, December 15, 1989.

29. George Bush, "Remarks Following the Swearing-in Ceremony for William J. Bennett as Director of National Drug Control Policy," The American Presidency Project, www.presidency.ucsb.edu/node/248477.

30. George Bush, "Remarks at a Republican Party Fundraising Dinner in New York, New York," The American Presidency Project, www.presidency.ucsb.edu/node/264831.

31. Peter Conrad and Valerie Leiter, *Health and Health Care as Social Problems* (Lanham, MD: Rowman & Littefield, 2003); Diana Dull and Candace West, "Accounting for Cosmetic Surgery: The Accomplishment of Gender," *Social Problems* 38, no. 1 (1991): 54–70, DOI: 10.2307/800638.

32. "Be All That You Can Be," *Poughkeepsie (NY) Journal*, July 31, 2004; Associated Press, "Pentagon Will Limit Cosmetic Surgery," *(Escondido, CA) Times Advocate*, July 11, 1990.

33. Mistretta v. United States, Oyez, www.oyez.org/cases/1988/87-7028.

34. Stuart Taylor Junior, "Supreme Court Roundup; Justices to Hear Case on Pocket Veto," *New York Times*, March 4, 1986.

35. "Beautifying Cons," *New York Times*, June 27, 1991.

36. Michael Daly, "The Devil and Clarence Thomas," *New York*, October 28, 1991.

37. Daly, "The Devil and Clarence Thomas."

38. Associated Press, "Group Offers to Crop Ears of the Devil," *(Bridgewater, NJ) Courier News*, March 19, 1992.

39. *The Regulatory Plan and Unified Agenda of Federal Regulations, Department of Justice Semiannual Regulatory Agenda* (Washington, DC: U.S. Government Printing Office, 1994).

40. Lori Dorfman, "Off Balance, Youth, Race and Crime in the News," *Building Blocks for Youth* (April 2001).

41. Melissa Lee, "Washington's Three Strikes Law," Columbia Legal Services, 2010.

42. Katherine Q. Seelye, "The Crime Bill: Overview; House Approves Crime Bill after Days of Bargaining, Giving Victory to Clinton," *New York Times*, August 22, 1994.

43. "Justice in Focus: Crime Bill @20," Vera Institute of Justice, www.vera.org/justice-in-focus-crime-bill-20/time-line.

44. William J. Clinton, "Press Briefing by Dee Dee Myers," The American Presidency Project, www.presidency.ucsb.edu/node/269681.

45. Melissa Hickman Barlow, "Race and the Problem of Crime in *Time* and *Newsweek* Cover Stories, 1946 to 1995," *Social Justice* 25, no. 2 (1998): 149–83.

46. William J. Clinton, "Remarks at the Summer of Service Forum in College Park, Maryland," The American Presidency Project, www.presidency.ucsb.edu/node/217266.

## AFTERWORD: HOT MUG SHOT GUY AND THE FUTURE OF PLASTIC SURGERY IN PRISONS

1. Stephen Deere, "A New Look for New Life of Former Inmate; After Decades in Prison, Vicky Williams Gets Gifts of Plastic Surgery, Finds Building a Future Takes More," *St. Louis Dispatch*, January 8, 2012.

2. "New York Crime Rates 1960–2019," www.disastercenter.com/crime/nycrime.htm. In 1963 there were 548 murders in New York City, in 1972 there were 1,691, and in 1990 there were 2,245 in New York City and 2,605 across New York State. Albert Samaha, "The Rise and Fall of Crime in New York City: A Timeline," *Village Voice*, August 7, 2014.

3. "Time Line," Vera Institute of Justice, 2014, www.vera.org/justice-in-focus-crime-bill-20/time-line.

4. Bureau of Labor Statistics, U.S. Department of Labor, "The Economics Daily: Largest Occupations in Private and Government Sectors," May 2009.

5. Eric Markowitz, "Making Profits on the Captive Prison Market," *The New Yorker*, September 4, 2016; Nicole Lewis and Beatrice Lockwood, "The Hidden Cost of Incarceration," The Marshall Project, December 17, 2019; Lauren E. Glaze, "Correctional Populations in the United States, 2010," U.S. Department of Justice, December 2011.

6. Barack Obama, "Fact Sheet: President Obama Announces New Actions to Promote Rehabilitation and Reintegration for the Formerly Incarcerated," The American Presidency Project, www.presidency.ucsb.edu/node/323088.

7. Barack Obama, "Remarks Following a Visit at Federal Correctional Institution El Reno and an Exchange with Reporters in El Reno, Oklahoma," The American Presidency Project www.presidency.ucsb.edu/node/311405.

8. Barack Obama, "Interview with Maya Rhodan of *Time*," The American Presidency Project, www.presidency.ucsb.edu/node/331716.

9. Alyssa Dana Adomaitis, Rachel Raskin, and Diana Saiki, "Appearance Discrimination: Lookism and the Cost to the American Woman," *Seneca Falls Dialogues Journal* (2017).

10. Geoffrey Hughes, *Political Correctness: A History of Semantics and Culture* (Hoboken, NJ: Wiley, 2011).

11. Daniel J. Boorstin, *Cleopatra's Nose: Essays on the Unexpected* (New York: Knopf Doubleday, 2011), 58.

12. Personal communication, Daniel Hamermesh, 2018.

13. Dr. Bryan Mendelson, *In Your Face* (Melbourne: Hardie Grant Books, 2013).

14. Personal communication, Steven C. Hayes, 2020.

15. Nancy Ectoff, *Survival of the Prettiest: The Science of Beauty* (New York: Random House, 1999).

16. Tommy Simons, "Idaho Transgender Inmate Becomes 2nd in Country to Receive Gender Confirmation Surgery," *Idaho Press*, July 27, 2020.

17. South Carolina Department of Correction, HS-18.15, "Levels of Care," South Carolina Department of Correction Policy/Procedure, November 1, 2007.

18. Rachel Roth, "Obstructing Justice: Prisons as Barriers to Medical Care for Pregnant Women," *UCLA Women's LAW Journal* 18, no. 1 (2010).

19. TDCJ, "Contract between Texas Department of Criminal Justice and the University of Texas Medical Branch at Galveston for Correctional Managed Health Care Services FY2020–FY2021 Biennium," 12.

20. Mila Gumin, "Ugly on the Inside: An Argument for a Narrow Interpretation of Employer Defenses to Appearance Discrimination," *Minnesota Law Review* (2012): 1769.

21. Cherea Hammer, "A Look into Lookism: An Evaluation of Discrimination Based on Physical Attractiveness," (undergraduate honors capstone project, Utah State University, 2017); Santa Cruz Municipal Code, "Prohibition against Discrimination," chapter 9.83, www.codepublishing.com/CA/SantaCruz/html/SantaCruz09/SantaCruz0983.html.

22. Personal communication, Joyce Pequeno, 2020.

23. Stephen Deere, "A New Look."

24. Rachel Hosie, "The 'Hot Felon' Who Went from Prison to Fashion Week," *Independent*, June 19, 2017.

25. Liana Satenstein, "'Hot Felon' Jeremy Meeks Makes His Runway Debut at Philipp Plein," *Vogue*, February 14, 2017.

26. Naci Mocan and Erdal Tekin, "Ugly Criminals," *Review of Economics and Statistics* 92, no. 1 (2010): 15–30.

27. Rey Hernandez-Julian and Christina Peters, "Student Appearance and Academic Performance," *Journal of Human Capital* 11, no. 2 (2017).

28. B. Teasdale and Bonnie Berry, "'Ugly' Criminals and 'Ugly' Victims," *Appearance Bias and Crime* (2019): 51–62, DOI: 10.1017/9781108377683.003.

29. Personal communication, Bonnie Berry, 2020.

30. Joni Hersch, "Colorism against Legal Immigrants to the United States," *American Behavioral Scientist*, December 17, 2018.

31. "I Am Not Your Villain: Equal Representation of Visible Difference in Film," Changing Faces, November 16, 2018, www.changingfaces.org.uk/i-am-not-your-villain-campaign-launches-today-in-the-telegraph.

32. Zack Sharf, "British Film Institute Vows Not to Fund Movies with Facial-Scarred Villains," *Indiewire*, November 30, 2018.

33. Julie Amthor Croley, Vail Reese, and Richard F. Wagner, "Dermatologic Features of Classic Movie Villains," *JAMA Dermatology* 6, no. 153 (2017): 559–64; personal communication, Vail Reese, 2020.

34. Paul Guerino, Paige M. Harrison, and William J. Sabol, "Prisoners in 2010," Bureau of Justice Statistics, 2011.

35. Correctional Association of New York, "People Incarcerated in New York: Population Profile and Recent Trends," CorrectionalAssociation.org, 2019.

36. New York City Council, "Rikers to Close," October 19, 2019, https://council.nyc.gov/data/closerikers.

# INDEX